REBUILDING
MILO

The Lifter's Guide to Fixing Common Injuries
and Building a Strong Foundation
for Enhancing Performance

Dr. Aaron Horschig
with Dr. Kevin Sonthana

Victory Belt Publishing Inc.
Las Vegas

First published in 2021 by Victory Belt Publishing Inc.

ISBN-13: 978-1-628604-22-1

Cover design by Eli San Juan
Interior design by Allan Santos and Charisse Reyes
Illustrations by Allan Santos

TC 0824

For Christine

TABLE OF CONTENTS

6   **Foreword by Dr. Kelly Starrett**

8   **Introduction**

14   **Chapter 1: Back Pain**

16   The Picture Isn't Always What It Seems

19   Back Injury Anatomy 101

36   How to Screen Your Low Back Pain

58   Classifying Your Back Pain

61   The Rebuilding Process

77   Bridging the Gap: Early Rehab to Performance

90   The Bridge to Performance

95   Should You Wear a Weightlifting Belt?

98   Cautionary Exercises for Low Back Injury Rehab

104   Does Stretching the Hamstrings Fix Low Back Pain?

120   **Chapter 2: Hip Pain**

121   Hip Anatomy

128   Hip Injury Anatomy 101

139   How to Screen Your Hip Pain

148   The Rebuilding Process

170   **Chapter 3: Knee Pain**

172   Knee Injury Anatomy 101

184   How to Screen Your Knee Pain

195   The Rebuilding Process

234 Chapter 4: Shoulder Pain

235   Shoulder Anatomy

241   Shoulder Injury Anatomy 101

250   How to Screen Your Shoulder Pain

265   The Rebuilding Process

312 Chapter 5: Elbow Pain

313   Elbow Injury Anatomy 101

320   How to Screen Your Elbow Pain

330   The Rebuilding Process

342 Chapter 6: Ankle Pain

343   Achilles Tendon Injury Anatomy 101

349   How to Screen Your Achilles Tendon Pain

354   The Rebuilding Process

374 Chapter 7: Don't Ice, Walk It Off!

377   Inflammation and Swelling

382   Using Muscle Contraction to Reduce Swelling and Facilitate Healing

383   Using NMES to Facilitate Healing When Movement Is Limited

384   Icing After Workouts

390 Acknowledgments

392 Index

Foreword

"We are drowning in information, while starving for wisdom. The world henceforth will be run by synthesizers, people able to put together the right information at the right time, think critically about it, and make important choices wisely." —E. O. Wilson

Aaron Horschig is a unicorn. He is that uncommon person who can simultaneously occupy the roles of user, teacher, and synthesizer. There is a trend today amongst the internet elite to do a lot of talking about problems without really ever having to live those problems on a daily basis. Don't get me wrong; not working in the trenches in real time is far easier. You can just talk about the world of others' work in a critical way. You don't really have to produce anything original, problem-solve in real time, work within the context of crazy professional/high-performance environments, or show any of your own work. If you could create a photonegative of this kind of phenomenon, the image would be of Aaron.

This book you are holding isn't actually that remarkable an achievement for the man behind Squat University. Don't mistake me here. This book is remarkable both for its content and for the paradigm shift that it represents. It is, however, altogether typical of Aaron and his drive to share his considerable success in helping people untangle the complexities of their pain and movement problems.

Perhaps it's the way our mentors and thought leaders engaged with us, or perhaps it's because it's the foundation of science, but "Test, Retest, Share" has been the mantra of every great thinker since the dawn of time. The E. O. Wilson quote is one of my favorites, but Dr. Wilson was always quick to point out that the ultimate goal of science was actually to improve the humanities. Think on that for a moment. Open your Instagram feed. Look at the educators who come up. Run their feeds through the filter that I use to try and make sense of what I'm seeing. Does what I'm seeing explain what's happening? Does it predict future movement behavior? Is the thinking reproducible and transferable? These are features of all good models. Good models aren't social media thirst traps. They aren't always that sexy, but they work. And they improve the lives of the people who use them.

If you look at the considerable amount of teaching Aaron has put into the world, you will see synthesis at its heart. This is a trait he shares with the entire crop of thought leaders who are driving the human movement train. Aaron was classically trained as a physical therapist, but he wears the mantle of a coach. This is his true superpower. He is a movement genius but trained as an expert in understanding the all-too-common problems of injury, pathology, and human durability. When Aaron teaches, he has one eye on going faster and heavier and one eye solidly on the problem of sustainability. Integrating these sometimes competing forces can require an iron stomach and a solid foundation in the complicated and always messy experience that constitutes any field that involves working with complex humans.

Don't be fooled by the casual way Aaron can spot the heart of a movement problem. Ultimately, no matter what's going on, you will be moving. Ergo, it's a movement problem. He's only going to be satisfied when he has fulfilled the last parts of both promises: share, and make sure you can see what he sees.

You are holding that promise in your hands. Test and retest it. Let us know what you find.

Kelly Starrett

Introduction

Behind many a legendary tale, there is a hidden lesson to be learned. Those who incorporate weight training with the goal of improving their physique, strength, or power should look to the story of Milo of Croton.

Milo was an ancient Greek Olympian and the poster child for athletic excellence in his time. Legend has it that at a young age, Milo started his strength journey by lifting a small calf and carrying it on his shoulders every day. As the calf grew over the years, so did Milo's strength, until one day he was hoisting a full-grown bull! Although it is unlikely that he was able to lift a 1,500-pound bull, like any good story, the legend sprang from humble beginnings.

The 2,500-year-old story of how Milo built his heroic strength set forth the training principle that all athletes adhere to. That principle is now known as "progressive overload." Within Milo's story is the idea that hard work combined with consistency can lead to legendary feats of strength and awe-inspiring athletic performance.

Deep inside each and every one of us is an innate desire to become our own version of Milo. The idea of building incredible strength and meeting our physical goals is why so many of us push our bodies day in and day out. While at surface level the story of Milo may seem simple, the reality is that the process of building extraordinary strength is as much about grit, hard work, and determination as it is about science.

You see, our bodies adhere to a scientific "code," a simple framework of rules governed by the laws of biology and physiology. The code is simple. To develop strength, you must strike a balance between stress and recovery. Every time you perform a set of squats, pick up a heavy deadlift, or press a barbell overhead, you place a stress on your body. The harder your training session, the more stress you accumulate. To progressively develop more and more strength, the demands of your training must not exceed the adaptive capabilities of your body. Therefore, training must be balanced with recovery for the body to adapt, rebuild itself, and gain strength. If you follow this code, the sky is the limit for athletic performance.

Sounds simple enough, right?

Not so fast.

In our pursuit of amassing strength, we all push the envelope. Our inner competitor drives us to complete one more rep, put 10 more pounds on the bar, and take one more attempt at setting a personal record on a lift. This kind of determination is vital if you want to excel as a strength athlete. However, it can just as quickly become a double-edged sword.

When we push our bodies to their physical limits and ignore the code, they eventually push back. I have never met a strength athlete who didn't have a nagging injury at some point in their career. Sometimes these injuries interfere with their training. When we push our bodies to the max and don't focus on sufficient recovery and/or lack ideal technique, injuries will occur. As fate would have it, in our quest to become our own version of Milo, we wind up falling short of our destination.

I want to share two stories with you.

Josiah O'Brien was like many powerlifters. He was a hard worker who was loyal to his friends and family, and he loved lifting heavy weight in the gym with death metal blasting. He never used a foam roller and thought mobility work was a waste of time. When parts of his body started to hurt, he ignored the pain. He lived by the mantra "no pain, no gain." Unfortunately, this lifestyle eventually caught up with him.

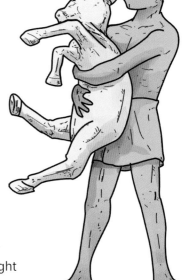

On October 22, 2016, Josiah entered a competition at 22nd Street Barbell in Des Moines, Iowa. The meet started like any other. After successfully completing his second of 3 squat attempts at 638 pounds, he decided to go for 655, a feat only 5 pounds heavier than his personal best at the time.

After unracking the massive weight, he took a few steps back and set his feet. To his surprise, the bar felt "light" on his back. However, as he descended into the squat, disaster struck. He heard and felt both legs snap. The weight came crashing down, pinning his legs behind his body as he crumpled to the floor.

That day, Josiah ended up tearing almost every supporting ligament and tendon (quad and patellar) in both knees. He was rushed to the nearest hospital in the bed of his friend's truck, unable to sit in the back seat, as the massive amount of swelling and pain wouldn't allow him to bend his knees. This was only the start of his troubles. Josiah ended up developing rhabdomyolysis, a serious condition in which the kidneys start to fail because the muscle damage to the body is so severe.

In the following weeks after Josiah was stabilized, he underwent extensive surgery to repair the torn ligaments and tendons. He then was placed in straight leg braces (unable to move his knees whatsoever) for 12 weeks. Eventually, in early 2017, he came to me to start physical therapy.

It would be an understatement for me to say that this was the most challenging case I had ever seen. By this time in my career, I had helped hundreds of athletes rehab knee injuries ranging from meniscus repairs to ACL reconstructions. The damage inflicted on Josiah's body that day in October 2016 was on a whole different level. After all was said and done, rebuilding his body required over 100 physical therapy visits spread out over nine months. He had to completely relearn how to walk, jump, and run.

He hobbled into my clinic that first day, unable to walk normally, and left with the ability to deadlift over 600 pounds, jump over 24-inch hurdles, and run without any issues. He even returned to the competition platform on August 12, 2017, less than a year after the devastating injury, and successfully squatted 195 pounds. While the weight on the bar was a far cry from the 600-plus pounds he was used to moving, he proved to himself that this injury hadn't redefined who he was. He was a powerlifter, and powerlifters never quit.

The second story is my own. As an aspiring weightlifter, I always dreamed of the day I could compete on the same stage with the best in the United States. While my ambition far outweighed my athletic talent and strength, I was able to qualify for the 2011 USA Weightlifting Senior National Championships in the 85-kilo (187-pound) weight class.

Leading up to the competition, I decided to turn up the heat in my preparation. I started to pull two-a-day training sessions. I would wake up at 6 a.m. to get my squats and pulls in before heading to grad school classes for the day. I would return later to finish up whatever snatches, cleans, or jerks the program had in store. There was no way I was going to pass up my chance to perform at my very best on the national stage.

A few weeks before the competition, I developed severe pain in my left knee. Every time I went into a deep squat, it felt like a knife was being jabbed into my patellar tendon. So I did what every physical therapy student would do: I went to my professors for guidance. The advice I received was the same unfortunate advice that many athletes in my situation are given: "Just stop lifting so often."

Seriously? They knew I had a huge competition coming up soon. I couldn't just *stop* lifting.

So I resorted to doing what most athletes do in this situation. Before each training session, I would pop three or four Advil and slather Icy Hot all over my knee, and I iced my knee at the end of each day. While I was able to make it through the rest of my training cycle without further injury, I was frustrated by how the competition went. I placed sixth in my weight class, but I knew I could have performed better if my training hadn't been interrupted by this injury.

I tell you these stories to remind you that *all* strength athletes deal with pain. While Josiah's life-threatening injury is the exception rather than the rule, the underlying theme of both stories remains true. When you train hard and don't give your body enough time to recover, the stresses of training begin to accumulate. And when you mix in less-than-perfect lifting technique, they add up even faster. Eventually, these stresses culminate in injury. Ninety-nine percent of the time, the pain you experience as a strength athlete is not a severe medical emergency like Josiah's, but minor aches and pains like mine that disrupt your training and limit your performance.

Unfortunately, most athletes don't have the basic knowledge of how to perform simple maintenance on their own bodies. From an early age, athletes are told that pain is a normal part of training. This mindset has created a cycle where athletes continue to lift and push through pain until they literally break. It is not until the pain affects *performance* that athletes finally seek help. We must put a stop to this broken system of *lift, lift, break.* While it is impossible to eliminate all aches and pains from weight training, we can have better control over it.

Today's society tells us that pain is a medical problem. I don't believe this is correct. You see, the way in which many in the medical community address pain is to treat the *symptoms* of pain and not the *cause.* While the "solution" of painkillers and anti-inflammatories might satisfy your craving for a quick fix, it is not going to help you in the long run. On the other hand, restoring optimal movement through subtle improvements in strength, mobility, and coordination is the key to solving pain and returning to a high level of performance.

Using temporary quick fixes to address pain is like putting a piece of tape over a hole in your car's tire. This isn't to say that these fixes have no value. Sometimes you *need* that piece of tape to get your car to the mechanic. But covering it up doesn't change the fact that there is a hole in your tire.

If you still have pain after you've completed this book, I recommend that you seek professional care. I encourage you to take this book with you to consultations so that you and the rehabilitation professional are on the same page about your recovery and your desire to fix the cause of your pain rather than just cover it up.

There is always a reason for pain. It doesn't develop out of thin air. It not only hinders your performance but also changes the way you move. Pain affects your coordination and the efficiency of your technique. It limits your mobility and diminishes your strength—all of which are part of your body's effort to protect itself from further injury.

If you've picked up this book, you know what I mean. You've likely already experienced a problem. Being unable to lift like you want without pain is frustrating and straight-up maddening. Trust me, I've been there. I get it.

I'm here to tell you that there is hope. David Viscott once wrote, "The purpose of life is to discover your gift. The work of life is to develop it. The meaning in life is to give your gift away." I have made it my life's purpose to help every single person who walks into a weight room get back to doing what they love to do *without pain.* The information contained in this book is the culmination of my life's work as a performance physical therapist, and I want to share it with you.

Now, the ideas presented in these pages may challenge some of your beliefs about how to address pain. I want to put *you* back in control of your body and what you're feeling. The majority of the aches and pains we experience are not serious medical issues. Fixing them doesn't require a visit to the doctor or an expensive surgery. As physical therapist Kelly Starrett says, "You wouldn't bring your car to the mechanic to put air in your tires or call an electrician to change a light bulb." Simply stated, you should have the ability to perform basic maintenance on your own body.

Through these pages, you'll be guided along a path to uncover the *why* behind your injury. Each chapter is built around a specific site of pain (low back, hip, knee, etc.). You will learn about the specific causes of pain, from disc bulges to patellar tendinitis. You'll learn how to evaluate your strengths and weaknesses with simple-to-perform tests and assessments. Once you've uncovered the precise cause of your pain, you can immediately apply the suggested exercises and strategies in your training to help decrease your pain and build a strong foundation for enhancing your future performance.

To maximize the effectiveness of this book, I recommend that you choose a chapter to start with and read that chapter in its entirety. Take mental notes the first time through to understand the differences between the injuries. The text contains the most up-to-date science on injury and rehabilitation, but I explain it in a way that anyone can comprehend. The more you understand the *why* behind your symptoms, the more empowered you will feel to take control of your recovery and stay consistent with the recommended rehab plan.

The second time through the chapter, perform the diagnostic tests and suggested rehabilitative exercises. Go slowly through each movement and listen to your body. The journey to become pain-free will take discipline and commitment.

In 1997, Apple released the iPod. For the first time in history, you could have "1,000 songs in your pocket." This creation gave you instant access to all of your favorite artists and songs. In a similar manner, I designed this book to give you direct access to the knowledge that elite physical therapists and performance coaches possess.

No matter whether you're a world-class powerlifter who has fallen on hard times or a 35-year-old avid CrossFitter who just wants to return to training with your friends, the lessons found within these pages will put you on the right path to rebuilding yourself into a modern-day Milo.

Let's begin.

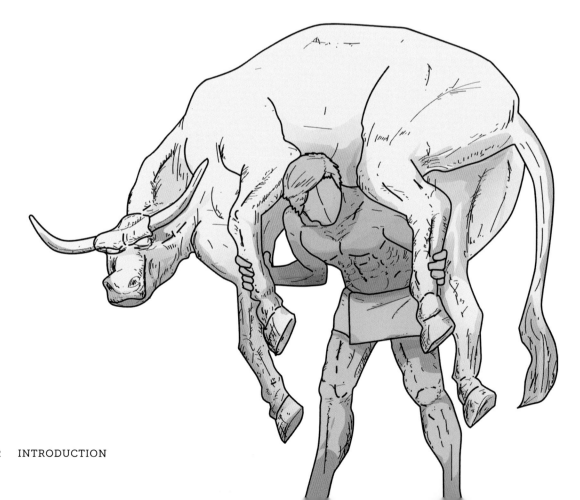

Equipment Used in This Book

To do the rehabilitative exercises described in this book, you will need to have access to some simple equipment:

- Barbell
- Double lacrosse ball "peanut"
  - → Home alternative: two tennis balls taped together (see page 265)
- Dumbbells
- Foam roller
  - → Home alternative: 3- to 4-inch PVC pipe
- Hip circle bands from MarkBellSlingShot.com
  - → Orange Grippy Hip Circle®
  - → Hip Circle® Sport Pack
- Kettlebell
- PVC pipe
  - → Home alternative: broomstick
- Rogue Monster Bands
  - → #4 Black (1.75-inch width/100-pound resistance) for joint mobilizations
  - → #5 Purple (2.5-inch width/140-pound resistance) for Spanish squat exercise (see page 213)
- Single lacrosse ball
- Suspension trainer
- TheraBand resistance bands
  - → Can substitute a light resistance band loop

If you're dealing with pain associated with swelling, you may want to consider an additional investment item: a neuromuscular electrical stimulation (NMES) unit. This device helps pump excess fluid/waste out of the injured area through the passive lymphatic system and dilates your blood vessels to bring nutrients and other helpful white blood cells to enhance the healing process. My favorite units are the Marc Pro, PowerDot, and Compex. (See pages 383 and 384 for more on NMES devices.)

CHAPTER 1

BACK PAIN

Of all the injuries a strength athlete can sustain, low back pain is often the most frustrating and debilitating. Not only does an injury to your back instantaneously drain you of power and strength, but it can also have an intense psychological effect that leaves you feeling like a shell of yourself.

If you've ever had a back injury, ask yourself if this story sounds familiar.

Ryan is a 24-year-old CrossFitter. During a recent competition, he felt a small "pop" in his low back while finishing up his round of 30 clean and jerks at 135 pounds. He struggled through the rest of the competition and has since been dealing with debilitating pain every time he bends over. Even little tasks such as picking up a sock off the floor and tying his shoes have become extremely difficult to perform.

After two months of dealing with this aggravating pain and feeling frustrated that his training had started to stagnate and decline, Ryan decided to see someone about it. His doctor told him that he needed an MRI scan of his spine. So Ryan made another appointment and waited patiently, hoping that the end of his pain was in sight.

Unfortunately, his journey was just beginning.

After another two anxious weeks, the day of his next appointment finally came. Over six short minutes of face-to-face time, the doctor looked at the scans of Ryan's spine and gave him a diagnosis of a "bulging disc." He wrote up a prescription for heavy pain medication and told Ryan to stop weight training and take it easy for the next few weeks.

After six weeks of rest, Ryan's pain had started to decrease, so he did what every athlete would do: he went back to the weight room. However, after only a week, the pain returned. Heartbroken, he went to see his doctor again, who gave him the fateful prognosis that surgery was likely the best option.

Have you found yourself in a similar situation? If so, you're not alone. Year after year, millions of people around the world are stricken with back pain. Research has shown that up to 80 percent of adults will experience low back pain at some time in their lives.[1] An even more troubling statistic is that many of them will experience recurring episodes.[2]

Lifts like the squat, deadlift, and Olympic lifts place tremendous forces on the low back.[3] It should not be surprising, then, that low back injuries are among the most prevalent injuries sustained by strength athletes,[4] as Ryan found out the hard way.

Unfortunately, the way traditional medicine approaches back pain today leaves many athletes and patients addicted to painkillers. Worse, some undergo multiple back surgeries when their injuries could have been resolved with much more conservative measures. Finding the solution to a serious back injury can be tricky, but it is certainly possible without injections, addictive pain meds, or operations.

Next, I am going to walk you through every step of Ryan's experience. I want to expose the holes in it and show you how our medical community largely treats low back pain the wrong way. Then I am going to show you how things *should* be done, with a step-by-step plan that you can use to empower yourself to understand and fix your pain.

Let's start with the first problem in Ryan's story: the idea that a doctor can determine why a patient has back pain just by looking at an MRI.

The Picture Isn't Always What It Seems

Have you heard the expression "a picture is worth a thousand words"? It means that something can be summed up better with a single image than a lengthy description. This phrase shouldn't have any place in the diagnosis of back pain.

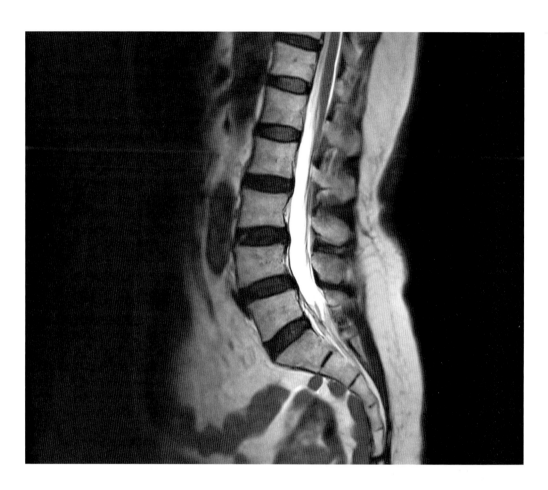

An MRI of the spine can't tell us everything we need to know.

Ryan's doctor gave him the diagnosis of "back pain caused by a bulging disc" simply by looking at an expensive "picture" of his spine. Many medical doctors seek out "abnormal" findings (like a bulging disc) on an MRI scan, interpret them to be recent developments, and presume these specific tissues to be the source of pain. Basically, if something looks off on the scan, it is assumed to be the exact cause of the newly developed pain.

This presumption that "abnormalities" on imaging can be directly linked to the cause of pain is flawed for many reasons, including these:

- Results on imaging show poor correlation to symptoms of pain.[5]

- The MRI scan cannot show if the damage is a new "wound" or an old "scar."

- Pathology does not necessarily drive treatment.

- The MRI shows only anatomy, not function.

What if I told you that disc bulges are fairly common and often show up on lumbar spine MRI scans? It's true! Many people are walking around with disc bulges but have zero back pain.

Research has estimated that almost a third of healthy, pain-free 20-year-olds have a disc bulge in their spine.[6] This number increases by 10 percent for every decade of life, meaning that half of all 40-year-olds likely have a disc bulge yet are not experiencing back pain.

In 2006, a group of researchers collected MRI scans of 200 individuals without any history of back pain.[7] Those who developed severe pain during the study had new MRIs taken, and their results were compared with the previous scans. You may be surprised to hear that in 84 percent of those who developed pain, there was zero difference in their spines from their original scans. Some people even had *improved* markers compared to their first MRI! Clearly, research has shown that just because a scan picks up an "abnormality" does not necessarily mean that it is the root cause of pain.[8]

When a radiologist sees a bulging disc on an MRI scan, they have no way to determine whether it is due to a recent event (a wound) or is 20 years old (a scar). This is because disc bulges can heal over time and no longer cause pain, even if they are still visible on an MRI.

It's also important to understand that an injury to the spine is different from an injury to the knee or hip. A spine injury sets off a cascade of events.[9] For example, when the spine is compressed under load, a healthy disc helps distribute that load evenly across the entire vertebral bone. When a disc bulge occurs, the load is no longer evenly distributed but instead is shifted to the posterior aspects of the spine (the facet joints). Just like a flat tire on a car, the injured disc loses stiffness and pressure, leaving the car to drive a little unevenly on the road.

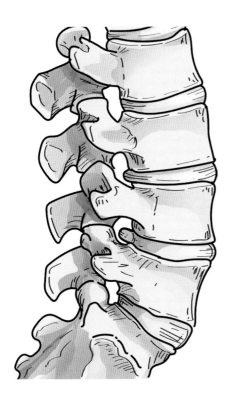

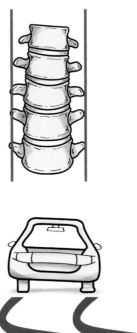

While the pain from a disc bulge may "burn out" in a few weeks or months, the mechanics of the spine are instantly changed. How the spine carries load from then on is affected at that particular segment, and forces are shifted to the facet joints. Therefore, if someone with back pain receives an MRI, there is no way a radiologist can determine whether an observed disc bulge is a new "wound" generating symptoms. It is very possible that the "abnormality" is a "scar" that is no longer creating pain, and the true source of pain is an issue at the facet joints. Proper rehab that instills sufficient core stability limits this cascade of events.

Even if the anatomical structure causing pain is identified, this knowledge does little to guide the clinician in finding the best fix for rehabilitation.[10] A problem like a disc bulge could be due to a number of causes. For this reason, doing a simple Google search for "5 best exercises for a disc bulge" would be of no benefit. In the end, the only person who benefits from this knowledge is the surgeon who attempts to "fix" the presumed cause of pain.

Moreover, an MRI scan is a picture of your anatomy in only one particular posture. It would be naïve to think that a mechanic could look at a picture of a race car and know exactly why it's making a weird noise when shifting from third to fourth gear above 60 mph. However, while you may be quick to question a mechanic who would attempt to diagnose your car troubles in this manner, we are hesitant to do the same with medical doctors attempting to interpret the results of an MRI.

To make an accurate diagnosis of a car's issue, a skilled mechanic must take the car for a spin, rev the engine, and test the capabilities of the machine. Simply put, the mechanic must establish context for what is creating the problem. The same goes for the human body. We need context from a thorough examination to uncover which specific movements, loads, and postures trigger pain. Only after completing this process can we turn to imaging if we want to look deeper and know which specific tissues are likely driving symptoms.

Here's an example of how you should view the results of an MRI. Going back to Ryan's story, let's say he has pain only when getting into the bottom of a deadlift. After further observation, it becomes apparent that his low back is fully flexed/rounded in that position. Ryan also mentions that he has no pain when standing upright or walking. If having him perform that same deadlift while focusing on limiting excessive flexion in his low back decreases his pain, we can come to the understanding that the movement of flexion under load is the trigger of his pain.

If Ryan's MRI shows an active disc bulge, we can say with more confidence that his painful low back flexion coincides with that finding. When Ryan rounds his lumbar spine excessively, the forces are unevenly distributed, causing the inner nucleus to seep its way through the outer ring of the disc and triggering pain. Without the context found through the examination, however, there is no way to determine if the findings from an MRI are truly the cause of pain.

Ryan's story took a turn for the worse the moment he met with a doctor whose only form of evaluation was to ask him some questions and order an MRI. The evaluation process is the most crucial part in fixing back pain because it establishes the foundation on which the entire treatment plan is based. Ryan's evaluation was built on the rocky assumption that a picture is worth a thousand words.

Back Injury Anatomy 101

One of my biggest pet peeves is when doctors and other practitioners neglect to take the time to educate patients about the basics of anatomy and why their injuries occurred (called the *injury mechanism*). I want to briefly go over the anatomy of the low back and cover some of the most common injuries that occur in this region.

The Spine

Your spine is not just a stack of bones. It's a slightly curved "tower" of small bones called *vertebrae,* separated by discs. These discs provide cushioning for the vertebrae as they move, much like airbags. Each vertebra is connected to the others through small joints in the back called *facets,* which give the spine tremendous movement options. You can flex your spine as you bend over to tie your shoes, extend it to place a box on a high shelf, twist it to drive a golf ball down the fairway, or do any conceivable combination of those to perform the latest dance move.

NEUTRAL SPINE

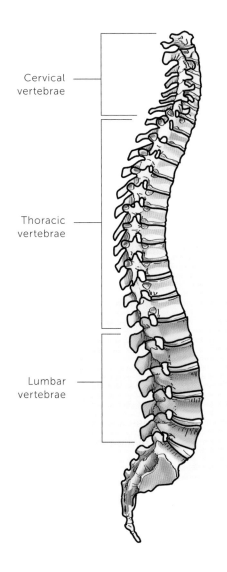

Cervical vertebrae

Thoracic vertebrae

Lumbar vertebrae

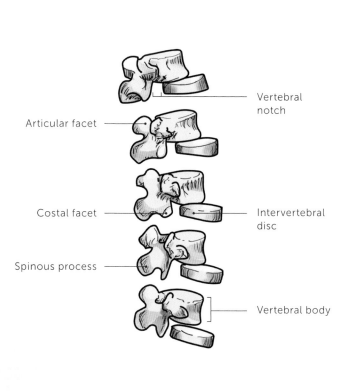

Articular facet

Costal facet

Spinous process

Vertebral notch

Intervertebral disc

Vertebral body

When you stand with good posture, your spine assumes its "neutral" alignment. This is not a completely straight position; as shown on the previous page, it has three distinct curves in the cervical (upper), thoracic (mid), and lumbar (lower) regions. Contrary to popular belief, *neutral* doesn't describe a singular static position; it describes a small range of motion or zone around the neutral posture.[11] Within this zone, load placed on the body (such as when squatting a barbell) is equally distributed across the discs and vertebrae. However, if the spine is loaded outside of this neutral zone, the forces are unevenly distributed, and the risk of injury increases.[12] Let's discuss specifically how this injury may be created.

How Back Pain Occurs

Since starting the Squat University podcast, I have had several opportunities to speak with one of the world's most renowned experts on back pain, Stuart McGill. I can say with confidence that in my career as a physical therapist, few people have had a greater impact on how I approach treating low back injuries than Dr. McGill. He has dedicated his life's work to researching the spine and has written extensively about back injuries and core stability in books such as *Ultimate Back Fitness and Performance*[13] and *Back Mechanic,* as well as countless professional journal articles. I highly recommend checking out his website, www.backfitpro.com.

In one of our conversations, Dr. McGill laid out a simple way of understanding how injuries occur at the spine. It often comes down to one simple equation:

Power = Force × Velocity

The first part of this equation is pretty straightforward. *Force* is an energy that manifests in effort or exertion. You place more force on your spine when deadlifting 600 pounds than you do when deadlifting 100 pounds.

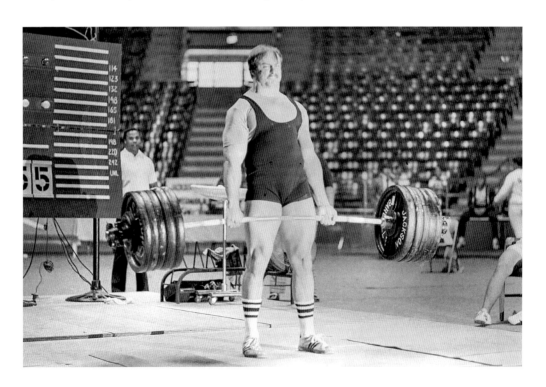

Heavy deadlift. *John Kuc, ©Bruce Klemens.*

Velocity is simply the speed at which something moves. Every time the spine moves, it moves at a certain velocity. Twisting slowly to grab a glass of water sitting on a table to your right creates very little velocity compared to the speed at which Tiger Woods rotates his torso as he swings a golf club.

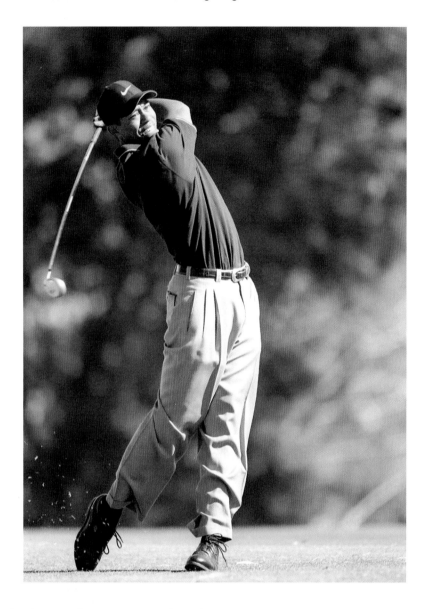

Because golf clubs are lightweight, golfers like Tiger Woods can safely twist their spine with tremendous speed. *©Jerry Coli | Dreamstime.com*

Your body is resilient to injury when the power generated at your spine remains low. Ask yourself this simple question:

"Does the action I want to perform require spinal movement?"

If the answer is yes (as is the case with swinging a golf club), you don't want to generate a lot of power at your spine.

Think about it like this: A golf club is fairly lightweight, which allows a golfer to twist their spine over and over again with tremendous speed without a great risk of injury because it requires little force. However, imagine how your back would feel if you tried to swing a 10-pound golf club over and over again!

As soon as you add load to the equation, things change. Think of a powerlifter attempting to deadlift 600 pounds. Obviously, the load is very high, and therefore the force needed to complete the movement is significantly higher than the force needed to swing a golf club. If the athlete locks their spine and doesn't move it as they lift the weight, the overall power generated at the spine remains relatively low.

If you load your body and *then* move your back, the power generated at the spine increases, as you have high force *and* high velocity, raising your risk of injury.[14] Therefore, the idea is quite simple. If you want your spine to move, you want to move it under minimal load. This is how dancers, MMA fighters, and golfers can safely compete in their sports. Similarly, if you want to lift heavy weight (placing load on the spine), it is best not to move your spine and keep it within the neutral zone. Lock it in place and keep it stiff while you move at the hips.

Now, many variables influence the timeline of exactly *when* an injury may occur. Even though the prior equation is simple in theory, the reality of how injuries happen is more complex. There is no "*X* number of movements" that one can safely perform under a certain load before a disc herniation develops. But the mechanism for injury remains the same. With this understanding in mind, let's dive a little deeper into some of the common forms of back injury sustained by strength athletes.

Disc Bulges and Herniation

What exactly is a disc bulge? Many healthcare professionals explain this injury using a jelly donut as an analogy.

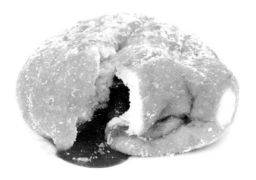

The nucleus pulposus (the gel-like center of a spinal disc) is kind of like the jelly inside a jelly donut.

Between each pair of vertebral bones lies a disc. Like a jelly donut, each disc of the spine has an inner gel-like center called the *nucleus pulposus*. If there is too much compression on the spine, the vertebrae will be squeezed together, and, like the jelly in a donut being smashed, the gel will be forced out of the disc that lies between those vertebrae.

However, this isn't as good of an analogy as many think. Here's why.

Barbell training places a considerable amount of compression on the spine, but most of that compression actually comes from the back muscles. As you pull a barbell from the ground, for example, the muscles that surround your spine tighten down to create enough stiffness to keep your spinal "tower" from buckling. The contraction of these muscles (along with the force of the weight being lifted) compresses the spinal column.

NEUTRAL SPINE SIDE VIEW

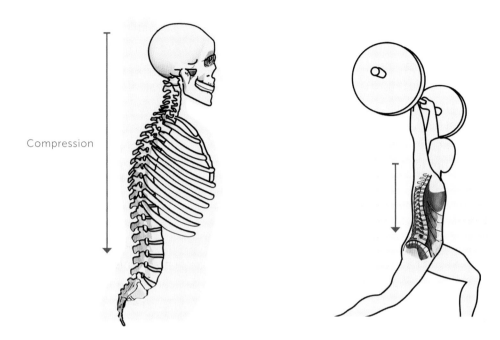

Compression

The nucleus pulposus is surrounded by many ringlike layers of a strong material called *collagen.* While you can easily push the jelly out of the center of a donut by smashing it with your hands, the collagen rings that surround the nuclei of your spinal discs are extremely tough. As the nucleus of the disc becomes pressurized by load, the tough collagen rings contain its jellylike material. This is why a disc bulge is rare when the spine is compressed in a neutral position; the power generated at the spine remains relatively low when force is high but velocity is low.[15]

HEALTHY INTERVERTEBRAL DISC

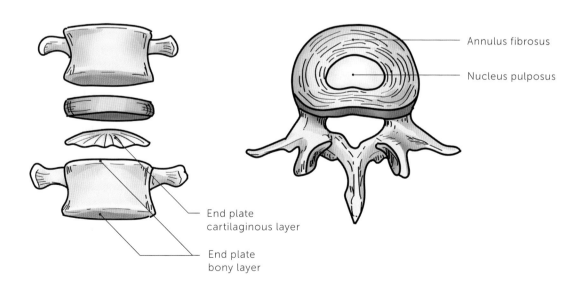

Annulus fibrosus

Nucleus pulposus

End plate
cartilaginous layer

End plate
bony layer

However, if the spine is loaded and *then* moved, the story changes. When power increases at the spine (through a combination of load *with* movement in and out of flexion), the collagen layers of the disc slowly begin to crack and break apart; this process is called *delamination*.[16]

FLEXED LUMBAR SPINE

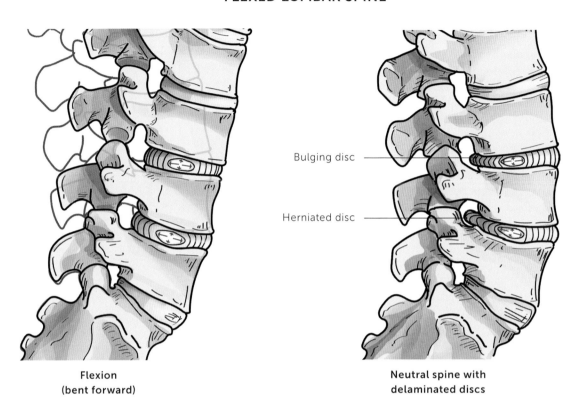

Bulging disc

Herniated disc

Flexion
(bent forward)

Neutral spine with
delaminated discs

DISC DELAMINATION

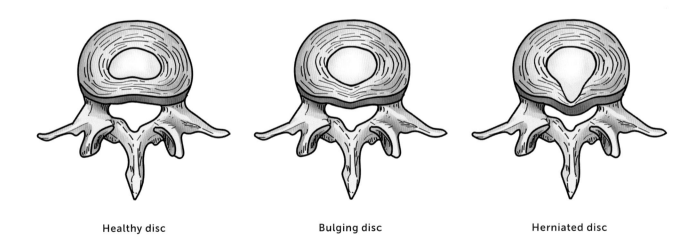

Healthy disc

Bulging disc

Herniated disc

When the collagen rings of a disc break apart or "delaminate," the disc loses its ability to withstand load. If the combination of load and movement at the spine continues, the pressurized inner gel of the disc (aka the jelly) will be forced through these newly formed cracks in the surrounding collagen.[17] This seepage of the inner gel of the disc is called a *bulge,* and if it's severe enough, it can lead to debilitating back pain and nerve irritation, causing pain to radiate down one or both legs.

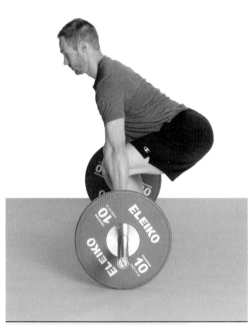

DEADLIFT WITH NEUTRAL SPINE

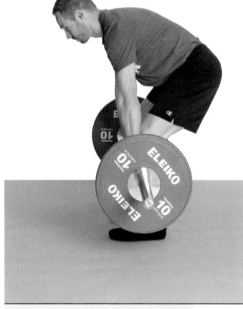

DEADLIFT WITH ROUNDED SPINE

In the weight room, a combination of load and movement occurs when an athlete allows their back to move when deadlifting or allows their lumbar spine to round at the bottom of a squat (known as "butt wink"). I often hear discussions across the internet where people claim, "Butt winking is *not* dangerous!" If the spine were composed of ball-and-socket joints like the hip and shoulder, I would agree. But spinal joints are different. The hip joint is designed to create power through a full range of motion; the spine is not.

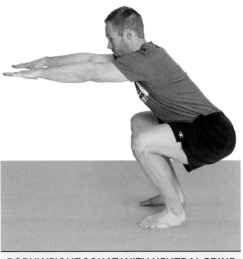

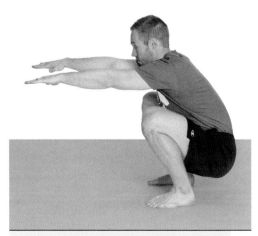

BODYWEIGHT SQUAT WITH NEUTRAL SPINE **BODYWEIGHT SQUAT WITH BUTT WINK**

Now, if you are just performing a few bodyweight squats and butt winking occurs, it's likely not a big deal. Minimal power is generated at the spine during a normal-tempo air squat. However, as soon as you add a barbell, things change. If butt wink-ing continues under load, the power generated at the spine increases at one or two specific joints of the lumbar spine (usually L4/5 and L5/S1). Therefore, when you have a stress concentration of power at one or two lumbar segments, injury risk increases. The more load and the more repetitions that take place, the higher the risk.

Does this mean every rounded-spine lift will create a bulging disc? Not necessar-ily. Many factors play into this discussion. Every athlete tolerates the forces of bend-ing their spine differently. This is why elite gymnasts can bend themselves in half over and over, yet attempting the same movements would eventually spell disaster for an elite heavyweight powerlifter. Here's a great way to understand this principle.

Some tree branches are slender and bend easily over and over again. Other branches are thicker and begin to snap in two after a few bends. Every body is different. Depending on a number of factors, such as your anatomy, genetics, the amount of weight lifted, and the degree of poor technique, your body may be more or less resilient to developing a disc bulge.[18]

This doesn't mean you should fear flexion of the spine. However, you must under-stand that the mechanism that creates a disc bulge *includes* flexion. If the force applied to the spine as it flexes is low, power generation remains low, and so does injury risk. This is why the cat-camel exercise (moving the spine through a full range in and out of flexion but under low load) is a great option for many people. It is not until we introduce force into the equation that things begin to change. Flexion by itself isn't the problem.

This is one reason why performing high-repetition Olympic lifts to the point of fatigue can lead to injury. The snatch and clean and jerk are amazing lifts *if* you don't break form. Elite weightlifters spend years perfecting their technique, often with low-repetition sets (1 to 3 lifts in a single set). However, consider a CrossFitter who performs 30 repetitions of the snatch lift as fast as possible in a fatigued state. While the quality of the first few reps may be high, fatigue can slowly deteriorate form. The back starts to round slightly in the deep reception of the lift, increasing stress on the disc and creating a pathway for a potential bulge. Every spine has a breaking point, and the quickest way to find it is to load your spine with a ton of compression and perform rep after rep with poor technique.

But what about elite powerlifters who deadlift with a rounded back?

Because lifting the most weight is the goal for competitive powerlifters, it is common to see a small degree of back rounding during max-effort deadlifts.[19] This is more often seen in those who use a conventional-style pulling technique versus a sumo-style deadlift (this is because the wider stance used during the sumo-style deadlift allows the lifter to have a more upright trunk position comparatively). However, some elite powerlifters have been known to hunch or round their backs purposefully.[20]

But doesn't this go against everything we just learned? Yes and no. To start, elite powerlifters who lift with this technique aren't usually allowing their back to move into more flexion as the lift is pulled. They're instead bracing or "locking in" their spine with a slight curvature in the spine, maintaining that degree of flexion and moving about the hips to complete the deadlift. The late Konstantin Konstantinov was a great example of this; you can find many of his legendary lifts on YouTube.

During one of my conversations with Dr. McGill on this exact topic, he had the following to say: "In terms of spinal stress and resilience, locking the spine in a neutral posture and moving entirely about the fulcrum of the hip would be the most resilient for the spine. However, you can flex without creating a stress concentration at a single level but create a gentle curve (and some of the great powerlifters have quite

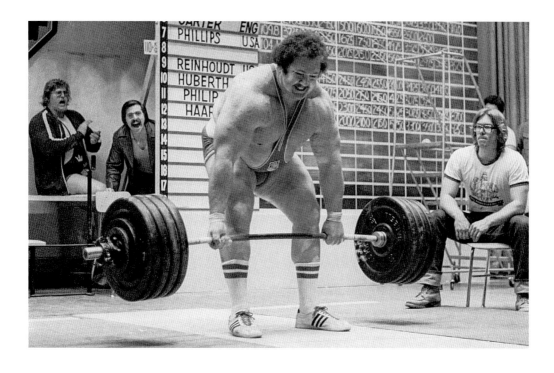

Elite deadlifter with rounded back.
*Don Reinhoudt,
©Bruce Klemens.*

a bit more in the thoracic spine) to allow the mechanics to pull around the knee. So it's a little bit of flexion, and then they lock it in place. When you measure this, the motion is still around the hips. This is the second best in terms of spinal stress and resilience to injury. For some lifters, it creates a mechanical advantage."[21]

So, by not allowing any back *motion* to occur, powerlifters can limit the extreme amount of concentrated stress that would be transferred to the spine if it were to be moved into more and more flexion.[22] The rationale is that starting with a slightly rounded spine decreases the amount of force the low back extensor muscles need to generate to perform the movement. If you want to go into the science of it, the rounded back shortens the moment arm between the shoulders and lower lumbar joints.[23] When discussing lifting mechanics, the moment arm is the length between a specific joint and the vertical line of gravity pulling down on the barbell. A shorter moment arm theoretically demands less from the body to lift the weight from the floor.

This same rationale is what allows a strongman to lift the giant Atlas Stone safely. After stiffening their spine over the stone and locking the spine into place, they can concentrate the majority of the movement of the heavy lift about the hips, keeping the power generated at the spine relatively low.

You should certainly take advice to start rounding your back to add a few more pounds to your deadlift with extreme caution. While some lifters can get away with this less-than-ideal technique, many will not adapt and fall prey to a disc bulge injury. Therefore, you must weigh the risks and rewards of lifting with this technique.

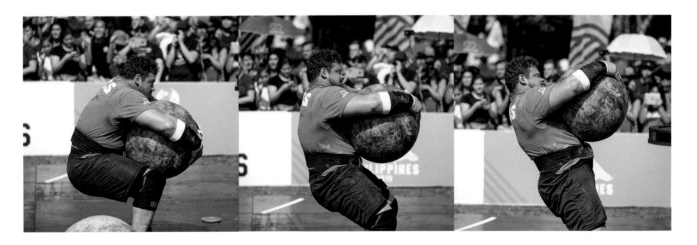

Atlas Stone lift.
Martins Licis, © SBD

Vertebral End-Plate Fracture

Your vertebrae aren't solid bone. If you sawed one in half, you'd see an intricate network of spongelike struts called *trabecular bone* that branch throughout and connect.[24] This complex arrangement creates a stiff framework to support the bone, allowing it to bear weight and resist being crushed by compressive loads.[25]

Just like your muscles, your bones can respond negatively or positively to the loads and frequency of loading they experience. Astronauts who are weightless for long periods in space commonly find that they have lost bone density when they return to Earth. If we deload the body, the bones respond negatively and lose strength.

TRABECULAR BONE OF VERTEBRAE

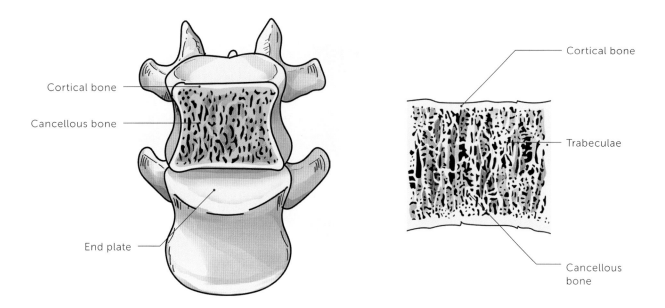

Lifting heavy weights, however, can cause your spine to adapt and the trabecular struts within your vertebrae to thicken over time.[26] This is why research has shown elite powerlifters (who experience spinal compressive forces of up to 16 times their body weight) to have some of the densest vertebral bones seen in humans.[27] However, we must not be quick to assume that all loading is good loading.

The cells of your bones respond to the stimulus of load by building more bone (a process called *osteogenesis*).[28] However, this process does not follow the "more is better" mantra. If you load your spine with heavy training over and over again, you will eventually reach a stage of diminishing returns where the response to lifting begins to stagnate. If you continue to push past this point, your bones will begin to break down.

When this happens, the spine sometimes develops tiny fractures. It is not uncommon for these microfractures to occur in strength athletes who continue to push their bodies to the max with heavy training year in and year out. In his book *Gift of Injury*, Stuart McGill writes that he has never seen an elite powerlifter who did not have evidence of a history of microfractures in their spine.[29]

These fractures usually start at a layer of tissue that is part bone and cartilage and separates the vertebra from the underlying disc, called the *end plate*. The end plate has two jobs. First, it has to be strong to handle compressive forces placed on the spine and prevent the inner gel of the disc from bulging into the bone above. Second, it must be porous or soft enough to allow nutrients and blood to flow to and from the disc below.

VERTEBRA END PLATE

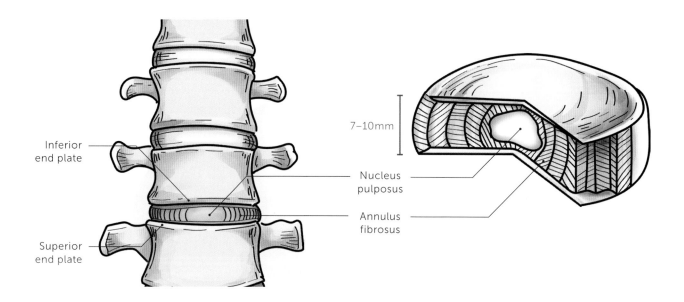

Inferior end plate

Superior end plate

7–10mm

Nucleus pulposus

Annulus fibrosus

When a lot of compression is applied to the spine, the end plate is stretched across the bone it covers, like someone spreading plastic wrap across a bowl.[30] Excessive compression can eventually overwhelm this plate and cause it (along with the underlying trabecular bone of the vertebra) to crack.

END PLATE FRACTURE

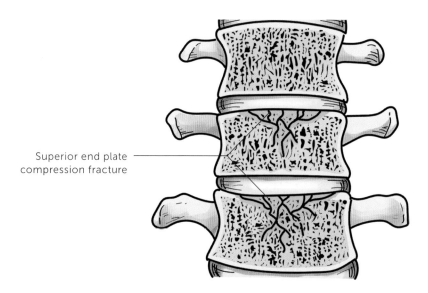

Superior end plate compression fracture

If given time to adequately recover after being overloaded during a heavy training cycle, the body can adapt and replace a microfracture with stronger bone. Think of this process like calluses developing on your hands to keep them stronger and more resilient to gripping the barbell. However, if there is insufficient recovery—like jumping back into another heavy training cycle without taking a deload week or two—the pressure placed on the spine will accumulate and push the bones past the tipping point. This is when these once-small fractures turn into a big problem.[31]

Facet Injury

Another reason pain can develop at the low back is an injury to the small joints on the back side of the spine called *facets*.[32] In fact, some research studies have estimated that between 15 and 40 percent of chronic back pain is due to a facet joint injury.[33]

FACET JOINT MOBILITY

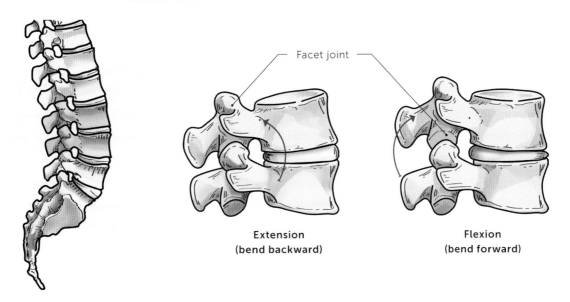

Facet joint

Extension
(bend backward)

Flexion
(bend forward)

Injuries to the facet joints occur for a few reasons.

Much like a glove that fits tightly over your hand, each of your facet joints is surrounded by a strong capsule. This capsule is highly innervated, meaning it has a ton of nerves running through it that help sense spine position, movement, and pain.[34] Much like a disc bulge, a facet joint injury is not often caused by one specific event but instead can be traced back to repetitive strain or microtrauma over time.[35]

The interesting thing about facet joints is that their shape can change depending on the spine level. Some facet joints can help create and limit excessive rotation of the spine, while others are set up to do the same for backward and forward bending.

For this reason, these joints can be injured during a number of different movements. For example, when the spine is extended to extreme end ranges (like an athlete who overarches their back while pressing a barbell over their head), a large amount of pressure shifts to these small joints of the lower spine (lumbar spine), which stretches the surrounding capsule.[36] If the body cycles too often into this position, it can irritate these joints and the surrounding capsules, leading to pain and eventual arthritis.

Research has also shown that facet joint irritation can be caused by combining either flexion or extension of the spine with rotation.[37] Let's take, for example, a weightlifter who has uneven hip mobility. If they move under the bar to catch a heavy clean, a mobility asymmetry in the hips could lead to a small twist in the pelvis, resulting in excessive stretch to the capsule of the lifter's lower spinal facet joints. If this side-to-side difference isn't addressed and fixed, over time the small technique problem may lead to irritation of a facet capsule/joint and eventual pain.

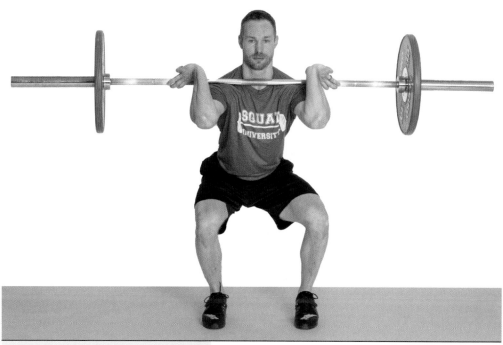

BARBELL CLEAN WITH TWISTED HIPS

As discussed earlier, an injury to one part of the spine often sets off a cascade of events. If an athlete has a history of a disc bulge, load is no longer evenly distributed across the vertebrae. Instead, when the spine is loaded, forces at that particular vertebral joint shift to the posterior aspects of the spine (the facet joints). Over time, this overload of the facet joints could lead to arthritis and the development of pain. As you can see, the facet joints can be injured in many ways.

Spondylolysis

Another possible injury to the structures on the back side of the spine is spondylolysis. Historically, this is one of the most serious back injuries for strength athletes. Spondylolysis is a fatigue stress fracture of the spine. It occurs at a very small part of the vertebra called the *pars interarticularis*, which is right next to the facet joint.

SPONDYLOLYSIS

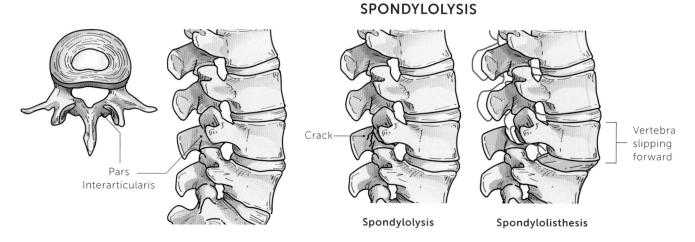

Pars Interarticularis

Crack

Vertebra slipping forward

Spondylolysis   Spondylolisthesis

Mechanically, this area absorbs a significant amount of force, especially if the low back is in an overextended or arched position (called *lumbar lordosis*). Much like a facet joint injury, repetitive loading of this area with an extended spine over time is thought to be the main cause of spondylolysis. If left unchecked, this stress fracture can lead to the more serious problem known as *spondylolisthesis* (anterior sliding of the spinal vertebra). This injury is most commonly found at the L5 vertebra.

Spondylolysis was once thought to be prevalent in strength athletes. A number of research articles suggested that weightlifters and specifically powerlifters were at high risk for sustaining this type of fracture.[38] For example, after following 26 Japanese weightlifters for several years, researchers found 24 of them to have recurrent back pain. Eight of these athletes (31 percent) were found to have spondylolysis.[39] Another group of researchers studied 27 weightlifters and 20 powerlifters and found 21 (44 percent) to have spondylolysis.[40] No significant difference was found between the weightlifters and powerlifters in this study.

However, there are a few things to take into consideration when looking at these numbers. First, research has shown that spondylolysis is strongly influenced by a person's genetics.[41] This means some of us are unfortunately predisposed to this injury, and the sport itself isn't necessarily the main culprit.

Second, every one of the studies that observed this injury among weightlifters did so before 1972. In that era, the clean and press was an official lift used in competition; it was removed in 1972. The pressing portion of this lift was usually performed with considerable extension of the lower back (out of the "neutral zone"). Performing this repeated motion while pushing tremendous weight likely led to the high percentage of documented spondylolysis injuries.[42]

Nevertheless, while this injury may not be as widespread among strength athletes as previously reported in research, this spinal stress fracture can occur if you repeatedly arch your low back and place it in a very extended position while performing any exercise (such as a squat, push press, or even a snatch from the hang position).

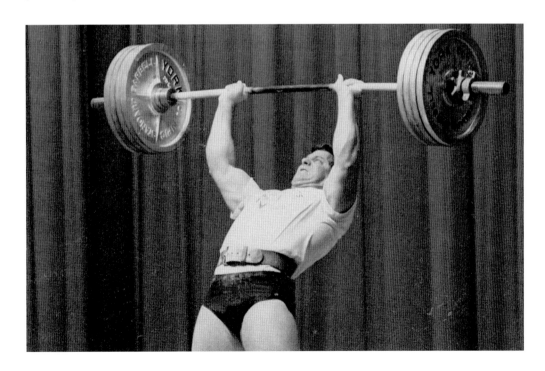

Barbell push press with extended spine.
Bob Kemper, © Bruce Klemens.

Nerve Pain

Do you have a stinging or burning pain that shoots down your legs? What about numbness in your thighs or feet? These symptoms are caused by irritation of nerves.

Think of your spinal cord as a major highway. Much like the small roads that branch off a highway, you have many nerves that exit your spinal column through tiny openings and travel throughout your body, providing a constant stream of information (like the sensation of pain, touch, or movement) to your central control center for processing.

When an injury in the spine occurs (from a bulging disc or degrading arthritis in the facet joints of the vertebrae), the nerves that run close by can be pinched. When this happens, pain can shoot down the entire length of the nerve.[43]

If you have experienced pain that radiates down the back of your thigh, it is likely sciatica (irritation of the sciatic nerve). This type of pain can be caused by a disc bulge, a narrowing of another canal of the spine, or an entrapment of the nerve by the piriformis muscle much lower at the hip. Pain that is felt traveling down the front of the thigh is caused by irritation of a different nerve, called the *femoral nerve*. Regardless of which nerve may be at fault, the first step in decreasing nerve-related pain is to change the way you move by avoiding motions that are associated with symptoms and replacing them with movements that are more sparing of the spine (something you'll learn about later in this chapter).

Muscle Pain

Have you heard the term "lumbar muscular sprain or strain"? It's one of the most common diagnoses medical doctors give to anyone who has an acute episode of low back pain. However, some experts are starting to agree that this is rarely the main cause of the injury.[44]

An injury to the back (due to a disc bulge, end plate fracture, facet irritation, or spondylolysis) creates a chemical reaction called *inflammation*. This leads to a secondary contraction or spasm of the muscles surrounding the injured site, likely as a compensation reaction of the body to stabilize around the injury.[45]

While a muscle strain injury may be common elsewhere in the body (like the hamstrings), any sensation of pain or tenderness in the muscles of your low back are likely only referring pain from the real problem that lies much deeper.[46]

The Mechanism of Injury

Only a few skilled master clinicians have the ability to diagnose which specific anatomical structure is causing back pain. Doing so requires expert assessment skills and expensive spinal scans. To make matters even more difficult, it is not uncommon for more than one structure to be generating pain (such as an active disc bulge and facet arthritis). Fortunately, you don't need to spend hundreds or even thousands of dollars to take the first steps to understanding and addressing your pain.

When someone asks, "What causes low back pain?" the simplest answer is that pain is the result of cumulative microtrauma on the structures of your back caused by three things:

- Specific movements
- Excessive training loads (too much compression on the spine)
- Sustained postures or body positions

Every part of your body, from the small bones and joints to the large muscles that span them, has a certain amount of force or load that it can tolerate before it fails and breaks. Athletes who can push themselves to the brink of this tipping point without going overboard often find massive success in improving their strength and performance. However, if that threshold is exceeded, injury occurs, and pain sets in.

Sometimes the mechanism that creates injury is blatant. Take, for instance, a powerlifter who allows their back to round into more and more flexion while deadlifting and all of a sudden feels a shot of pain. Other times the trauma is slowly applied over months or years through micromovements you cannot see with the naked eye.[47]

Although pain may strike at one specific moment (as Ryan from our previous story felt with the "pop" in his back during his last clean and jerk), the injury itself for most strength athletes is the result of something that has been building for some time. The signs of injury are often present even *before* symptoms appear. This means that while you may have "thrown your back out" while bending over to tie your shoes or performing your last set of clean and jerks, the cause of injury has actually been building for a while.

Keep Your Head Up

As you have read, the spine and its surrounding tissues can be damaged in many ways during weight training. While each injury is different, you may have noticed a similar theme underlying them all: the quality of your technique and the manner in which you load your body during training are the most important factors in determining whether your body adapts positively and becomes stronger or fails to adapt and ultimately finds injury.

If you have been told that you have one of the injuries described in this section, don't hang your head. There is hope! While you may be in pain, the good news is that your spine can heal from these injuries—and without surgery!

In the next section, we'll start the process of fixing your injury by diving into how to screen your low back. An efficient screening process is more valuable than an MRI scan that costs thousands of dollars.

How to Screen Your Low Back Pain

Back pain doesn't just appear out of thin air, and it's not "all in your head." There is always a reason for back pain. To remove it, you need to figure out why it started in the first place.

In my career as a physical therapist, I have spent countless hours reading, researching, and implementing many methods and techniques from experts around the world. I did not invent the screens and tests described in this section; they are a blend of ideas and techniques from experts including Gray Cook, Dr. Stuart McGill, Dr. Shirley Sahrmann, and Dr. Kelly Starrett. I have molded this wealth of information into my own approach to evaluating and treating patients. It is due to the wisdom and hard work of these experts that I can share it with you.

Most injuries that occur in the weight room are due to poor movement/technique or inappropriate loads. Over time, poor movement and/or loading habits create tiny amounts of trauma to your body that accumulate and eventually lead your body over the proverbial tipping point into injury. The framework for this theory has been called the *kinesiopathologic model*, or KPM.[48] While most of you will never have to remember the fancy name, the idea behind it is the key to fixing your pain. The idea is to start by finding out which movement problems led to the development of the injury in the first place.[49] Pretty simple.

The model is so different from the traditional medical approach because it focuses on the *why* behind your pain (which is typically poor movement or excessive load). The traditional way is typically to treat the specific tissue or part of the spine where the pain is located (e.g., disc bulge, symptomatic facet joint, or end plate fracture).[50] Basically, the goal is to take a giant step back and view how the body moves from head to toe rather than look at the injury through a microscope or with an MRI alone. This movement model does not dismiss or assume a specific anatomical problem as the cause of pain but instead treats any particular findings as "pieces of the pie" in the decision-making process. By stepping back, you avoid tunnel vision with low back injuries. Treat the person, not the injury.

Here's a brief example of this concept at work. Amy is a 21-year-old weightlifter who was referred to physical therapy with a diagnosis that reads, "Low back pain due to spondylolysis at L5." Spondylolysis is the specific anatomical cause of pain that her orthopedic doctor would like to fix. Through the examination, I found that Amy had difficulty performing any of the Olympic lifts from the hang position without moving into excessive lower back extension. Any time she arched her back in this manner, she felt extreme low back pain. With some proper coaching and cueing, she was able to correct her lumbar spine position during the hang position of a clean and reduce her symptoms.

Screening and classifying based on movement problems that cause pain (extension intolerance) is a more useful driver of the treatment process than trying to fix the pathoanatomical diagnosis. If we concentrate on the fact that Amy has a spondylolysis, then we miss the big picture, which could be movement dysfunction or strength/mobility deficits. Knowing that someone has a stress fracture of the spine doesn't necessarily tell us *why* they have pain or *what* needs to be corrected.

Therefore, instead of labeling Amy as a person with spondylolysis injury, I would classify her injury as "low back pain due to extension intolerance." By switching the focus to a movement diagnosis, we can then address her deficits and correct her technique/movement.

During the screening process that follows, I want you to think about which of the following categories your back pain fits the most:

- Flexion intolerance

- Extension intolerance

- Rotation with extension intolerance

- Load intolerance (due to dynamic and/or compressive loading)

Gather clues from each screen and test to help you figure out what type of posture, movement, or load triggers your back pain. The understanding and knowledge you receive from this self-assessment will empower you to take control of your injury and become your own best advocate for alleviating your pain.

Step 1: What Triggers Your Pain?

The first step in screening your low back is to do an in-depth self-analysis of what triggers your pain. You need to find out exactly *what* causes your pain. These are the activities, movements, and postures you assume throughout the day that bring out your symptoms. Think hard and write down your answers on a sheet of paper, as the answer is rarely "everything I do." Also write down which activities, movements, and postures you can perform without pain. Here are a few examples and things to keep in mind as you compile your list.

Excessive movement of the low back in training and on the competition stage are often huge predictors of the type of back pain strength athletes will experience. Think about all of the repetitive lifts or movements you do in the gym that create pain, either during or after.

Once you've placed your finger on the one or two things that lead to pain, can you find a common movement or position your back is in during them? For example, I often request athletes in pain to videorecord their lifting. I once worked with a weightlifter who came to me with back pain in the bottom of his squat. In the videos of his lifts, I noticed that he had excessive butt wink at the exact moment his pain came out. Therefore, we can use this clue to consider that his excessive spinal motion into flexion during squats was a possible trigger of pain (therefore categorized as flexion intolerance).

The amount of weight you attempt to lift could also be a trigger for pain. An athlete who experiences pain only when lifting over 70 percent of their one-rep max is likely placing excessive compression or shear forces on their spine. This would be labeled "load intolerance." If this sounds familiar, not only write down the amount of weight at which you start to experience symptoms but also analyze the motions and postures you are assuming during that specific exercise.

Along with your assessment of the gym movements that trigger your pain, the postures you assume and the movements you put your body through during the other 22 to 23 hours of the day outside of training are just as important to evaluate. The accumulated microtrauma that has caused your current back pain may not be due solely to training.

Think to yourself whether rounded or extended postures create or alleviate pain in your back. For example, I have many patients who complain of back pain after sitting all day at work yet have no pain if they are up and walking (this would point to flexion intolerance). However, some people may have pain when walking/running for 15 minutes that is relieved with they sit or bend forward (this is common of someone with an extension or load intolerance). Do either of those situations sound familiar?

Is your pain also associated with quick-tempo movements such as sneezing or jogging? If so, you may be dealing with load intolerance due to spinal instability. Often these pains can be modified by introducing spinal stability exercises (I'll go over these later in the chapter).

After doing your self-assessment, did you find a common motion, posture, or load that triggers your pain? Did you also notice any specific movements that you can do without pain? If you found a pattern to your pain, you should breathe a sigh of relief. You just took the first step in eliminating your pain.

Step 2: Screening Tests

To give you an even better idea of the cause of your pain, you will now perform a few tests. Again, the goal is to identify postures, motions, and loads that trigger your pain *and* those that you can perform without pain.[51] By pinpointing these problematic factors and making the invisible visible, you can then work to decrease your symptoms and return to lifting pain-free.

Posture (aka "Position") Assessment

As the great Yankee Yogi Berra once said, "You can observe a lot by watching." One of the first things I do as a physical therapist when working with a patient with back pain is to watch how they move. This part of the screening process is often referred to as a posture assessment.

When most people hear the phrase "posture assessment," they think of a clinician who stands in judgment of the way you stand, shaking their head at your rounded shoulders or slight anterior pelvic tilt. This is because many of us have been taught to appraise posture as either good or bad. However, this is *not* how we're going to do things. I want you to take a step back and look at your body through a different set of lenses.

Dr. Kelly Starrett once told me that the Latin root of *posture* is *position.* The goal of this part of the assessment is to see if you can link specific positions of your spine to your symptoms. This allows you to create better context around which spinal positions trigger your pain *and* which ones don't.

STANDING

Start by assessing the position of your spine when standing. Just stand as if you're waiting in line at the grocery store. Have a friend take a photo of you from the side, front, and back.

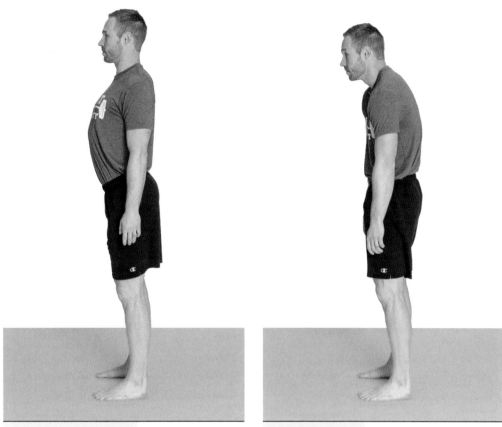

OVEREXTENDED SPINE   **ROUNDED SPINE**

Then ask yourself, "Do I have pain while in this position?" If the answer is no, move on to the next part of this examination. But if the answer is yes, see if you can figure out why and if you can modify the symptoms you're experiencing.

What do you notice about your standing position? Are your shoulders rounded? Is your chin poking out in front of your body? Is your low back flat, or does it have an excessive arch? Do you feel certain muscles of your back flexing or contracting hard?

Certain standing positions, such as slumped-forward shoulders, can cause some muscles to remain "on" and active during the day. Many people who report back pain while standing often adopt postures that don't allow the low back muscles to relax.

If this is you, try to change your posture right now by using the cue "stand tall" and see how it affects your low back stiffness. Did anything change? The goal is to teach your body a new way to stand that is pain-free and alleviates tension. If changing the way you stand has already modified your pain levels, you have found a strategy to modify and wind down your symptoms!

ADDING LOAD

Next, assess how your body responds to different postures or spinal positions when you add a compressive load to the equation. This test is one I picked up from Dr. Stuart McGill, and I have found it very helpful in the evaluation process with my patients.

Start by sitting on a stool with your arms by your sides. Assume a good postured "tall" position with your spine in neutral. There will be a small arch in your low back. Next, grab the stool with your hands and pull upward to compress your spine. What did you feel? Did this action create pain in your back? Next, round your lower back and perform the same pulling motion. What happened this time? Did you have pain in your back after adding a bit of compression in the rounded position? Do the test one more time, but with an overly arched back (spinal extension). Write down what you find.

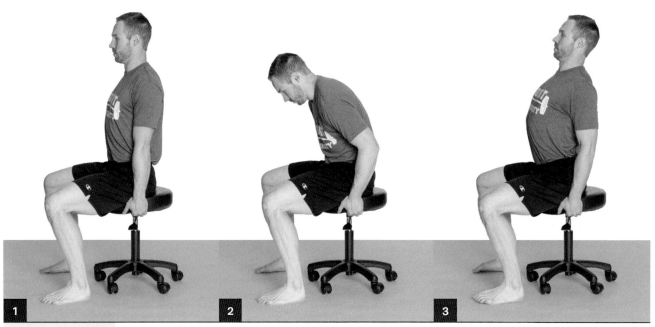

SEATED PULL TEST

If you found pain presented when sitting with good posture during this screen, you can conclude that certain loads trigger your symptoms. Even when lifting with good posture, the added compression (that largely comes from muscle contraction) is too much for your back at this time, and you must stop lifting heavy for the time being if you want your back to heal.

If instead you had pain that presented when you rounded or extended your back under compression, you can assume postures out of "neutral" triggered your back injury. We refer to these problems as flexion intolerance if your pain was brought out when rounding your back or extension intolerance if it was with the overly arched back.

Next, lie flat on your stomach on a bed or the floor for a minute or two. If this position starts to hurt, stand up and move to the next assessment; you likely have an extension intolerance that makes lying on your stomach painful. If this position causes you no pain, remain lying on your stomach for a few minutes. Afterward, stand up without letting your spine round; push up from your hands.

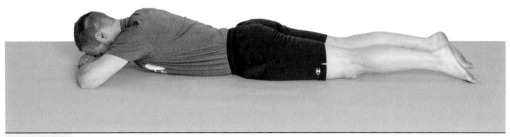

PRONE LIE

Did you notice anything different? If your pain was reduced after lying on your stomach for a few minutes, we can assume that you have flexion intolerance. In the prone position, you probably felt better because your spine is unloaded (no gravity compression) and your back is slightly extended when you're on your stomach. If this sounds like you, I recommend spending a few minutes every day lying on your stomach as a way to decrease your pain.

Next, while in that same prone position, raise one leg at a time off the bed or floor; make sure to keep it completely straight. It doesn't need to move far, but most of us should have around 10 degrees of hip extension. Assess both legs and compare how much movement occurs at each hip and whether the movement produces any pain in your low back.

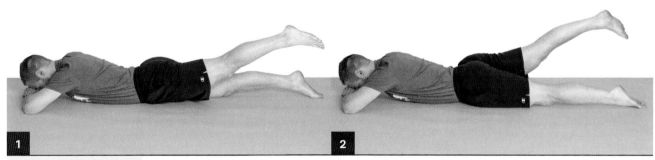

PRONE HIP EXTENSION

If extending your leg off the bed or floor (the movement of hip extension) produced pain, place a pillow under your stomach. Try the same test again, but this time brace your core muscles like you're about to get punched in the stomach, and don't allow your opposite leg (the one that remains flat on the bed or floor) to push into the bed or floor (the movement of hip flexion).

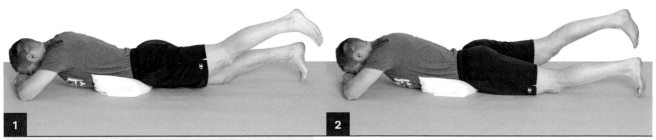

PRONE HIP EXTENSION WITH PILLOW UNDER STOMACH

When you raised your hip off the bed or floor this time, did your symptoms change? If so, this suggests extension intolerance with a rotational component, meaning that your low back is sustaining uneven forces when one leg moves behind you. This may be a clue as to why you have pain when moving into a weightlifting split jerk position or when running.

If you fall into this category, you may benefit from improving hip extension range of motion with an anterior pull banded joint mobilization. Kneel on the ground with the leg you want to mobilize in contact with the ground. Place a band around the down hip just under your glutes. You want the pull to be going forward toward the rig to which the band is attached. Brace your core and lock your lumbar spine in neutral, and then squeeze your glutes as you slowly shift your hips forward and backward.

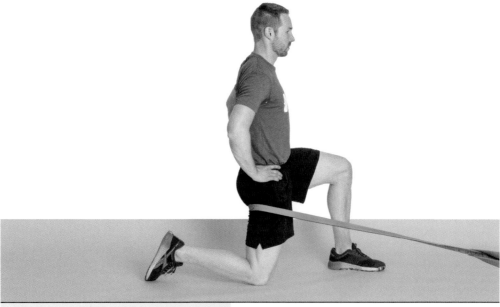

ANTERIOR BANDED JOINT MOBILIZATION

The idea behind this mobilization is to help assist the joint through this movement and free up any restrictions that are limiting hip extension. Perform a set of 10 to 20 repetitions and then recheck the prior prone leg-lift screen and see what you find.

Did the mobilization improve your hip extension mobility so that you could move about your hips and not your low back? Was the movement less painful? If so, you have found a helpful tool for addressing your individual movement problem and decreasing your pain.

Movement Assessment

After you perform the posture assessments, I want you to perform a few common movements. Start by doing a deep bodyweight squat and hold the bottom position for a few seconds. If pain-free, perform the same movement with a barbell on your back. Have a friend observe what happens to your low back as you reach the deepest portion of the squat.

Those who have pain in the deeper portions of the squat often show a posterior pelvic tilt that creates an excessive rounding motion in the low back—aka butt wink. This motion is often created at the hip joint.

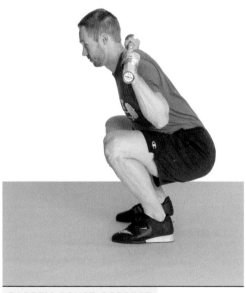

BARBELL SQUAT: CORRECT

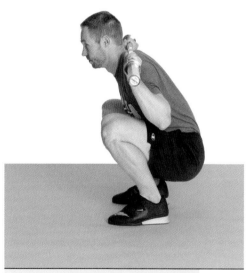

BARBELL SQUAT WITH BUTT WINK

You see, during the descent of the squat, the thigh bone (femur) rotates in the hip socket (acetabulum). As the depth of the squat increases, the femur can eventually come into contact with the front rim of the socket. The timing of this contact depends on the size and orientation of the femur along with the depth of the socket (anatomy we can thank our parents for). Often, the deeper the hip socket, the earlier this potential collision occurs.

HIP SOCKET DEPTH

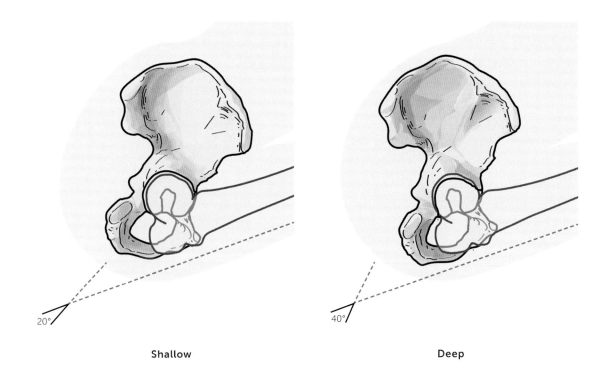

20°

Shallow

40°

Deep

Because the femur can no longer move at this point, the pelvis must reflexively rotate under the body to continue the descent of the squat, which brings the low back into a rounded position as well.

BUTT WINK

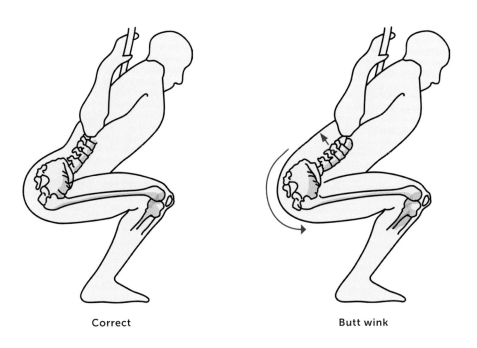

Correct

Butt wink

Is having butt wink automatically a sign of impending back pain? Not necessarily, but it is not encouraged when lifting weights. Think back to the equation power = force × velocity.

While your hip joint is meant to move under load, your spine is not. As discussed previously, the fibers that make up your vertebral discs begin to break apart when the spine is loaded and moved in and out of flexion, a process called *delamination.* Because the amount of flexion created at the lumbar spine during the butt wink motion is often small and takes place at only a select few segments (L4/5 and L5/S1, for example), it creates a stress concentration. Therefore, the butt wink motion not only moves the spine in and out of flexion but does so under load when you are lifting—the exact mechanism that leads to disc bulges.

If this motion creates pain for you, does eliminating butt wink by modifying your stance and depth so that you can maintain a more neutral spinal alignment during the squat alleviate your symptoms? If so, you can link the movement of your pelvis under load to your symptoms, and you likely have a flexion intolerance problem. Your first step is to be cognizant of how much butt wink your body has when squatting or dropping under a clean or snatch. The second step should be to check out the mobility of your ankles.

Why does ankle mobility matter when it comes to low back pain? When the ankle becomes stiff and immobile (particularly in the movement of dorsiflexion), the knee is unable to push forward over the toes during the deepest portion of the squat. This means that if you continue to descend, another part of your body (your pelvis and low back) has to give way and move excessively.[52]

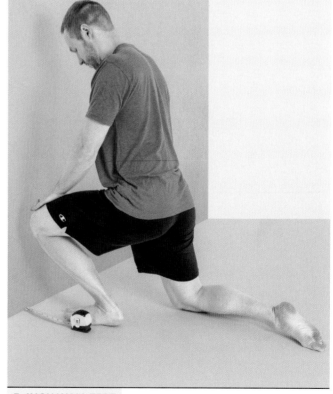

The 5-inch wall test is an easy way to screen for ankle mobility problems.[53] Find a wall and kneel close to it with your shoes off. Use a tape measure and place your big toe 5 inches from the wall. From this position, push your knee forward, attempting to touch the wall with your knee and keeping your heel in contact with the ground.

If you were unable to touch your knee to the wall, you have an ankle mobility restriction. It could be a soft tissue restriction, a joint mobility problem, or both! Make sure to check out the mobility exercises (foam rolling/stretching of the calf and joint mobilizations) discussed in the Ankle Pain chapter. Working every day to improve ankle mobility should be a priority if you wish to return to deep squatting pain-free!

5-INCH WALL TEST

For the next test, stand with an unloaded barbell on your back. Push your hips back and tip your pelvis forward (moving your back in and out of an arched position). Did this movement bring out pain? If it did, you are intolerant to the movement of spinal extension, and you will need to limit this position to avoid pain.

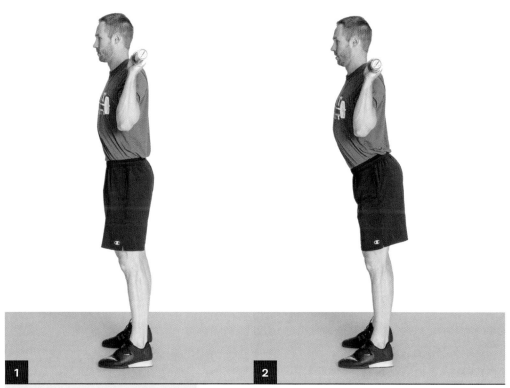

BAR ON BACK SPINAL EXTENSION

Take the barbell off your shoulders and hold it at your waist in the hang position. Bend forward and let the barbell drop to the middle of your shins as if you were performing a Romanian deadlift (RDL). If you don't have a barbell (or just holding one in your hands creates back pain), simply mimic the motion with your hands by your sides.

Hold this position for a few seconds and then return to the start position. What did you experience? If you felt pain while bending forward, try the motion again, but this time brace your core and start the movement with a proper hip hinge. Move entirely about your hips; don't let your back move at all. Did your symptoms change? If so, you probably have signs of flexion intolerance.

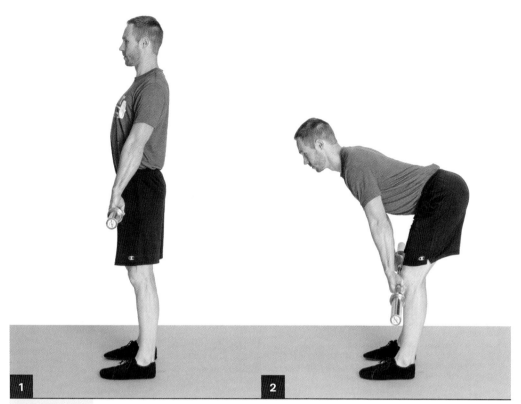

BARBELL RDL

If you didn't have pain while bending over but had pain while returning to a standing position, try a similar correction cue. Athletes who have pain upon returning from this forward position frequently move from the low back and *then* the hips (lumbar extension followed by hip extension). Try the movement again, but this time, squeeze your glutes while driving your heels into the ground on the ascent. Try to move entirely about the hips, and don't let your back arch. Was the movement pain-free this time? If so, it's a sign of an extension intolerance problem.

If these corrections modified your back pain even slightly, you must adopt a new way of moving to decrease your pain. The idea of moving about the hips and not the back applies to movements in the weight room and throughout your day (e.g., picking up a basket of laundry from the floor). At this time, your back is sensitive to certain movements, and the best way to decrease your pain symptoms is to adopt new strategies to work around your individual pain triggers.

Next, perform a single-leg squat on each leg while barefoot. Have a friend observe how you move on each leg, or take a video with your phone for self-analysis. The goal is *not* to see if you can perform a full-depth pistol squat, but instead to see if there is a side-to-side difference in how well you can control a single-leg squat *and* if this movement re-creates your pain.

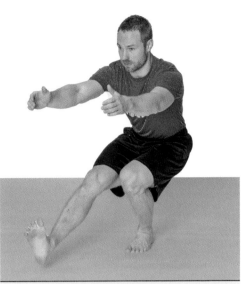

SINGLE-LEG SQUAT WITH GOOD CONTROL   **SINGLE-LEG SQUAT WITH POOR CONTROL**

While you may not perform single-leg squats as a part of your training in the weight room, you should have the ability to perform a quality single-leg squat to at least a parallel position for two reasons. First, think about what happens when you walk down a flight of stairs. You're moving on one leg. Every step you descend requires you to eccentrically lower your body under control (aka a single-leg squat). The same thing happens every time you run or hop.

Second, an imbalance in movement control during a single-leg squat will cause problems in double-leg movements (squat, clean, deadlift, etc.). If your lower body control is not symmetrical during barbell movements, forces will be unevenly transferred up to your spine. These subtle differences (which are often too small for the naked eye to see) are easily exposed with the single-leg squat assessment.

If the single-leg squat re-created your pain on either side, try using these cues to see if you can modify your symptoms. Stand on one leg and brace your core slightly. Grab the ground with your feet, creating the tripod foot (see page 201). Your body weight should be spread evenly across the entire foot, not all in the heel! Hinge at your hips by pushing your butt back and bringing your chest forward. If you do this correctly, your center of gravity will remain in the middle of your foot. Squat down slowly without allowing your knee to waver.

Did your symptoms change? If so, it is a sign that working on proper movement sequencing with single-leg stability drills will be an important part of your rehab plan. I highly recommend checking out the touchdown progression from the Knee Pain chapter (see pages 206 and 207).

Load Testing

A simple way to determine whether load, or the weight you are lifting, is triggering your pain is to perform the weighted front raise test.[54] Start by holding a light dumb-bell or kettlebell by your stomach; anything between 5 and 15 pounds works great.

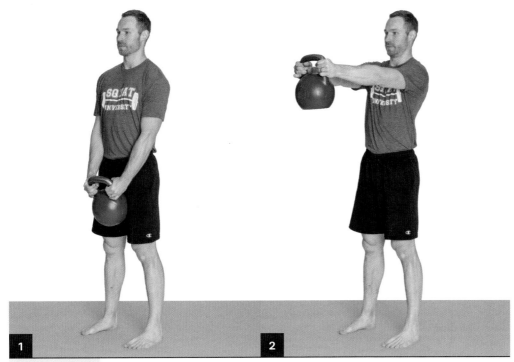

LOAD TESTING

Raise the weight out in front of you without bending your arms. Make sure to take a few deep breaths in and out while you hold the weight in the extended position. What happened to your pain level? If extending the weight triggered back pain, try the same motion again, but this time brace your core muscles and then move the weight. Did you notice a difference?

If bracing your core before extending the weight eliminates or significantly decreases your pain, you can assume that the loads you are lifting in the gym are contributing to your pain (also called *load intolerance*). Learning to stiffen your trunk anytime you move a load (picking up a box off the ground or squatting a barbell) needs to be your first priority. Ingraining this needed stability with purposeful core exercises will be key to your recovery.

However, if you still had pain even when bracing your core, your body is extremely load intolerant and sensitive to lifting any weight at this time. This means you need to eliminate weight training and heavy lifting outside of the gym (moving furniture around the house, picking up multiple bags of groceries at a time, etc.) for the time being to allow your back symptoms to calm down.

The last screen, called the heel drop test, looks into how your body deals with a rapidly applied load.[55] Start by standing with your abdominals completely relaxed, rise up on your toes, and then quickly drop down onto your heels. Your feet should hit the ground hard as if performing a power snatch or clean. Do this twice, once with both legs and again with one leg.

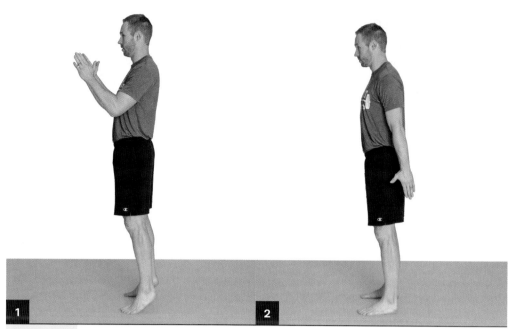

HEEL DROP

Did this jarring motion to your spine cause pain? If so, you can assume you have a load intolerance. It could be due to either excessive compression on the spine or instability (micromovements of the spine that occur because of an inability of the surrounding muscles to effectively stabilize against quickly applied force).

Now, repeat this test with a small brace of your core. Did you notice anything different?

If bracing your core when performing the heel drop eliminated your pain, you have uncovered a possible reason for why you have pain when performing movements like box jumps or when catching a clean or snatch, or when running. Your core muscles are doing a poor job of stabilizing your spine when load is rapidly applied to your body. This allows micromovements to occur and trigger pain. You should make it a priority to work on bracing your core and improving stability in your spine when performing fast-tempo movements.

However, if bracing your core while performing the heel drop test still led to an increase in symptoms, it probably indicates dynamic load intolerance due to excessive compression. You could have an end plate fracture. If you failed the drop test, it is imperative that you eliminate barbell training and dynamic activities such as running and sports to allow your spine to recover and heal. Sometimes, training through a back injury does more harm than good; this is definitely one of those situations where you should hit the pause button on training.

Hip Extension Coordination

Have you heard the term *gluteal amnesia*? Decades ago, a renowned clinician named Vladimir Janda began to notice patterns in patients with back pain. Specifically, he noticed that these patients had signs of inhibited weak glutes. At the time, there was little research to back up his theories as to why this inhibition occurred, but research now shows that pain can inhibit the activation of the glutes.[56]

In 2013, Stuart McGill and his team observed this inhibition happening in real time.[57] They started by measuring glute activity in study participants who performed glute bridge exercises. They then performed a therapeutic procedure called *capsular distension arthrogram,* which temporarily creates a ton of pain in the hip joint. When they immediately retested the bridge, they found the activity of the glute max on the side of the painful hip to be significantly reduced. Dr. McGill termed this phenomenon gluteal amnesia.[58] It's not that the glutes turned off completely; instead, gluteal amnesia means that the brain is diminishing neural drive and inhibiting the glute muscles from firing appropriately due to pain (a process called *arthrogenic neuromuscular inhibition*).

Here is a test to see if you may be dealing with gluteal amnesia. The goal is to see how your body coordinates hip extension, the movement that occurs at your hip joint when you stand up from a squat, pull a barbell from the floor, or propel your body forward during a sprint. For your back to remain healthy when lifting heavy, your hips must have the ability to generate the appropriate amount of force and fire at the appropriate time (called an *optimal motor recruitment pattern*). This screen looks into just that and assesses how the muscles that surround your hips (primarily your glute max) work with the low back.

While lying on your back with your knees bent, straighten one leg and perform a single-leg bridge. Hold your hips in the air for 10 seconds and feel for which muscles are working hard to keep you up *and* if this movement brings out any back pain.

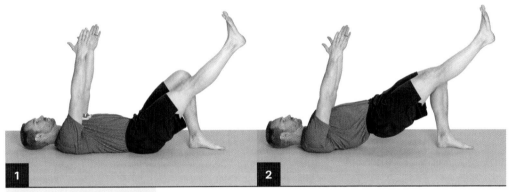

SINGLE-LEG BRIDGE TEST

Which muscles were working hard to keep your hips up? If anything other than your glutes (butt muscles) were the primary muscle group, you have a coordination issue in how your body is producing hip extension (aka gluteal amnesia).

Did this movement produce pain? As you bridge on one leg, pain is a response to the uneven forces being placed on your back. This is due to the inability of the glutes to kick on appropriately and contribute to hip extension, which means the erectors of your low back have to pull double time. When this happens, a ton of force is placed on the spine, which leads to pain.

If this was you, try performing a double-leg bridge. Jam your feet into the ground and squeeze your butt muscles as you raise your hips. Make sure to keep your low back from overarching; don't raise your hips too high off the ground. Was there less pain than before? If your pain decreased, you need to incorporate glute exercises into your rehab program. Strengthening and recoordinating the glutes to be able to do single-leg bridges with proper glute activation will be an integral part of your rehab program to help re-establish a proper muscle recruitment pattern.

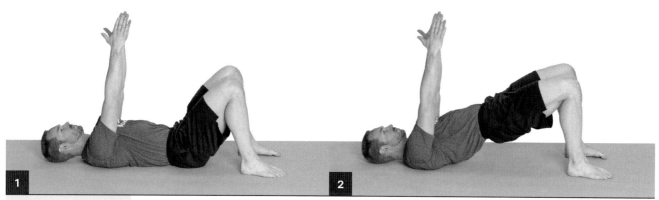

DOUBLE-LEG BRIDGE

Hip Mobility Assessment

Stiff hips affect the role of the joint complex directly above: the low back. Restrictions in hip mobility or significant differences from one side to the other can lead the low back to move out of the desired neutral spinal alignment when lifting. For this reason, a thorough evaluation of a back injury must include an assessment of hip mobility.

Research has shown that the rotation of the hips (especially a lack or a difference from side to side) is a large risk factor in the development of back pain.[59] If an athlete has a significant deficit in rotation on one side of the body, the low back will sustain uneven forces as the body drops into the bottom position of a squat, clean, or snatch.

To screen for hip rotation problems, start by lying on your back. Have a friend grab your leg, bend your knee, and lift your thigh to a 60-degree angle from the bench or floor.

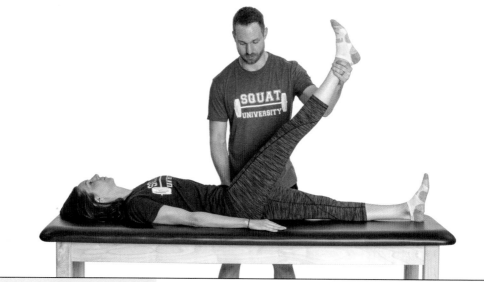

HIP FLEXION TO 60 DEGREES

From this position, your friend can rotate your lower leg away from the midline of your body to assess the amount of internal rotation you have and toward the midline of your body to assess the amount of external rotation you have. Perform the same movement on both legs. If one leg moves a few inches more in one direction than the other, you have a significant difference in side-to-side rotation.

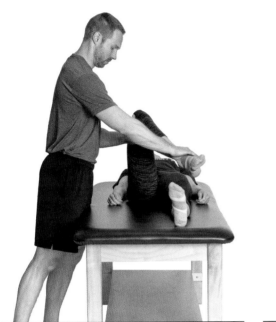

HIP EXTERNAL ROTATION

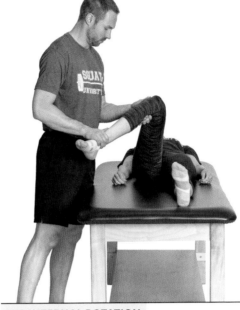

HIP INTERNAL ROTATION

If you uncovered an imbalance, banded joint mobilizations can be helpful for restoring lost motion. Start by placing a long resistance band around your thigh, getting it as high as you can toward your hip. Put a ton of pressure on the band as you assume a half-kneel, with the hip you want to work on in the forward position. The band should be pulling laterally away from your body.

Once in the half-kneeling position, use your hand to pull your forward knee across your body and back to the start position. After holding for a few seconds, drive your knee out to the side and squeeze your lateral glutes. Keep your foot firmly planted into the ground during this motion; don't let your foot roll onto its side!

Perform this movement of pulling your knee in and holding for a few seconds before pushing it out to the side and squeezing your glutes 20 times before retesting your hip mobility. Always recheck your hip mobility directly afterward to see if you were effective in creating the change you desire.

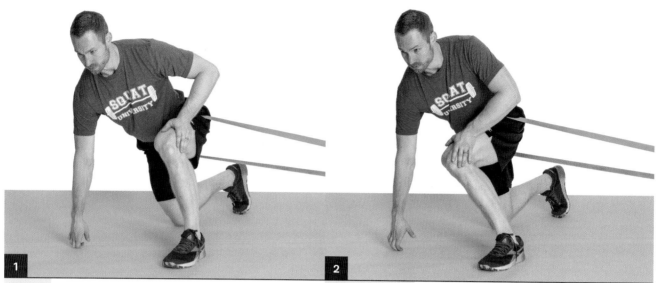

1
SETUP

2
MOVEMENT IN

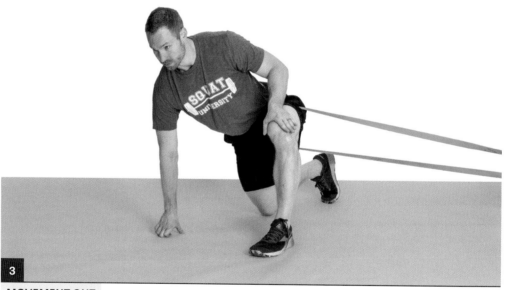

3
MOVEMENT OUT

Next, turn to the Hip Pain chapter and try the Thomas test (see page 144) and the FABER test (see page 142). You must address any uncovered hip mobility restrictions as a part of your comprehensive rehab program.

Thoracic Spine Mobility Assessment

Just as limited hip mobility can lead to excessive stress on the low back, mobility restrictions in the thoracic spine (mid-back) or shoulders can lead to unwanted stress in the low back. Poor mobility in either the thoracic spine or the shoulders often causes the low back to move excessively as compensation when the arms are raised overhead, such as when placing a box onto a high shelf, pressing a barbell, or performing a snatch. If you have found your back pain to fit into the "extension intolerant" category, I recommend the following tests.

While assessing thoracic spine extension can be tricky without the help of an expert clinician, the seated rotation screen is a good self-diagnostic test that can give you a good idea of how well this part of your back is moving.

Tape an "X" on the ground with the pieces of tape intersecting to form 90-degree angles. Sit in the middle of the "X" so that the tape forms a "V" in front of you. With a PVC pipe across your chest, rotate as far as you can to the right and then to the left. Ideally, you should be able to rotate your T-spine 45 degrees each way, which will align the pipe with the tape on the ground.[60] If you are unable to rotate to at least 45 degrees each way or you have a significant imbalance in either direction, you have uncovered a potential factor contributing to your low back pain.

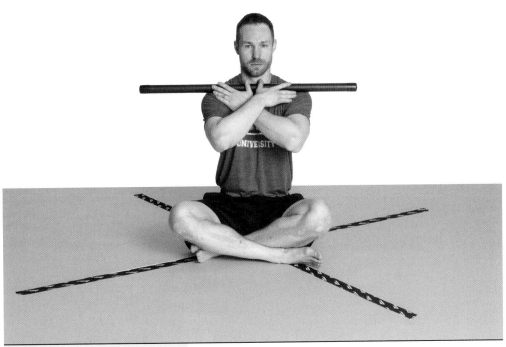

**T-SPINE ASSESSMENT SETUP
WITH PVC PIPE ACROSS CHEST**

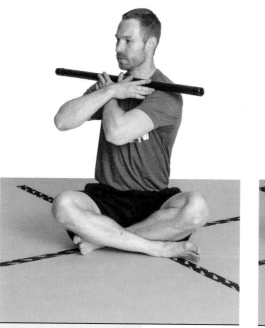

ROTATE TO RIGHT: GOOD

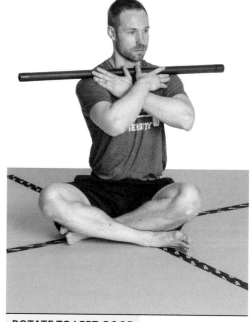

ROTATE TO LEFT: POOR

To assess your shoulder mobility, start by sitting against a wall. Your head, upper back, and hips should be in contact with the wall, and your lower spine should be neutral; you don't need to jam your low back into the wall.

With your arms extended in front of you and your palms facing the ground, raise your arms as high overhead as you can. If you'd like, you can do this test with a PVC pipe and the same grip you would use for a clean and jerk or an overhead press. Keep your core braced and your ribs from flaring out as you perform this movement.

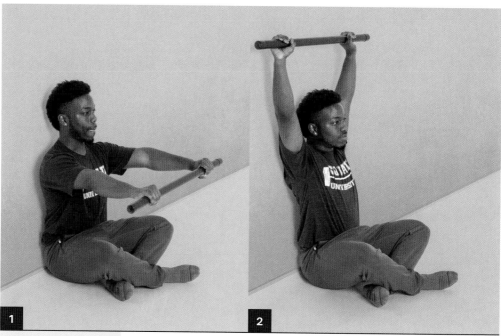

PVC PIPE WALL TEST

Ideally, you should be able to finish with your arms close to your ears, in a position similar to the narrow grip of an overhead press. This motion should be effortless and shouldn't require much force to complete. If you passed, congratulations; you have adequate overhead shoulder mobility. If not, you have uncovered another potential factor contributing to your back pain.

If you found limitations in either of the prior screens, the foam roller prayer stretch is a great go-to for improving overhead mobility. Start in a kneeling position with your hands on top of a foam roller. Sit your hips back on your heels and push your hands out in front of you (with your arms parallel, as shown, or with one hand on top of the other). Next, let your chest drop to the floor. Continue to reach overhead with your arms together while you slowly let out your breath. Try to sink your chest toward the ground.

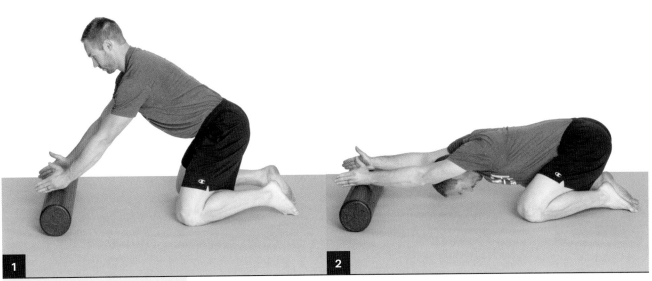

FOAM ROLLER PRAYER STRETCH

If you have a stiff mid-back, this exercise should bring out a good stretch in your spine. Those who also have poor lat flexibility may feel a good stretch on the sides of the back where these muscles run and attach to the undersides of the arms, near the armpits. I recommend doing 3 or 4 sets, holding the stretch for 30 seconds (about 5 deep breaths in and out).

Classifying Your Back Pain

Despite what some in the medical field say, there is no such thing as "nonspecific back pain." By now, I hope you have been able to find the exact trigger(s) for your pain. Understanding how your injury presents will help you figure out what you need to do *and* what you need to avoid in the short term to decrease your symptoms.

Nearly all back pain can be controlled and altered by changing the way you move. However, there is no one-size-fits-all approach to fixing pain. Everyone will respond differently based on their cause for pain. What may decrease pain in one person may increase it in another. However, the screening process you just went through should have helped you distinguish the specific postures (aka spinal positions), motions, and loads that aggravate your pain. From here, you need to make some small adjustments to your day-to-day movement habits to desensitize and "wind down" your pain levels.[61]

For example, if you feel pain when your spine is rounded or loaded in a bent position (i.e., flexion intolerance), you may be able to alter your pain throughout the day by moving about your hips (like an RDL) or even kneeling to the ground every time you bend over to pick something up. If your pain is reduced during the heel drop test by bracing your core (a classification of load intolerance due to core instability), learning to maintain sufficient stability when moving during the day and in the gym will be the first step in altering your pain levels. Modifying and eliminating these particular motions, postures, or loads that cause back pain in the short term and replacing them with those that feel good is the first step in fixing your pain. This is simply a matter of moving differently throughout the day.

Eventually, you will notice longer periods of pain-free time, but be aware that these changes won't happen overnight. This is because injury often heightens sensitivity to pain through a neurologic overreaction of the brain.[62] Think about how it feels when you stub your big toe: it becomes overly sensitive to forces placed on it. This is why every small step you take directly afterward hurts like crazy. This happens to a greater extent in those who have chronic back pain, and it is why the smallest movements, like bending forward to pick up a bag of groceries or turning over in bed, may set off tremendous pain. Identifying the triggers that influence your pain and completing the screens in the previous section put you on track to resolving your back pain.

Unfortunately, some claim that this idea creates fear of specific movements. This is far from the truth! Instead, I find that teaching and showing clients how specific movements can influence pain empowers them to understand their bodies better and ultimately take control of their injuries. After the tests you just performed, you are in the driver's seat, and how you use your body throughout the day will determine whether or not you have pain!

Stuart McGill once told me, "During recovery, what you *don't* do is often just as important as what you *do* do." Remember this motto as you begin your journey to eliminate your pain and return to the activities you love. Below, I have laid out some suggestions based on the movement diagnosis that you may fall under. These are general guidelines and certainly not hard rules.

Flexion Intolerance

Your pain tends to come out when your spine is in a flexed position or moves into flexion.

GUIDELINES:

In bed: Don't sit straight up when getting out of bed. Roll to your side and then push up with your arms. If lying on your stomach feels good, remain on your stomach for a few minutes two or three times a day.

Sitting: Place a small rolled towel under your low back to keep it from rounding. Sit up tall and don't slouch!

Standing: Make sure you're standing tall and not slouching throughout the day.

Picking things up: Instead of bending over to grab something (like clothes out of a laundry basket), kneel down to keep your back from rounding. Also learn how to hinge at the hips while maintaining a neutral spine. This will keep your low back from entering into too much flexion when picking objects off the ground.

Extension Intolerance

SIGNS & SYMPTOMS:

Your pain tends to come out when your spine is in an overarched position or moves into extension.

GUIDELINES:

In bed: If you're a stomach sleeper, place a pillow under your belly. If you sleep on your back, place a pillow under your knees. Both will help decrease the amount of extension in your low back to make sleeping more comfortable.

Sitting: Relax your back against the back of a chair. Don't sit on the edge, which may cause you to overarch your spine.

Standing: Check your posture in the mirror (lateral view). Make sure your low back is in neutral and not excessively arched.

Picking things up: Think about moving from your hips more than your low back (emphasize hip extension over low back extension). Kneeling or squatting down to pick something off the ground is also helpful.

Rotation with Extension Intolerance

SIGNS & SYMPTOMS:

Your low back becomes painful when extension is coupled with a rotational or twisting movement.

GUIDELINES:

In bed: If you're a side sleeper, place a pillow between your knees to limit excessive rotation at your spine and hips. When getting out of bed, roll your legs and trunk together.

Sitting: Try not to cross your legs. Also avoid leaning or shifting your weight excessively to one hip.

Standing: Stand with normal posture, but make sure you are placing equal weight through both legs. Having one foot forward and one foot back may cause unwanted rotation at the hip/spine.

Picking things up: Limit excessive rotation in your trunk. Move with your hips/legs, not with your back.

Load Intolerance (Dynamic or Compressive)

SIGNS & SYMPTOMS:

Your pain comes out when lifting something heavy or when performing physical tasks that load your spine rapidly, such as performing Olympic lifts or running.

GUIDELINES:

- Avoid running or any other task that places a load or shock through your body.
- Limit your lifting in the gym to pain-free tasks at this time! Don't be a tough guy and push through pain; it will only stretch out the time it takes to become pain-free.

Can I Still Lift?

During these next few weeks and possibly months, you must consider limiting your heavy training and exercising only with movements that do not create pain. Pain not only is an annoyance but also changes the way you move.[63]

This means the back pain you are experiencing is hindering your ability to use good technique when lifting. Not only does this have direct implications on your performance, but training through pain and loading your body with compromised technique can worsen the injury.

I have worked with many athletes who have continued to push through heavy programming while dealing with back pain. It does not end well. If you want to eliminate your pain and return to high-performance lifting, you must tone down any lifting that creates pain at this time. This doesn't mean you should stop working out! You must change how you are lifting in the short term to allow healing to take place.

When Is It Time to See a Doctor?

If none of these strategies works, or if your pain is progressively getting worse, please seek out a skilled clinician (physical therapist, chiropractor, or orthopedic doctor who specializes in back pain). If you are experiencing a recent unintentional loss in weight, incontinence, pain, or numbness in your abdomen or pelvic floor, I highly recommend you make an appointment to see your medical doctor.

The Rebuilding Process

By now, you should have a good idea of which specific triggers cause your pain. You should also have an understanding of which postures and movements you can perform pain-free. It is time to start addressing a common weak link in almost all cases of back pain: core instability.

Think about the last time you went to your family doctor with a complaint of pain. There's a good chance the doc uttered these words: "I recommend not lifting for a few weeks." Sound familiar? Many people find some short-term relief of their symptoms by following these orders. It makes sense on paper. If deadlifting causes your back to hurt, not deadlifting will likely decrease your pain! Problem solved, right?

Wrong.

Chances are the pain will eventually return because you never addressed *why* the problem started in the first place.

Eliminating the movement, posture, or load that causes your pain is only half the battle in fixing any injury. Anyone can tell you to stop doing something that hurts. Eliminating symptoms and building your body to become more resilient to injury requires a different and more active approach.

To kick-start this active approach, let's learn about the core and how it relates to both the cause and the fix for low back injuries.

Core Stability

Imagine a symphony orchestra. Just as every musician in an orchestra must play their instrument in a united manner despite constant changes in tempo and volume, your body must coordinate every muscle to create purposeful and sound movement.

The muscles that surround the spine—the front and side abdominal muscles, the erector muscles of the back, and even the larger muscles that span multiple joints, like the lats and psoas muscles—are considered the "core" of the body. It may surprise you that the glutes are also an important part of the core (something you'll learn about very soon!). These muscles must work together to enhance the stability of the spine.

Spinal stability is something Dr. McGill has been able to define and measure in his work. First, when muscles contract, they create force and stiffness. It is the stiffness that is important for stability. Think of the spine as a flexible rod that needs to be stiffened to bear load. This is the role of the muscles. Through his research, he has measured athletes who failed to obtain appropriate muscular stiffness around the spine by coordinating muscle activation and their subsequent injuries and pain.

Second, the body functions as a linked system, and distal movement requires proximal stability. Consider trying to move a finger back and forth very quickly—the wrist needs to be stable; otherwise, the entire hand would move. Now, using the same principle, consider the action of walking. The pelvis must be stable in relation to the spine; otherwise, the left hip would drop as the left leg swung forward to take a step. This core stiffness is non-negotiable to enable walking. Thus all body movement needs appropriate coordination of muscles. To move, run, or squat requires spinal stiffness and core stability.

When the core fails to meet the stability demands placed on the body during certain lifts, parts of the spine are overloaded with forces that increase injury risk, and performance suffers—much like a bad musician who is playing off-pitch or off-beat, which would quickly affect the rest of the orchestra. Each muscle that surrounds or attaches to the spine must play in concert with others to produce safe, efficient and, when needed, powerful movement.

Where Do We Start?

There are two general approaches taken to address the core. The first and more common method (which you'll see in fitness clubs across the world) is dynamic strengthening exercises such as crunches, back extensions, and Russian twists. Traditionally, coaches and medical practitioners have used these exercises that build strength through movement with the mindset that a stronger core will give the spine less chance to buckle and break under tension.

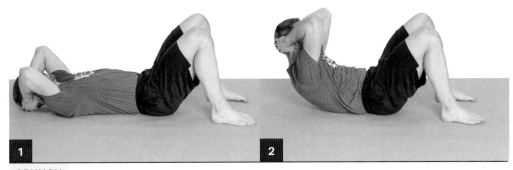

CRUNCH

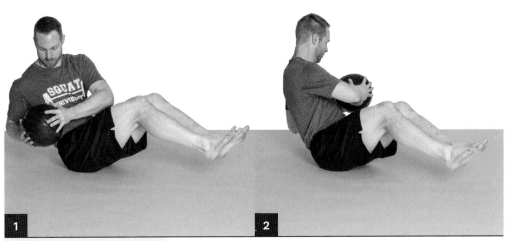

RUSSIAN TWIST WITH BALL

To a point, this is true. Each muscle that surrounds the spine does need a sufficient amount of strength to contract and "turn on." When the muscles of the core contract, stiffness is created. Much like guy-wires that attach to and hold up a radio tower, each muscle that surrounds the spine must provide a certain amount of tension and stiffness to maintain the strength of the spine as a whole and keep it from buckling and becoming injured.

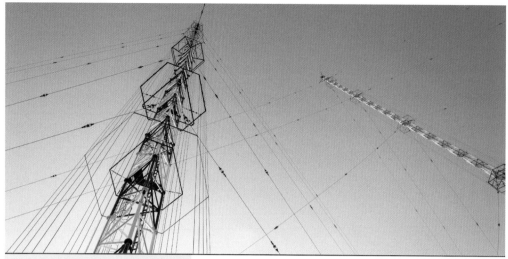

RADIO TOWER WITH GUY-WIRES

ANATOMY OF CORE

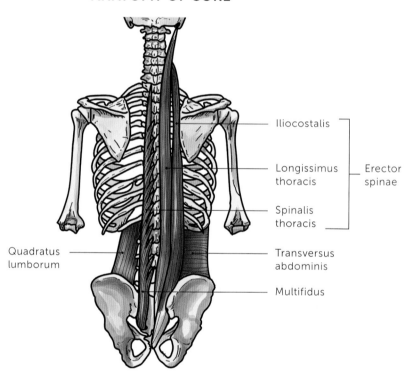

Quadratus lumborum

Iliocostalis
Longissimus thoracis — Erector spinae
Spinalis thoracis

Transversus abdominis
Multifidus

However, here's what most people don't understand. Many people who develop back pain already have strong backs![64] While exercises like Russian twists, sit-ups, and back extensions from a GHD machine may be great at increasing strength, they do little to increase core stiffness.[65]

To enhance the quality of stiffness, you must train the core differently. This comes through the second approach of using isometric exercises built to enhance muscular endurance and coordination.

An isometric describes when a muscle or group of muscles are activated and contracted, but there is no change in the joints they cross. For example, during a side plank, the lateral oblique and quadratus lumborum (QL) muscles are very active, yet the spine and hips remain still and do not move. Research has found that isometric exercises to enhance muscular endurance are far superior when compared to dynamic strengthening exercises in enhancing spinal stiffness and stability (making them ideal not only for rehabilitation of back injuries but also in the training and enhancement of athletic performance).[66]

QL IN SIDE PLANK

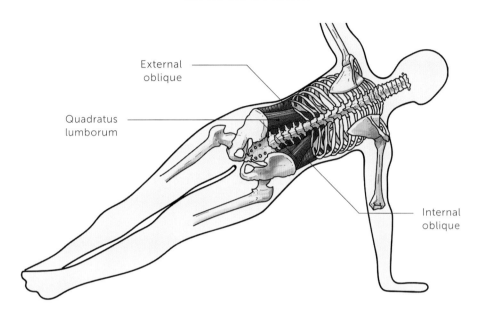

External oblique

Quadratus lumborum

Internal oblique

Have you ever pushed your body to the max while performing a high-volume squat session and ended up failing to complete the set? I have many times during my lifting career. You're tired, and while trying to grind out three more reps, you come up one short and have to drop the bar to the ground. Sound familiar? If this is something you've experienced, go back and review that specific set, but instead of analyzing the failed last rep, check out the one right before it. Often, the "smoking gun" is a drop in core stability—you became a little loose in your ascent, your spine rounded ever so slightly, or your hips shifted a bit to the side.

As soon as your brain senses a loss in core stability, it shuts down "neural drive" to your muscles, making it much more difficult to squeeze out another rep. Without the core functioning correctly, your body has two choices. The first is to allow technique to falter even more as you grind out the last rep (allowing for even more spinal rounding or hip shifting). While you may "get the job done," your risk for injury dramatically increases. The second option: fail the rep, drop the barbell to the ground, and live to squat another day.

You see, your brain shuts down how hard your body can push through that next repetition as a protective mechanism. The way to train your body to withstand this breakdown and maintain a high "neural drive" to your muscles is to address the failure mechanism head-on (the *why* behind the collapse): core stability endurance.

The definition of stability is the ability to limit excessive or unwanted motion. Therefore, the traditional way the fitness and rehab world has approached addressing the core for years has been completely backward! This is why someone can have a ripped six-pack and yet easily experience technique breakdown when it comes to deadlifting or performing a squat.

To stiffen the torso and limit excessive motion, every muscle of the core must co-contract or work together. **When this is done correctly through a bracing action, your body creates its natural "weightlifting belt."** Not only will this stiffen your spine and keep it safe when performing heavy lifts (like a squat or deadlift), but it will also help transfer force throughout your body. For example, a weightlifter performing a jerk requires sufficient core stability to transfer the power he or she generates from their legs through the core and into the upward drive of the barbell.

All for One and One for All

Much like the symphony orchestra analogy from before, every muscle of the core has a role to play, but none is more important than the others. For this reason, proper stability training should not focus on one specific muscle. For decades, medical practitioners were incorrectly taught to focus on and isolate certain muscles such as the transverse abdominus (TA), multifidus, or QL to enhance core stability. This method is flawed for a number of reasons.

First, research has shown that it is impossible for an individual to activate only one specific muscle of the core. Despite what your physical therapist or doctor says, you cannot train your multifidus, your QL, or even your TA muscle in isolation.

TRANSVERSE ABDOMINALS

Iliocostalis
Longissimus thoracis
Latissimus dorsi
Serratus posterior inferior
Quadratus lumborum
Gluteus maximus

Pectoralis minor
Pectoralis major
Rectus abdominis
Transversus abdominis
External oblique
Internal oblique
Quadratus lumborum

Even if it were possible to target a specific muscle of the core (as some would argue is possible through exercises like abdominal hollowing), methods like this have been shown to be far less efficient in creating stability for the spine compared to abdominal bracing (contracting all of the core muscles together).[67]

The Big Three

Now that you know which types of exercises are superior for rehabbing most back injuries, it's time to discuss which exact exercises to start with. There is unfortunately no one-size-fits-all approach when it comes to core exercises because there is no one universal movement that equally stresses all of the muscles that surround the spine. For this reason, we must utilize a battery of exercises to work all of them efficiently.

Technically, *any* exercise can be a "core" exercise if it is performed with sufficient attention to creating and maintaining a stable spine. It all depends on the objectives of the exercise and the individual's needs. One key to fixing injured backs is to use exercises that enhance stability but place minimal stress on the spine while the exercises are being performed.

In his years of studying the spine, Dr. McGill has found three exercises that efficiently address all of these areas without placing excessive stress on the parts of the back that may be aggravated or irritated due to injury. This group of exercises has become known as "the Big Three":

- Curl-up
- Side plank
- Bird-dog

Mobility First

Before you begin core stability training, I recommend addressing mobility restrictions at the hip and/or thoracic spine.

If your mobility in either of these areas is limited, it can lead to movement compensations at the low back. For example, if there is limited hip mobility during the squat motion, the pelvis can be pulled underneath (posterior pelvis tilt), causing the lower back to leave its neutral position and round.

For this reason, if you perform only core stability work but don't address any significant mobility restrictions in joints above or below the lumbar spine, the stiffness you created will always be compromised.

After addressing mobility restrictions in those areas, Dr. McGill recommends that you perform the cat-camel before the Big Three to reduce low back stiffness and improve motion of the spine. Unlike other stretches for the low back that can place harmful stresses on the spine, this exercise emphasizes mobility in a spine-friendly manner.

Assume an all-fours (quadruped) position. Slowly arch your entire spine and hips into a flexed or rounded position as high as possible without pain. You should end with your head looking down toward the ground. This is the camel position. After pausing for a few seconds, move into the opposite downward extended position with your head looking up (the cat). Make sure you move into a *light* stretch for each position; do not force your spine into any pain.

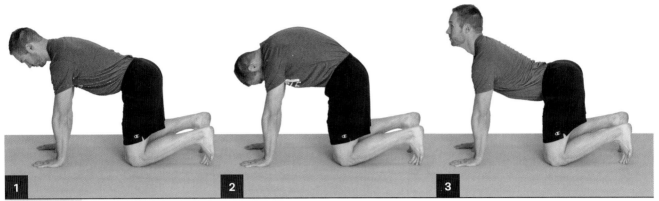

CAT-CAMEL

Perform five or six cycles of this exercise before moving on to the Big Three, starting with the curl-up.[68]

Curl-Up

When most people perform what they have been taught to be a curl-up, they bend or flex their entire spine and attempt to bring their chest toward their knees. While this exercise does activate the anterior core muscles to a great degree (especially the rectus abdominis, or six-pack muscle), the "crunch" motion does a few things that aren't so appealing, especially for those dealing with back pain.

First, the motion of the classic curl-up places a large amount of compression on the spine that can flare up symptoms for those who are "load intolerant."[69]

Second, the motion pulls the spine out of its neutral slightly arched position and flattens it into a bit of flexion. If your low back symptoms increase when you bend your spine ("flexion intolerance"), you should avoid this motion for the time being.

The traditional curl-up also relies heavily on the psoas muscle of the anterior hip to pull the torso toward the thighs. So, while you think you may be isolating and sculpting that sexy six-pack by doing endless crunches, you're actually doing a really good job of strengthening your hip flexors.[70]

We can home in and focus our attention on improving the stabilizing ability of the anterior core muscles in a more efficient way by performing a modified curl-up.

Step 1: Lie on your back with one knee bent and the other straight. If you have pain that radiates down one leg, keep that knee bent and straighten the other against the ground. Place your hands under your low back (this will ensure your spine remains in a neutral slightly arched position during the next step).

Step 2: Lift your head only 1 inch off the ground and hold that position for 10 seconds. If you're resting your head on a pillow, imagine it as a scale and lift your head enough to make the dial read zero.[71] The goal is to perform the curl-up without any movement in your low back! If you raise your head and shoulders too high (like a traditional curl-up or crunch), your low back will round, and excessive forces will be transferred to the spine that could increase your symptoms.

Step 3: After a 10-second hold, relax your head back down to the resting position.

You can progress this exercise by bracing your abs before moving your head or raising your elbows from the ground to decrease your base of stability.[72]

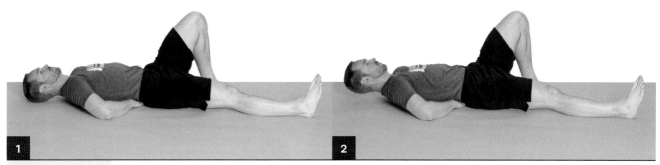

MCGILL CURL-UP

Unlike training for pure strength or power, the endurance component of stability requires the body to perform many repetitions of an exercise to see improvements. Dr. McGill advocates for using a descending pyramid rep scheme with 10-second isometric holds to enhance stability without fatiguing or overworking the body.

An example program would be to perform 5 reps, then 3, and finally 1 to end (each with an 8- to 10-second hold). Rest for 20 to 30 seconds after each set. As this rep scheme becomes easier, increase the number of repetitions rather than the duration of the holds to build endurance without causing muscle cramping.[73] This can be freely modified to suit your current level of endurance and goals: for instance, using a 6-4-2 or 8-6-4 rep scheme.

During these 10-second holds, focus on your breathing. Inhale and exhale slowly (about 5 times in a row for each repetition). As you breathe, concentrate on maintaining the contraction of your abdominal muscles. The cue to take "small sips of air in and out" (as if you are breathing through a straw) will teach you how to create sufficient core stability while moving throughout your day. You wouldn't hold your breath when climbing stairs or while performing a 10-repetition set of squats! Learning how to breathe and maintain sufficient core stability for the task you're going to carry out is a vital step in the early rehab process for low back pain.

The McGill Big Three has been highly effective since I started using it with my patients who come in for low back physical therapy. I have also found the Big Three beneficial in my own training as a weightlifter. I perform these core stability exercises before all my lifts.

Side Plank

Now that we've addressed the anterior core muscles, let's move to the sides of the body. The side plank is a unique exercise because it activates the lateral oblique and QL muscles on only one side of the body, making it an excellent choice for addressing weak links in stability while placing minimal force on the spine. It also engages an important stabilizer of the hip/pelvis on the lateral hip: the glute medius.[74]

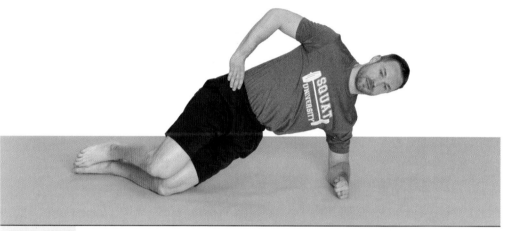

SIDE PLANK

Step 1: Lie on your side with your knees bent and your upper body supported through your elbow. Place your free hand on your opposite hip or shoulder.

Step 2: Raise your hips so that only your knee and arm support your body weight. As you lift your body from the ground, push your hips forward with the cue "squat your hips up."

Step 3: Hold this position for 10 seconds before returning back down. Push your hips back using the cue "squat your hips down." Perform the same descending pyramid rep scheme for each side.

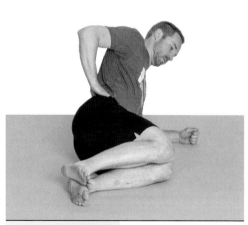

SQUAT HIPS DOWN

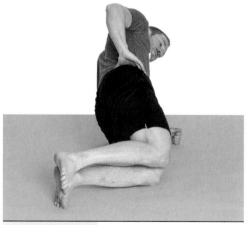

SQUAT HIPS UP

You can do a number of progressions with this exercise. You can start by moving your hand placement from your opposite shoulder to the top of your hip or even move to a full side plank, with your body weight supported by your feet and elbow.

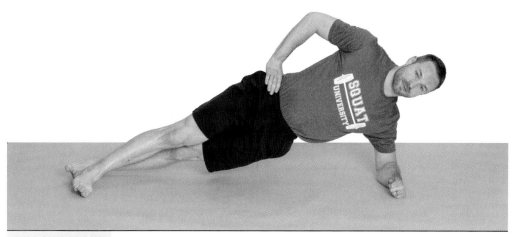

FULL SIDE PLANK

If you are unable to accomplish even the modified side plank (bridging from the knees) due to shoulder or arm pain, you can perform a side-lying leg lift. Lie on your side, brace your core muscles appropriately, and raise both legs together off the floor a few inches. Hold for 8 to 10 seconds before relaxing down.

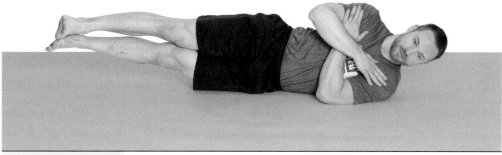

SIDE-LYING LEG LIFT

Bird Dog

The last of the McGill Big Three is the bird dog. This is an excellent exercise to promote a stable core while movement occurs at surrounding joints. The combination of movement occurring at the hips and shoulders while the low back remains stable allows this exercise to have excellent carryover to movements you perform throughout the day and in the weight room.

Step 1: Assume an all-fours (quadruped) position with your back in a neutral alignment. Remember, a neutral position is slightly arched, not completely flat.

Step 2: Without allowing any movement to occur at the low back, kick one leg backward while simultaneously raising the opposite-side arm until both limbs are fully straightened. A helpful cue to make sure the leg movement doesn't create an overarching of your back is to think about kicking the heel of your foot straight back. Making a fist and contracting your arm muscles as you hold it in the extended position can also increase the muscle activity of your core, especially of your erector spinae muscles.

   If you are unable to perform simultaneous arm and leg movement without pain, or if you find that you're losing balance, try the modified version with only leg movement.

Step 3: Hold each extended pose for 10 seconds before returning to the all-fours position. You can also "sweep" your arm and leg back underneath your body between repetitions. Don't let your back round during this motion; instead, maintain a neutral spine and allow motion to occur only from the hips and shoulders! Perform the same descending rep scheme as in the previous two exercises. You can progress this exercise by drawing a square with only your outstretched hand or both your hand and opposite foot.

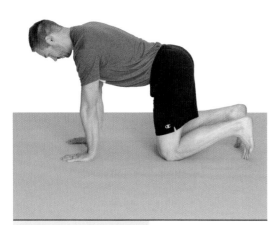

BIRD DOG QUADRUPED

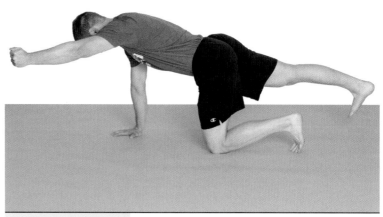

EXTENDED BIRD DOG

While performing the bird dog, pay special attention to the position of your back as you move your arm and leg. Research shows that those suffering from low back pain often have a decreased ability to sense spinal movement (diminished proprioception awareness).[75] Always start this exercise by stiffening your core *before* moving your limbs. Focus on your breathing and on maintaining sufficient abdominal contraction during your 10-second pose *and* during the "sweep" motion in between.

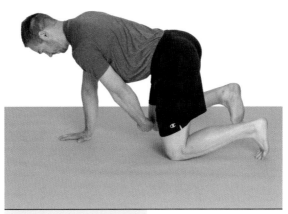

SWEEP UNDER & TOUCH

What About Back Stretching?

If you didn't notice, the prior exercises to kick-start the rehabilitation process do not include any stretches for the back! Early in my career as a physical therapist, it was common to prescribe certain stretches for back pain, like pulling the knees to the chest while lying on your back.

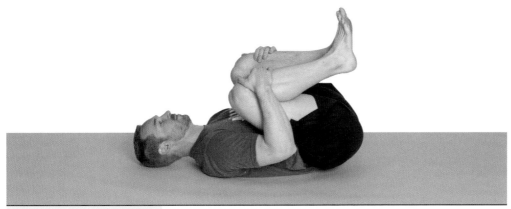

KNEES TO CHEST STRETCH

At the time, this exercise made sense. Those who had difficulty standing for long periods or lying flat on their back often felt better in a flexed position. Many who complained of low back stiffness and pain found instant relief of their symptoms after performing a few of these stretches.

However, after reading and studying with Dr. McGill, I realized that for most people, this relief is only temporary. Stretching the low back stimulates the stretch receptors deep inside the muscles, giving the perception of pain relief and the feeling of less stiffness.

Most of the muscle pain and stiffness you feel in your back is a consequence of a chemical reaction called *inflammation* that occurs from the real injury located deeper in the spine (disc bulge, facet irritation, etc.).[76] This underlying injury is what causes the secondary contraction or spasm of the surrounding muscles.

For this reason, a large majority of athletes should aim to stabilize the core and restore proficient movement in order to successfully rehab a back injury. Stretching the low back only treats the symptoms and does not address the true cause of the pain.

Reawaken Those Sleeping Glutes!

It is common to see athletes with back pain also have an inability to properly activate and coordinate their glute muscles. Simply put, the butt muscles can fall asleep.[77] When this happens, the body naturally starts to use the hamstrings and low back muscles more to create hip extension; both are problematic in creating efficient movement and place excessive stress on the spine.[78]

If the single-leg bridge test (see page 51) exposed a problem in how your body coordinates and turns on the glutes, the following exercises should help.

Bridge

Step 1: Lie on your back with your knees bent.

Step 2: Squeeze your butt muscles *first* and *then* lift your hips from the ground. Squeeze your glutes as hard as you can for 5 seconds before coming back down. Eventually, work your way up to a 10-second hold.

If your hamstrings start cramping, two modifications can help. First, bring your heels closer to your hips. Doing so shortens the length of the hamstrings and puts them at a disadvantage to contribute to the movement (a concept called *active insufficiency*).[79] You can also jam your toes into the ground and think about pushing your feet away from your hips. This will turn on your quads slightly, which in turn will decrease hamstring activity (a concept called *reciprocal inhibition*). The only muscles left to create hip extension with the hamstrings out of the picture are—you guessed it—the glutes!

Recommended sets/reps: 2 sets of 20 reps for a 5-second hold

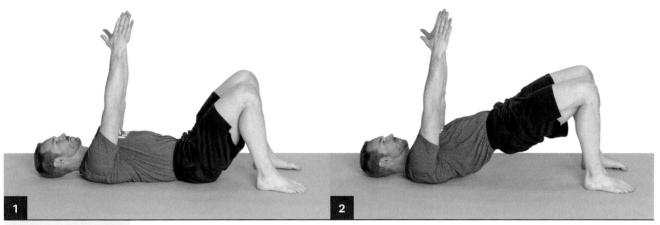

DOUBLE-LEG BRIDGE

If you still notice back pain when performing the bridge with the prior cues, try this modification. Position yourself with your head near a wall and push your hands into the wall prior to performing the bridge. Pushing into the wall engages your core, thereby increasing the efficiency of the bridge and hopefully decreasing your pain.

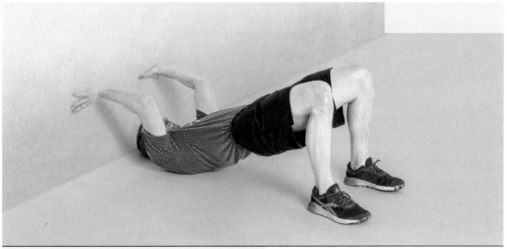

DOUBLE-LEG BRIDGE WITH HANDS INTO WALL

Deep Squat with Isometric Hold

Step 1: Hold a weight in front of your body and perform a deep goblet squat.

Step 2: Brace your core in this bottom position and drive your knees to the sides while keeping your feet in an arched position. This should turn on the outsides of your hips (glute medius muscles).

Step 3: Rise a few inches and squeeze your glutes like crazy. Hold for 5 seconds before sinking back down. This translates the glute activation from the previous exercise into something functional that mimics your squat technique. This exercise should be attempted only if you can perform it without any back pain.

Recommended sets/reps: 1 or 2 sets of 5 reps for a 5-second hold

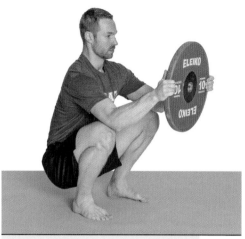

DEEP SQUAT WITH PLATE STRETCH

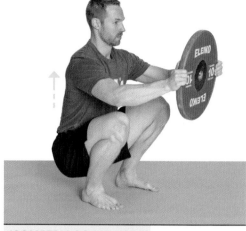

ISOMETRIC SQUAT HOLD

I recommend using these exercises not only as a foundation for your rehabilitation from back pain but also as a part of your weekly training program to prevent future injury once your symptoms have resolved.[80] The combination of these exercises should be safely performed daily if you are trying to recover from back injury but should not be performed directly after rising from bed in the morning, when the discs of your spine are the most hydrated and most prone to injury.[81]

The Early Rehab Plan

Now that you know your specific triggers for pain and have a good understanding of the McGill Big Three exercises, you can start to piece together a well-organized rehab program to follow.

Dr. McGill recommends coupling a regimented walking program with the Big Three exercises every day.[82] Getting up and walking throughout the day can be extremely helpful for maintaining the health of your spine and your base level of fitness after a small setback of a back injury. Start with smaller bouts of walking—5 to 10 minutes with a fast pace that causes you to swing your arms. The goal should be to eventually reach a 10- to 15-minute walk 3 times a day.

Do the Big Three every day for the first few weeks. You can then progress the frequency to twice per day while keeping your overall volume the same. For example, start by performing the 6-4-2 descending rep scheme once per day. Then progress to performing a 3-2-1 descending rep scheme of each exercise held for 10 seconds twice per day.

Bridging the Gap: Early Rehab to Performance

Resolving any kind of pain requires a three-stage approach. You must first eliminate the cause of the pain to decrease your symptoms and provide an optimal environment to kick-start your body's natural healing process. This means avoiding your individual triggers for symptoms at all costs! While this step seems easy, many athletes have a hard time complying with it. When I advise an athlete to stop squatting or deadlifting for the time being, I'm often met with the line, "I can't stop completely or I'll lose the gains I've made!"

Have some perspective and drop your ego. You will *not* lose all that you have gained by taking a few steps back in the short term. No rehabilitation plan or corrective exercise program will truly fix your pain and restore your body in the long term if you are too stubborn to deviate from a training plan that is creating pain. If certain lifts cause you pain, stop performing them for now. Have faith that you can and will return to them eventually.

The second stage of rehab is to address your body's weak links that led to pain in the first place. This includes a well-rounded approach of starting back-friendly core stability work like the McGill Big Three, doing mobility/flexibility exercises for restricted joints, and retraining poor movement patterns.

Learning the Hip Hinge

One of the most common reasons for developing back pain is an inability to use the hips properly.[83] From bending over to pick up a pencil off the ground to grabbing a loaded barbell, many who develop back pain have forgotten how to move about the hips and instead have allowed the lumbar spine to become unstable and move excessively. Therefore, learning to move from the hips and keep the spine stable (a movement called a *hip hinge*) is an essential part of the rebuilding process. This step is crucial for those who are "flexion intolerant."

To perform a proper hip hinge, stand with your hands straight out in front of you. Grip the ground with your feet (big toes into the ground) and feel for your body weight to be spread evenly across your entire foot. Next, drive your knees out to the sides to engage your lateral glutes, making sure to keep your feet firmly glued to the ground. Looping a small resistance band around your knees early on in the learning process can be a great way to teach your body how to create sufficient tension in your lateral hip muscles.

Start by pushing your butt backward and bringing your chest forward. (No motion should occur at your back.) Push your arms forward so that they're parallel to the ground; this will help counterbalance your hips going backward. Without allowing your knees to move forward, squat down a few inches and hold this position for a few seconds. If you did it correctly, you should feel tension building in your glutes and hamstrings.

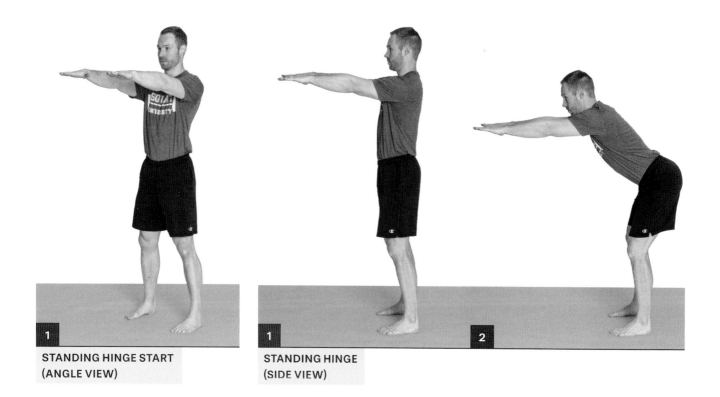

**STANDING HINGE START
(ANGLE VIEW)**

**STANDING HINGE
(SIDE VIEW)**

If you have difficulty performing this motion without allowing your knees to come forward (as if performing a normal squat), place a box directly in front of your toes. Your knees will be unable to translate forward without hitting the box, so you *must* hinge properly about the hips!

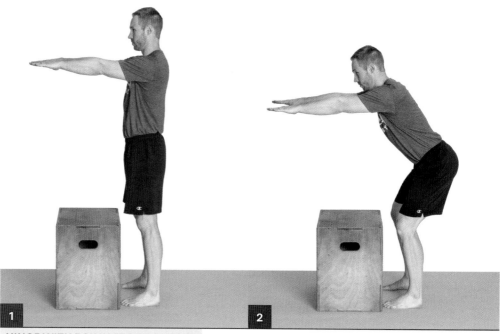

HINGE WITH BOX IN FRONT OF TOES

If you were unable to perform this motion without pain in your back, place your hands on the fronts of your thighs. As you push your butt backward and bring your chest forward, slide your hands toward your knees. Placing pressure through your hands into your thighs should create a small amount of stiffness in your torso and upper body. If you did it correctly, you should no longer feel any pain in your back.

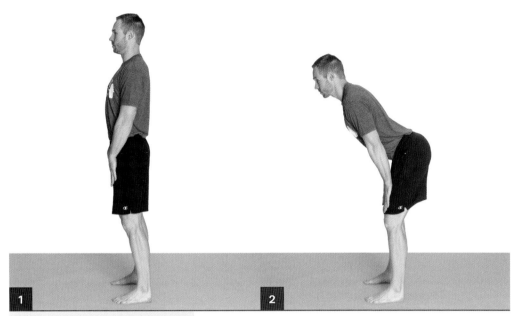

HINGE WITH HANDS ON THIGHS

Another helpful tool for learning a proper hip hinge is a weighted plate. Start by holding the plate against your glutes. While maintaining a slight bend in your knees, push your hips backward toward an imaginary wall behind you. Make sure your spine remains neutral throughout the entire motion. If you're doing it correctly, you should feel tension building in your hamstrings and glutes.

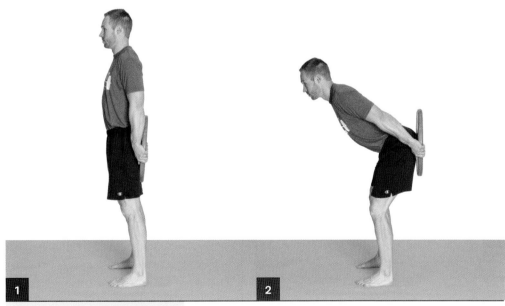

HINGE WITH PLATE ON GLUTES

Using this simple hip hinge with or without your hands pressing into your thighs can help you bend forward properly without creating pain symptoms. This means every time you grab food out of the fridge or pick up a sock off the ground, you should be hinging at your hips!

Building the Foundation

Assuming you have taken the right steps so far, you should be completely symptom-free at this point. It is time to progress to the third stage of the rehab plan and rebuild your body's capacity to handle the high demands of barbell training and competition. Unfortunately, there is no one universal exercise that stresses all of the muscles that surround the spine equally or places the same physical demand on your body. For this reason, we need to create a well-rounded training program that builds sufficient core stability through multiple planes of motion and movement patterns. The exercises in this third stage of rehab fall into four categories:

- **Push:** squat, sled push
- **Pull:** deadlift, inverted row
- **Carry:** suitcase carry
- **Anti-rotation:** Pallof press, one-arm row

Drawing from each of these categories will help you rebuild your body by forcing you to expose and address "weak links" that often go unnoticed in performance training. For example, a powerlifter will often perform exercises during training that fall into the push, pull, and anti-rotation categories (with exercises like the squat, deadlift, and bench press), but if they never perform any loaded carry exercises, they essentially leave their body open to potential injury because they fail to stimulate core stability in the frontal (forward and backward) plane of motion.

When returning from a back injury, you must take a careful approach during this third stage of rehab and choose exercises that facilitate healing without placing excessive load on your spine that re-creates your symptoms. For example, performing anti-rotation exercises before you can successfully squat with light weight often spells disaster. Exercises that create a twisting force on the body, like the Pallof press, can place upwards of four times as much compression on the spine compared to the same weight that attempts to create a flexion/extension force.[84]

The following is a logical progression of stability exercises that stress the body first through the sagittal plane (flexion/extension torque), then the frontal plane (lateral torque), and finally through the transverse plane (torsion torque). While there is no such thing as an ideal set of exercises for any rehabilitation program, these exercises can be a springboard for creating the plan that best suits your body and your goals.

As you work through each exercise, be cautious of how quickly you increase load. An efficient rehab program slowly applies load to the body. Too little and the body fails to adapt and remains fragile; too much and we overstep the adaptation process and pain returns. Listen to your body and remove your ego from the equation.

Squat

Once you can perform a hip hinge without pain, it's time to start rebuilding the squat. Start by performing bodyweight squats, increasing the depth as you are able to do so without pain. Depending on the severity of your injury, it may be a few weeks before you are able to regain a full-depth bodyweight squat without symptoms. When you can, it is time to load the movement.

The position of the load (on your shoulders versus on your back) and the amount of weight being lifted will dictate how much force is placed on your spine. For example, performing a goblet squat with a 30-pound kettlebell held by your chest places less force on your spine than a 135-pound front squat. In the same manner, a 135-pound front squat creates less torque on the lumbar spine compared to the same weight in a back squat. The more vertical torso assumed during the front squat to stay balanced provides a smaller moment arm (the distance from the vertical line of gravity pulling down on the barbell to the joints of the lumbar spine) than the relatively inclined torso of the back squat.[85]

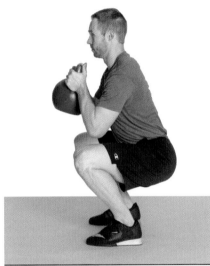 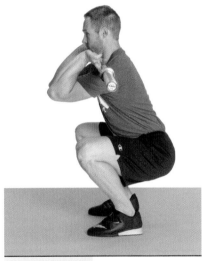 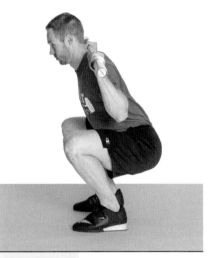

GOBLET SQUAT   FRONT SQUAT   BACK SQUAT

I recommend starting with the goblet squat (weight held by chest) before progressing to the front squat and eventually the back squat. Be cautious of how quickly you move through each pattern and how much load you choose to lift. Those who are impatient and return too quickly to lifting heavy weight can easily regress to injury. I have worked with many strong powerlifters who, during their rehab from back pain, used light goblet squats of only 30 to 40 pounds for a few weeks before returning to heavy barbell lifts.

Once you have returned to lifting ample weight in any of these techniques, focus on how you're breathing. When you're lifting heavy weight, it's not enough to brace your core; you have to learn how to breathe properly as well.

Contrary to what many medical and fitness professionals are taught, the line "breathe in on the way down and out on the way up" is not helpful for stabilizing the spine when lifting heavy weight. Think about what would happen to the spine of an elite powerlifter if they exhaled completely with 1,000 pounds on their back!

When attempting to lift heavy weight, I recommend taking a large breath in and then holding that breath throughout the entire repetition. When you combine this breath with a strong bracing of your core, your trunk will instantly become more stable and capable of handling tremendous weight. This is how you activate your body's natural "weightlifting belt."

To keep this increased pressure in your abdomen and your spinal stability high, you must forcefully stop your exhale from escaping; this is known as the Valsalva maneuver. By grunting or using a *tss* sound as you slowly exhale through a small hole in your lips, you can maintain a sufficient amount of stability in your core and keep your spine safe.[86]

This held breath should not be used for more than a few seconds during any lift, as doing so could increase your blood pressure to harmful levels and cause black-outs. If you have a history of cardiovascular issues, speak with your doctor before using this technique. For healthy athletes, however, a small temporary rise in blood pressure is not harmful.

Sled Push

Successfully pushing a weighted sled requires you to generate tremendous force with your legs and transfer it through a stiffened core into your arms and eventually the sled. If you are unable to create sufficient stability, your spine will move out of the ideal neutral position, causing energy to "leak out."

Start with your hands high on the sled poles. Before making any movement, grip the poles as hard as you can and drive your feet into the ground. Along with bracing your core, these actions will help create the spinal stiffness necessary to drive the sled with incredible power while keeping your back safe.

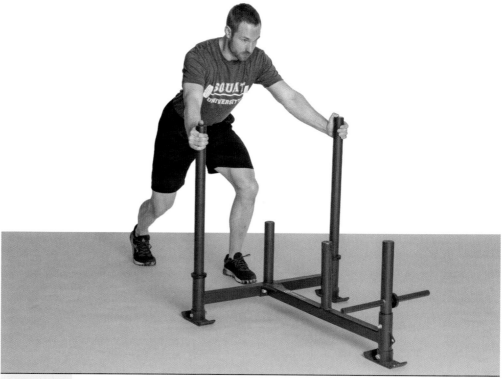

SLED PUSH

Deadlift

As you reintroduce the deadlift into your training plan, you want to do so in a spine-friendly way. Performing the lift off of a set of elevated blocks or stacks of weighted plates will place less shear force on your low back compared to pulling the barbell from the ground.

If we analyze the deadlift from the side view and "freeze frame" the movement at the moment the pull is initiated, we can calculate the amount of torque placed on the low back by determining the length of the moment arm (the distance from the vertical line of gravity pulling down on the barbell to the joint in question, in this case the joints of the lumbar spine).

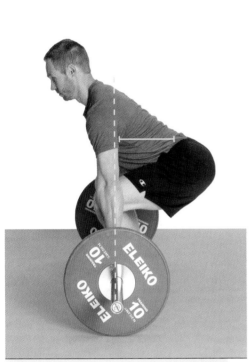
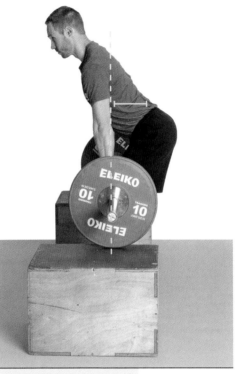

DEADLIFT START WITH MOMENT ARMS   **DEADLIFT FROM BLOCKS**

When performing a deadlift from the ground, the body naturally assumes a more forward-angled torso position than it does when pulling from the blocks. The more forward-angled trunk creates a longer moment arm for the joints of the low back and therefore places more load on the spine. Elevating the start position of the pull to knee height or slightly above therefore places less demand on the low back.

Performing the deadlift (either in a powerlifting competition or in training as an accessory lift like many weightlifters do) is all about finding the right balance of pushing your body weight into the floor and pulling up on the barbell. Many athletes who develop back pain when deadlifting do so because they fail to use their legs sufficiently and end up relying too much on their backs. As you pull yourself down into your start position stance, lock out your elbows and try to make your armpits disappear by squeezing your arms tight to your rib cage. This action engages your powerful lat muscles and creates a tremendous amount of core stiffness and upper body stability.

Next, engage the rest of your upper body by pulling upward against the bar—not moving it from the raised platform yet, but enough to essentially wedge your body against the bar like a "trust fall." If you're doing it correctly, you'll see the bar bend upward slightly—an action some call "taking the slack out of the bar."

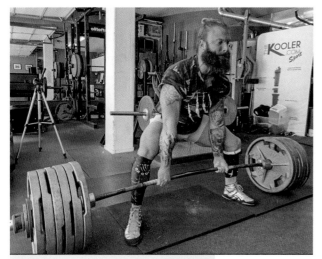 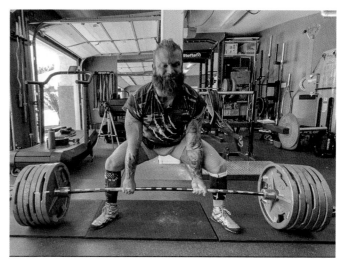

TAKING THE SLACK OUT OF THE BAR

Micah Mariano deadlift

While you're creating this tension with your upper body, you need to simultaneously do the opposite with your lower body. This means creating a tremendous amount of tension in your glutes and hamstrings as you drive your feet hard into the ground. Finding the right balance between pulling on the bar and pushing through the floor will help keep your back safe. As you progress with this lift, you can manipulate the different variables by adding weight or decreasing the height of the blocks.

Modifying your deadlift technique can also be helpful during the short-term rehabilitation process. For example, a sumo-style deadlift is often more friendly to the low back compared to the torso angle used during a conventional deadlift. The wider stance of the sumo deadlift allows you to keep the bar closer to your body and maintain a more upright torso position. Both of these factors shorten the moment arm on the lumbar spine and result in less overall load.[87]

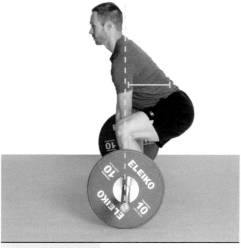 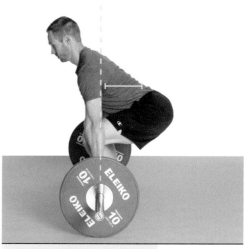

SUMO DEADLIFT   **CONVENTIONAL DEADLIFT**

Inverted Row

The inverted row, performed with a suspension trainer or gymnastic rings, has been shown in research to elicit a high amount of upper and mid-back muscle activation while placing minimal stress on the spine.[89] This makes this variation of the row a great exercise for the early stages of rehabilitation from a back injury. Make sure to focus on your breathing when performing this exercise. Take a big breath and brace your core, and *then* initiate the rowing movement.

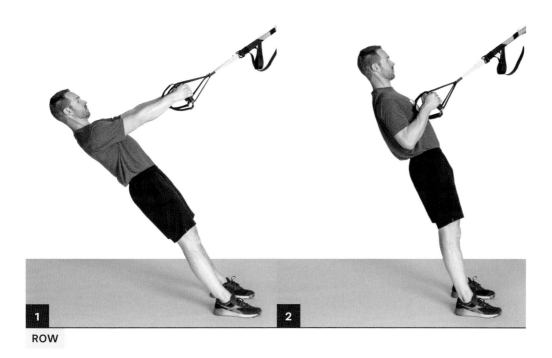

ROW

As you perform the row, your back should remain in a neutral braced position throughout the entire movement. As this exercise becomes easier for you to perform, walk your feet forward and angle your body closer to the ground. The end goal should be to assume a parallel position to the ground with your feet elevated on a bench or box, as shown in the photos on the next page.

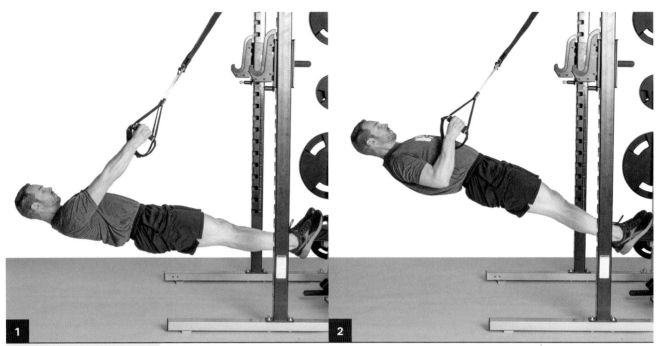

ROW WITH FEET ELEVATED

Suitcase Carry

Most of the lifts that are performed in the weight room occur in the sagittal plane of motion: you move the barbell along a relatively vertical path with both feet firmly planted on the ground. As athletes spend hours upon hours training these lifts, they can develop weaknesses in strength and stability in other planes of motion.

For example, the lateral musculature of the core (quadratus lumborum and obliques) is not sufficiently challenged during the classic lifts of the deadlift and squat and even the more dynamic movement of the Olympic snatch. If you cannot sufficiently activate these muscles to stabilize your body through different planes of motion, you leave yourself open to potential injury. Consider these two examples, for instance.

To perform a heavy squat, you must walk the barbell out of the rack a few steps before setting your stance. During the execution of a heavy snatch or clean, an Olympic weightlifter may stumble one foot forward quickly to recover an off-balance lift. In each case, every step forward or backward an athlete takes moves their body through the frontal plane of motion.

The suitcase carry challenges the core in the frontal plane and will help address this common imbalance for many athletes. To perform it, grab a lightweight kettle-bell or dumbbell (10 to 20 pounds to start) with one hand and hold it at your side. Brace your core and squeeze your arm to your side to activate your lats; use the cue "make your armpits disappear" to create upper body tension when setting up. Grip the kettlebell handle as tightly as you can before you start. As you walk, concentrate on limiting side-to-side leaning of your torso.

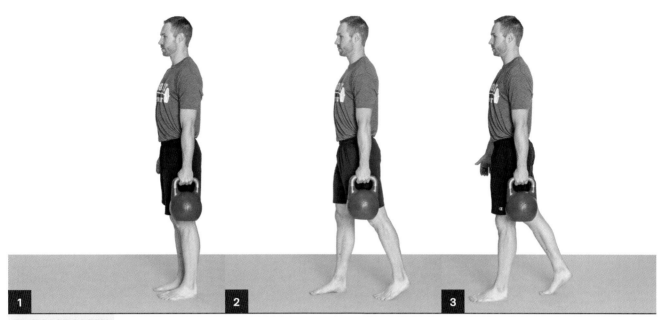

SUITCASE CARRY

Performing a suitcase carry with the weight in one hand is significantly harder and poses a greater challenge to your core than performing the exercise with weight in both hands. In fact, research has shown that carrying double the weight in each hand (using two 30-kilogram/66-pound kettlebells) places significantly less compression on your spine than carrying a single 30-kilogram/66-pound kettlebell in one hand.[90] This is because the effort to stabilize the uneven forces moving up your spine by holding the weight with one arm challenges your body to a greater degree.

You can increase the stability challenge to your core by holding the kettlebell in the upside-down position. Brace your core and *then* start your walk. If you want to progress this exercise one step further, lift your thighs and march in a slow, controlled manner.

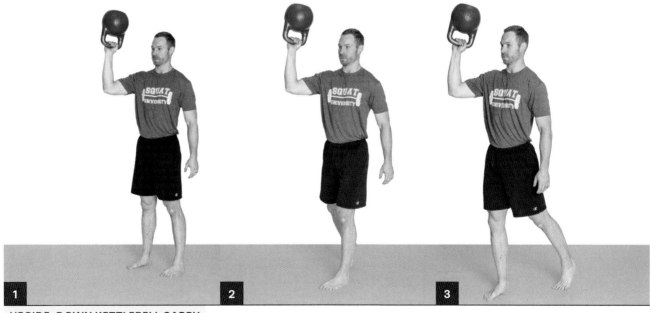

UPSIDE-DOWN KETTLEBELL CARRY

The upside-down kettlebell carry is one of the most challenging variations. If you struggle to keep the kettlebell from wobbling, you may want to blame your grip strength. However, it is often a lack of sufficient core stability that leads to the weight falling over while you walk.

Research has shown that back pain diminishes our sense of spinal position and postural control.[91] The more stable you can keep your core, the easier it will be to keep the kettlebell from wavering. Therefore, instead of focusing on the kettlebell, focus your attention on maintaining a braced core.

Pallof Press

The lateral banded press or Pallof press challenges the body's ability to resist a twisting motion. This provides a unique test for strength athletes who rarely encounter twisting forces during normal barbell training.

Begin in a standing position with your hands close to your stomach and holding a band/cable. The attachment for the band should be perpendicular to your side. Brace your core and push your hands away from your body. Hold this position for five seconds without allowing your body to twist.

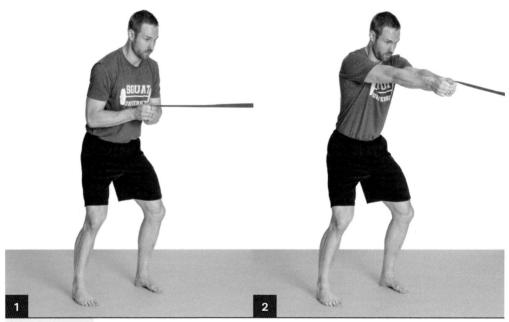

PALLOF PRESS

You can alter this exercise by assuming different positions, such as half-kneeling, tall kneeling, or even a split stance. You could also add a lift after the initial press and hold. Another variation is squatting while doing the press. You can play with different squat depths to challenge your core and hips at different angles.

Recommended sets/reps: 2 or 3 sets of 10 reps on each side

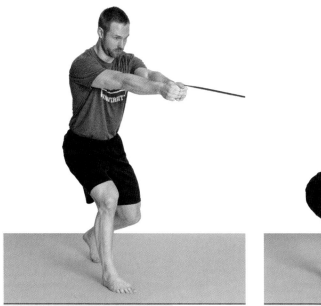

PALLOF PRESS SPLIT STANCE

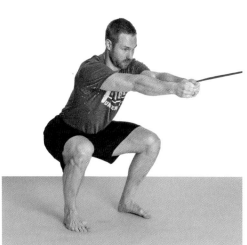

PALLOF PRESS IN DEEP SQUAT

One-Armed Row

At first glance, most people would classify the one-armed row (performed with a resistance band or cable machine) as a shoulder stability exercise to emphasize the strength of the upper back and posterior shoulder musculature. While this classification is correct, the one-armed row also provides an excellent challenge as an anti-twisting or rotation core stability exercise.[92]

Stand facing a cable machine or attach a band around a rig. Perform a row with one arm while maintaining a neutral spine. Don't allow your body to twist at all. After a two-second hold, extend your arm back to the start position. (Turn the page for photos of this exercise.)

You can perform this row in a number of positions, such as in a lunge or kneeling.

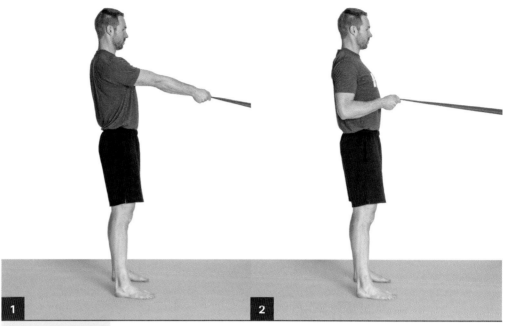

ONE-ARMED ROW

Recommended sets/reps: 2 or 3 sets of 10 reps

The Bridge to Performance

Once you have eliminated your pain and returned to your prior level of training, you must maintain your newfound core stability. This means performing the McGill Big Three and other core stability exercises from the prior section on a weekly basis. There is no right or wrong answer when it comes to choosing which of those exercises to include, but I recommend that you incorporate the ones that challenge your body in different planes of motion.

If you are a strength athlete looking to perform at the highest level, I recommend taking your core training one step further and using the following exercise modifications in your training.

Olympic Lifts

The Olympic lifts (the snatch and the clean and jerk) can eventually be added to the rehabilitation program. Due to their complexity and speed requirements, however, I do not recommend reintegrating these lifts into your program until you can easily perform a single repetition of both the squat and the deadlift at 70 percent of your prior 1-rep max without pain.

As with the deadlift, using blocks initially can help you to perform either Olympic lift with less load on your low back. Start with a block height that positions the barbell at mid- to low thigh (above the knee). Research has shown that assuming a more vertical trunk position as the barbell passes the knees places significantly less stress on the low back during either the snatch or the clean and jerk (meaning that the start of the full lift from the ground is the most demanding on the spine).[88]

As you progress this lift, you can manipulate the different variables by adding weight or decreasing the block height.

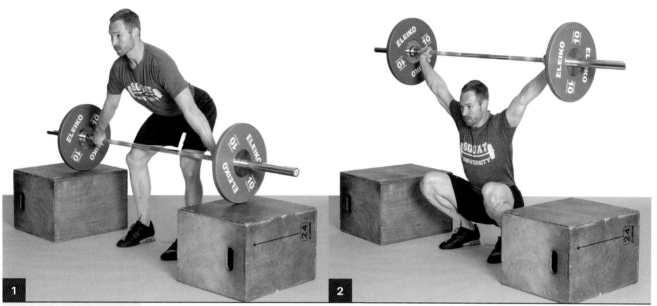

SNATCH FROM BLOCKS

Paused Deadlift

The paused deadlift is a great variation to reinforce proper pulling technique. To perform it, start with the exact same approach you would use for a regular deadlift. Take a huge breath, brace your core, and slowly pull the bar from the ground. You can perform two- to five-second pauses in a variety of positions, such as mid-shin, below the knee, and above the knee. I also like to add a pause at the knee on the way back down for an added challenge.

During the pause, feel your legs pushing hard into the floor. If you maintain sufficient core stability by holding your breath and bracing your core, you should not feel any recurring pain in your low back. Perform up to three reps per set.

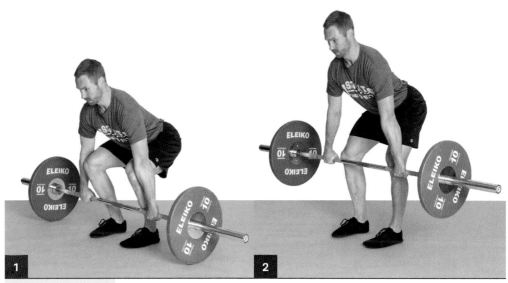

PAUSED DEADLIFT

Zombie Front Squat

When performing a front squat or a clean, you want to maintain as much of an upright trunk as possible. Athletes commonly hit a decent-looking bottom position with each rep but fail to maintain an upright torso on the ascent, allowing their backs to excessively round into flexion. The no-hands zombie front squat solves this problem.

Start by holding a barbell on your chest as if you were performing a front squat. Extend your arms straight out in front of you so that the barbell is resting solely on the tops of your shoulders and chest. Set your feet in a stable position by grabbing the ground with your toes. Take a big breath, brace your core, and begin your squat.

To maintain the bar on your chest and keep it from rolling off and onto the ground, you must keep an upright torso! Start with sets of one to three reps with light weight and progress in weight only as you can continue to maintain perfect technique.

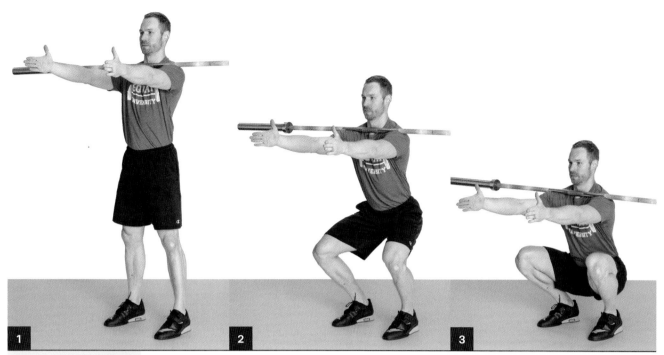

ZOMBIE FRONT SQUAT

Squatting with Chains

The use of chains has been a popular method in the powerlifting community for many decades since it was introduced by Louie Simmons of Westside Barbell.[93] The theory behind their use is to accommodate for how the body naturally responds to moving weights, called the *force velocity curve.*

For example, everyone can picture that one lifter who does quarter squats with a lot of weight on the bar but has zero chance of completing the same weight to full depth. This is because the body is able to generate much greater force at the top portion of the lift as compared to the bottom.

Let's say an athlete's one-rep max squat is 300 pounds. They could load a barbell to 220 pounds and hang two chains per side at 20 pounds each. The total weight at the top of the lift would be the lifter's max of 300 pounds. As they drop into the bottom of the squat, the chains hit the ground and pile up, which decreases the overall weight pulling down. Therefore, at the top of the lift, there are 300 pounds on the bar, but at the bottom there are only 220 pounds. During the ascent, the weight is then slowly reapplied to the barbell (this is called *accommodating resistance*).

With a regular barbell squat, the weakest position for most people is at the bottom. The closer you get to the top position, the easier the motion usually becomes. Using chains allows you to work with heavy weights at the top part of the squat and decreases your chance of failing a rep when you're coming out of the bottom. Refer to the next page for photos.

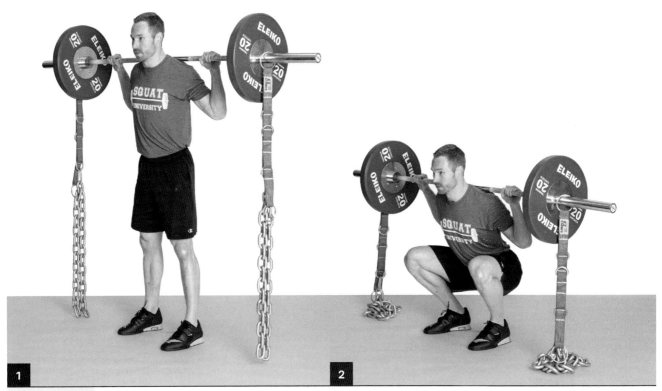

CHAIN SQUAT

This means using chains effectively accommodates for the body's natural force velocity curve during the lift. This method can help athletes improve their bar speed and power through the sticking points of the ascent.

Another less recognized benefit of using chains during lifts like the squat, and the reason I like them for athletes with a history of back pain, is to work on core stability by enhancing proprioception (sense of spinal position). The light swing of the chains as they hang from the barbell places an uneven and irregular stimulus on the lifter—a concept similar to using rhythmic stabilization drills to enhance neuromuscular control. To create this unstable environment, make sure your chains are hanging a few inches off the ground when you're in the standing position.

Remember, you must perform every part of the lift—from lifting the bar out of the rack to walking the weight back to your starting position—with intention. This is especially true for those recovering from back pain. As you walk the barbell out of the rack, the swinging chains will give you instant feedback as to whether you have a sufficiently braced core!

Should You Wear a Weightlifting Belt?

I once worked with a powerlifter who was trying to recover from a recent flare-up of back pain. During one of our sessions in which we were reintroducing the barbell back squat, he asked if he could wear his weightlifting belt. In his mind, a belt was to be used to keep his back safe anytime he touched the barbell. The belt was his reassurance that his back wouldn't "go out" the next time he squatted heavy.

What I told him next may surprise you. I've come to find that a large majority of athletes and coaches are using belts incorrectly, and many times for the wrong purposes. Let me explain.

Why Use a Belt?

Before I jump into the use of a belt in the context of a back injury, let's discuss why someone would wear a belt in the first place. Research shows that a weightlifting belt provides additional stability for the lower back.[94] It does so by aiding your core muscles.

When you get under a heavy barbell, you need to take a big breath and brace your trunk muscles so that the weight on the bar doesn't bend you in two. This action of breathing and bracing your core amplifies the pressure inside your abdominal cavity and creates tremendous stability. A helpful cue is to think "fill the tank" as you push your breath into your gut. If you do it correctly, you will feel your stomach rise and fall—not your chest. This breath should be held for the duration of a single repetition.

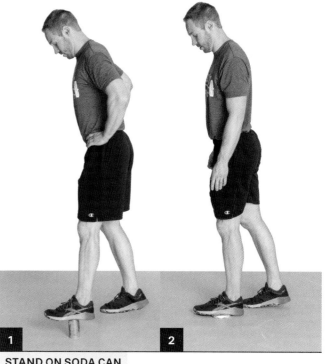

STAND ON SODA CAN

Essentially, the volume of your body's intra-abdominal cavity increases when you take a big breath. If you couple this expansion of your core with bracing your trunk muscles, the pressure inside your abdominal cavity grows because the volume can no longer expand. This is how intra-abdominal pressure (IAP) is created.

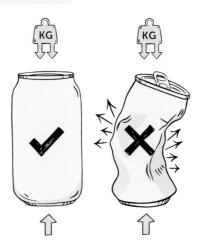

Think of IAP as an unopened soda can. If you place a full unopened can of soda on the ground and stand on top of it, it will remain strong and won't crumple under the weight of your body. The pressure inside the can gives it strength and stability.

It is common to hear coaches use the breathing cue "inhale on the way down and exhale on the way up." This advice is not appropriate if you are attempting to lift heavy weight. Can you imagine what would happen if a powerlifter started to exhale at the start of the squat ascent with 900-plus pounds on their back? If you let the air out too soon during the ascent (or if you don't take a big enough breath at the start), you have already begun draining your "tank," which will ultimately cause a loss of stability. This is synonymous with opening the can of soda, draining it, and then trying to stand on it. Obviously, the can will be instantly crushed under the weight of your body after the pressure inside is removed. To maintain the desired stability, hold your breath until you have passed the sticking point of the ascent (usually about three-quarters of the way up), and then slowly let it out.

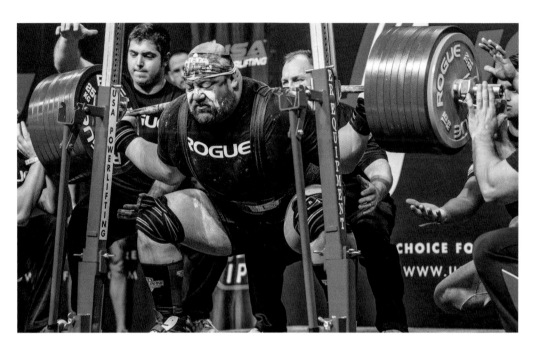

Squat with belt.
Blaine Sumner.

Proper breathing and bracing of your core muscles when lifting activates your body's "natural weightlifting belt." A weightlifting belt, therefore, just adds another "layer" to your body's "tank." The belt does not replace your core muscles, but rather acts as an additional restraint. Wearing one can be extremely helpful if your goal is to lift tremendous weight. In fact, research has shown that when the use of a belt is combined with a correctly braced core and held breath, IAP values can increase anywhere from 20 to 40 percent, which means more trunk stability.[95]

How to Use a Belt

When most people use a weightlifting belt, they use it incorrectly. Ask yourself if this scene sounds familiar. You look toward the squat rack and see an athlete struggling with all their might to fasten the belt as tightly around their stomach as possible as if they were donning an eighteenth-century corset.

Proper use of a belt involves much more than just wearing it tightly! To use a belt, you must breathe "into the belt." If you only cinch it tight, you will miss out on the benefits it has to offer. Always think about expanding your stomach into the belt and then bracing against it.

Research has shown that athletes who wear a belt correctly tend to lift heavier weight with more explosive power. They are also able to maintain their trunk stiffness for more reps during higher-rep maximum lifts like an eight-rep max attempt.[96]

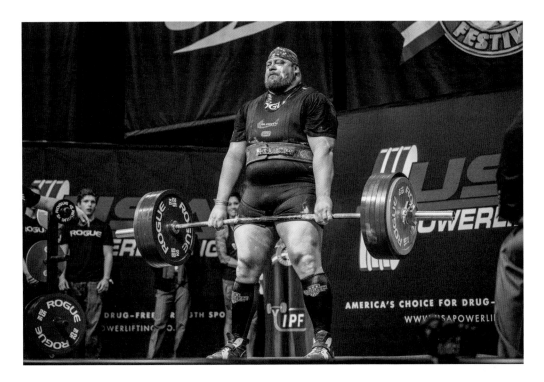

Deadlift with belt.
Blaine Sumner.

When to Wear Your Belt

Most athletes start wearing a belt for the following reasons:

- They observe elite athletes wearing them and think they need to wear one as well.

- They want to lift heavier weight.

- Their back is sore or starts to hurt, and they think a belt will help.

Just because an elite athlete (who has spent years training and competing) wears a weightlifting belt doesn't mean you need to wear one as well. First, ask yourself, "Am I competing in a strength sport like weightlifting or powerlifting?" If the answer is yes, I strongly encourage you to spend your first few years of training for that sport without using a belt. During these early years, it is crucial to home in on developing proper technique. Take this time to cultivate your "natural weightlifting belt." Doing so will help you build a solid foundation of stability so that if you do decide to use a belt when reaching for heavier weights one day, you can do so with better technique.

If you have no desire to compete in weightlifting or powerlifting and instead are using the weight room to train for other sports, such as football, basketball, or baseball, I highly recommend keeping belt use to a minimum. You wouldn't wear a belt while participating in any of these sports, so wearing one in the weight room is probably not the best idea. Instead, spend your time building a stable torso and lifting with pristine technique.

There is nothing wrong with the desire to lift heavy, but it should never come at the expense of technique. While wearing a belt can be very helpful on heavy lifts, the long-term use of a belt on *all* lifts can have harmful effects. If you use a belt all the time, your body will naturally start to rely on the passive support that the belt supplies. You can potentially weaken your core by relying on the belt as a crutch. Therefore, learning how to brace and create stability on your own with lighter weight should be the priority. For serious lifters, I recommend programming days of training with and without a belt so that you continue to build the capacity for maintaining stability with heavy lifting.

A belt should never be used with the goal of taking away back pain or soreness. Doing so is like covering up a hole in your car's tire with duct tape. It may give you some short-term relief, but it is not a smart long-term solution. Simply put, a belt has no place in the process of rehabbing back pain. Once the pain has been completely eliminated with proper rehabilitation and you have demonstrated the ability to maintain sufficient technique and stability while training with moderate weight, you can then introduce a belt.

We should always work to ensure that we are lifting safely and with the best possible technique. A belt can facilitate this, especially with heavy weights. Some athletes will not use a belt, even with maximum attempts. That's okay, as long as you maintain good technique. However, if you are going to use a belt, make sure you know how to use it correctly.

Cautionary Exercises for Low Back Injury Rehab

A few exercises that are common to strength athletes require some caution, especially in the context of recovering from a back injury. I want to briefly go over two of those exercises so that you may better understand their use:

- Hip extension "reverse hyper" machine
- Back extension machine or Roman chair

Hip Extension "Reverse Hyper" Machine

The hip extension or reverse hyper machine was created by famed powerlifting coach Louie Simmons of Westside Barbell. Many people are taught to simultaneously move their back through flexion and extension as they raise and lower their legs. When performed like this, the swinging action is created through contraction of the hamstrings and glutes (extending the hips) as well as the erectors of the low back (extending the lumbar spine).

While this exercise can be excellent for training hip extension strength, the muscular contraction that takes place at the low back when you allow it to move in this manner creates extreme posterior shearing forces on the spine. For some people (such as someone who is "extension intolerant"), this exercise may trigger back pain. However, I don't think we can jump to the conclusion that it is inherently dangerous for everyone or should be avoided in all cases of back pain. Instead, we need to have a better understanding of how and when this exercise should be used.

For example, to strengthen his posterior chain and rehab from back injury, world champion powerlifter Blaine Sumner modified this technique into a more "spine-friendly" variation. By propping himself up on the machine's platform and supporting his upper body through the elbows (instead of lying flat on his stomach), he found that he could limit low back movement and instead move solely about the hips.

As you support yourself on the platform, grab the handles and squeeze as hard as you can to create tension from your hands to your shoulders. Your pelvis should be resting on the edge of the platform, and your spine should be in a neutral position. Next, brace your core and stiffen your entire torso so that you can focus the motion solely about your hips. Raising and lowering your legs with your torso buttressed against the platform allows you to strengthen your hip extensors (glutes and hamstrings) while minimizing the harmful forces on your low back. This exercise can be performed by extending both legs or just one at a time.

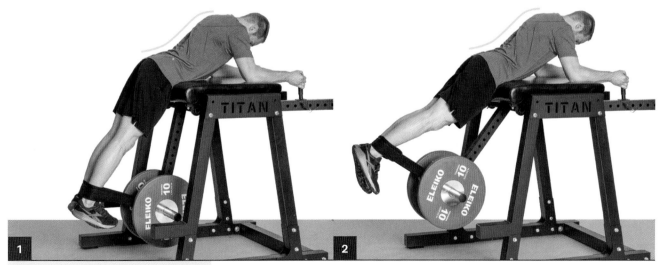

REVERSE HYPER: GOOD TECHNIQUE

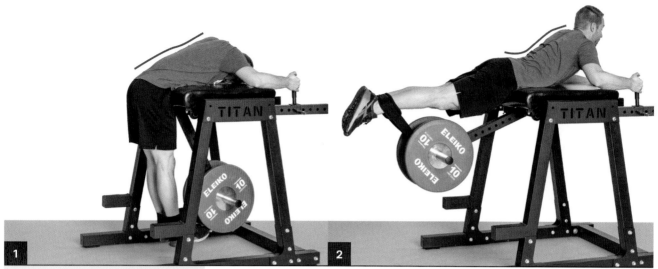

REVERSE HYPER: POOR TECHNIQUE

For those who do not have access to a specialized machine like the reverse hyper, a kettlebell swing is a great late-stage rehabilitation exercise that emphasizes and trains dynamic hip extension in a similar cyclical motion. Not only does a kettlebell swing train the posterior chain, but it does so in a manner that enhances full-body coordination. Every "link" in the body's kinetic "chain," from the stable foot grabbing the ground to the powerful hips working in sync with an unwavering spine, must work in harmony to produce a quality swinging pattern.

To perform the kettlebell swing, assume a good athletic stance, with your toes relatively straight forward and your feet about shoulder width apart. If you can, take off your shoes and socks and grip the ground with your toes. This allows you to create tremendous stability and limit unwanted rocking either forward onto the toes or backward onto the heels.

With the kettlebell resting slightly in front of your toes, hinge your hips (butt backward and chest forward) and lower yourself to the weight as if setting up for a deadlift. Your shoulders should be slightly higher than your hips, and you should be looking straight ahead, not down at the kettlebell. Brace your core in a neutral spinal position.

Next, drive your feet hard into the ground and lock your arms to pre-tension your entire body before any movement occurs. This is the same step-by-step process that should occur before any barbell lift from the floor.

Draw in a big breath before you pull the kettlebell back between your legs (like a center hiking a football to the quarterback). As this happens, you should feel the posterior chain muscles of your glutes and hamstrings tighten like a rubber band being stretched. Then drive your hips forward in a powerful, explosive manner, releasing the tension of the prestretched "rubber band." Release your breath powerfully as you swing the bell violently forward, similar to a boxer throwing a quick jab.

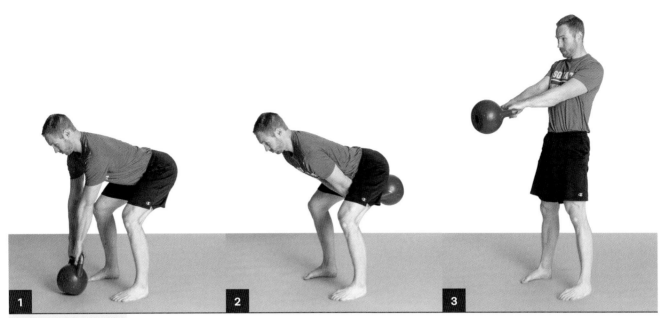

KETTLEBELL SWING

   Don't think about lifting the weight with your arms; rather, focus on producing force with your lower body, specifically your glutes. If you do this exercise correctly, the kettlebell will almost float forward to chest height. Make sure that your core remains braced for the entire movement. If you find that your shoulders are fatiguing, you are probably overusing your arms to complete the swing and are not generating power through hip extension.

   As the weight begins to descend back toward the ground, fill your lungs with air again. Keep your arms locked out as you hinge from your hips and allow the weight to swing between your legs. If you bend your knees too much at this time, the motion will turn into a squat; this is not what you want. If you do it properly, you will feel the tension rise in your posterior chain muscles as the "rubber band" is pulled back and readied for another release of violent energy in the next swing.

   Begin by swinging the weight to shoulder height. Eventually, you can work toward a higher swing if you prefer. For more on the use of kettlebells in training, I highly recommend checking out the work of Pavel Tsatsouline.

Back Extension Machine or Roman Chair

The back extension exercise from a Roman chair machine is used to strengthen the erector muscles of the back. The use of this machine dates back decades and is fairly popular in barbell sports like weightlifting. I remember seeing videos of famed Soviet weightlifter Vasily Alekseyev using the Roman chair machine as a staple of his training en route to setting over 80 world records in the 1970s.

A similar machine to the Roman chair is the GHD, or glute ham developer. While the name of this machine gives the impression that the focus is on the posterior chain, the GHD is often performed incorrectly, and many lifters end up using their spinal erectors to complete the exercise.

Caution must be taken when using both of these machines, especially when it comes to returning from back pain. Performing a back extension exercise places a high demand on the spinal erectors with little co-contraction involvement from the rest of the core muscles.[97] Just like the hip extension reverse hyper machine, this action could trigger back pain in some individuals.

Contrary to the exercise name, I recommend performing back extensions in a very hip-centric manner. Start by adjusting the machine so that the top of your pelvis is positioned slightly past the pad. This allows you to maintain your back in a stable neutral position (through isometric contraction) throughout the entire motion while your hamstrings/glutes work dynamically to lower and raise your trunk.

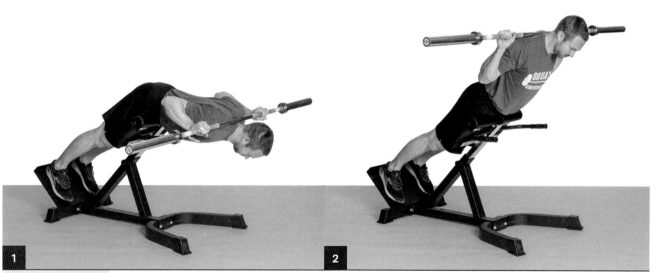

BACK EXTENSION

Why is it so important to limit back movement during this exercise?

Research has shown that those who develop back pain often have altered muscle recruitment patterns during movements that require the trunk to flex and extend.[98] When a healthy individual stands up after bending over to touch their toes (extending from a flexed position), the movement is largely accomplished about the hips.[99] However, those who have back pain often move with a "top-down" or "spine-dominant" strategy, meaning they over-rely on the low back compared to those without pain when performing a trunk extension movement.[100] It would therefore be unwise for someone with low back pain to perform an exercise that involves extending the spine from a flexed position, as doing so under load only strengthens the problematic movement pattern. By limiting motion from your low back during this exercise, you can hope to break this cycle and retrain your body to move in a more "hip-dominant" manner.

If you do not have access to a Roman chair or GHD machine, an RDL (Romanian deadlift) provides a similar training stimulus. Stand with a barbell or kettlebell held in front of you at hip level. Grab the ground with your feet and brace your core to create sufficient tension throughout your body. Your knees should be slightly bent. Begin the movement by hinging at the hips as you lower the barbell toward the ground. Lower as far as you can without losing the natural curve of your low back. Once you reach the lowest position of the movement, return to standing by moving only about the hips.

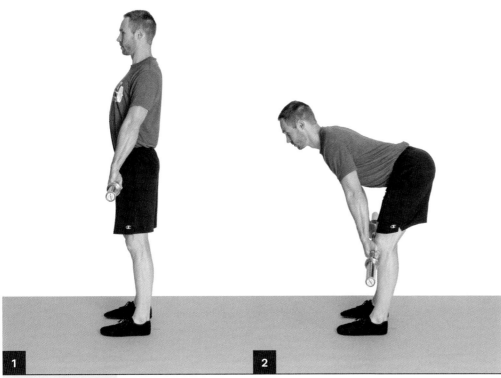

RDL WITH BARBELL

Exercises are only tools in our toolbox. If you are designing a program for rehab or performance, you need to choose the best tool to help you accomplish your individual goals. While the muscles of the low back do need to be strong, especially for those attempting to return to heavy strength training, I caution against doing any exercise that loads and then moves the spine.

Does Stretching the Hamstrings Fix Low Back Pain?

I've heard it from patients time and time again like a record on repeat: "My doctor told me I need to stretch my hamstrings because they're causing my low back pain." Many people in the medical and physical therapy professions hold the idea that low back pain is caused by tight hamstrings, and stretching them is the solution. When you glance at the research, this theory makes sense. If you do a simple Google search, you can easily locate a number of studies that link low back pain with "tight" hamstrings.[101]

However, while "tight" hamstrings may be common in those with low back pain, I've found in my years of treating patients as a physical therapist that it is *not* a direct cause. For this reason, I find the idea that every single patient who walks in the door with low back pain needs to stretch their hamstrings very misguided. In this section of the chapter, I want to walk you through exactly why that is.

How We're Taught to Assess Hamstring "Tightness"

One of the most common hamstring flexibility assessments performed in doctors' offices around the world is a passive straight-leg raise (SLR) test. Here's how you do it.

While lying on your back, relax your muscles and have a friend raise one of your legs as far as possible without your knee bending. If they can raise your leg to 80 degrees or more without causing you pain, you are considered to have "normal" hamstring flexibility.[102] However, if they are unable to lift your leg to 80 degrees without you feeling excessive tightness or pain in the back of your thigh, the limitation is usually attributed to "tight" or inelastic hamstrings.

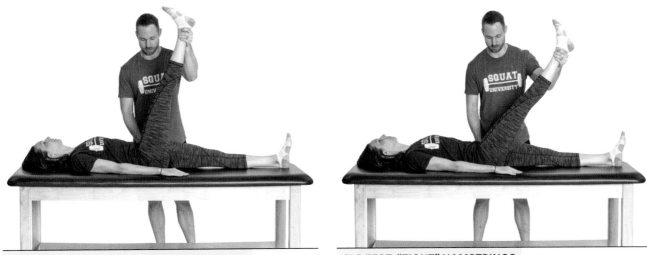

SLR TEST: NORMAL HAMSTRING FLEXIBILITY

SLR TEST: "TIGHT" HAMSTRINGS

Why We Stretch

Stretching is used to improve flexibility. In physical therapy school, we're taught to stretch muscles that are either stiff or short to restore them to normal flexibility. In the strength and conditioning and fitness worlds, stretches are used to promote better-quality movement, improve performance, and limit injury risk. Over the past few decades, a tremendous amount of research has been published demonstrating the effectiveness of stretching in both the medical and strength and conditioning fields.[103] But how does stretching really work?

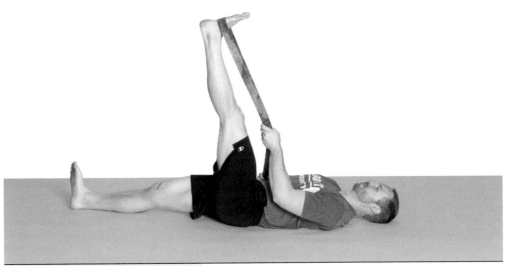

HAMSTRING STRETCH WITH BAND

When a muscle or group of muscles like the hamstrings are stretched (such as when you lie on your back and a friend pushes your leg to the sky), some short-term changes occur. The most obvious effect is improved flexibility (meaning you have more range of motion and can lift your leg higher during the next stretch); however, this effect doesn't always last long.

For example, one study showed that the improved hamstring flexibility seen after 5 rounds of a stretching protocol lasted only 6 minutes![104] Thirty-two minutes after the stretching stopped, the muscles had returned to their prestretch length. Other, more extensive stretching protocols have shown that the effects of stretching can last anywhere from 60 to 90 minutes.[105] This means both the amount of time spent stretching and the length a stretch is held affect how long the short-term benefits of improved flexibility last. Regardless, the improved range of motion often returns to baseline.

Theoretically, there are two ways to improve flexibility. The first model is the mechanical theory, which is based on the idea that if range of motion improves after stretching, that improvement can be due to either increased muscular length or decreased muscular stiffness.

Muscles are fairly elastic, meaning that they can stretch when a force is applied to them and then return to their normal length after the force is removed, similar to a rubber band. We can measure elasticity two ways:

- **Extensibility** is the ability of a muscle to elongate or lengthen. It is usually defined as the ability to extend the muscle to a certain end point (most often the point at which a person feels they can't tolerate any more stretch without pain). We can measure extensibility by looking at the angle at which a joint can be moved, as with the hip joint during the SLR test.

- **Stiffness** is how much force is needed during a stretch to elongate the muscles. It can be a tricky concept to define (and isn't at all how most people use the word today) because stiffness can change based on how fast a stretch is applied and the angle of the joint.

Most medical books that discuss stretching would have you believe that increases in flexibility are often due to the mechanical model, and the muscle itself is actually lengthening when stretched. There are three theories under this model that try to justify the changes in flexibility:

- **Viscoelastic deformation:** This is a fancy way of saying that muscles have both an elastic component (like a rubber band) and a viscous or gooey component (similar to honey). The idea is that as a stretch is applied, the force causes the muscle to relax, and flexibility improves. However, research has been quick to disprove this theory, as any changes seen because of viscoelastic deformation are likely short-lived. For example, one research study showed that a hamstring stretch held for 45 seconds had no significant effect on the next stretch performed 30 seconds later.[106] If the muscle really deformed and stayed that way, the researchers would have seen a significant difference.

- **Plastic deformation:** Another popular theory states that the increased flexibility observed after a stretch exists because the connective tissues that make up the muscle are stretched to a point where they become permanently lengthened. Research to support this notion, however, has been poor.[107]

- **Increased sarcomeres in series:** The third theory is based on the idea that the building blocks that make up muscle (called *sarcomeres*) increase in number in response to a stretch. Think of a sarcomere like a LEGO brick. A muscle is made up of thousands of muscle fibers, each of which is composed of a long block chain of sarcomeres. Based on a few animal studies, researchers found that if they created a long held stretch (by splinting or immobilizing a joint in a cast for a few weeks and holding the muscle in a lengthened position), the body would increase the number of sarcomeres (more LEGO bricks in a row) by upwards of 20 percent.[108] Basically, the block chain inside each muscle fiber is stretched to such a degree that the body decides to add more blocks to the chain to restore the prior "normal" balance. However, what most people don't understand about this adaptive change is that it appears *without* an overall change in muscle length! While there may be more blocks in the chain of sarcomeres, the length of each block becomes smaller. The blocks basically shrink! Also, these adaptive changes do not last long; the muscle returns to its prior "normal" number of sarcomeres within a few weeks.[109] So, while these few animal studies have shown there to be changes in the muscle architecture after four weeks of an immobilization stretch, it is a bit far-fetched to think that these same changes would be seen after an intermittent stretching program like the ones used by most athletes.

The second and more probable theory for how stretching improves flexibility is a change in sensation. The latest research has shown that much of the short-term increase in flexibility comes from improving your stretch tolerance (or pain tolerance), *not* from increasing your muscles' length![110] Basically, after stretching your hamstrings for a few sets of 30 seconds, you have more flexibility because of your ability to tolerate a greater amount of stretch before you tap out.

What Are the Effects of a Long-Term Stretching Program?

Unfortunately, almost all of the studies published on the effects of stretching have lasted only between three and eight weeks. The improvements seen in these short-term programs are a result of increased tolerance to muscle stretching. The research shows that there is no actual lengthening of the muscle fibers.[111]

For now, we are unsure of the long-term effects of stretching. It is entirely possible that individuals who partake in a rigorous stretching program for years actually can alter the extensibility of their muscles. In a few years, researchers may provide a concrete answer on the effects of long-term stretching (programs lasting several months to years).

If you want to see significant changes in flexibility of any muscle or group of muscles, you must be consistent with your stretching. It's easy to become frustrated with your lack of progress if you stretch only once every few days. As I mentioned before, the improved range of motion seen directly after a single stretching session often returns to baseline within minutes to hours. To find your potential for significant change, take 5 to 10 minutes every day to address your limitations.

The Back Pain–Tight Hamstring Connection

Let's switch gears and talk about why so many athletes are quick to stretch their hamstrings, especially those who have back pain. Here is a normal thought process that goes through the minds of many in the medical community when assessing someone who is experiencing back pain:

> When assessing the patient's straight-leg raise, they were unable to raise either leg past 70 degrees. We were taught in school that this means the person has "tight" or short hamstrings. Short hamstrings have been shown in research to be associated with low back pain. This means we need to stretch the hamstrings as a part of the rehabilitation plan to decrease the back pain.

Sound familiar?

In 2000, a group of researchers from the Netherlands conducted a study in which they looked at a number of factors among three groups: those with flexible hamstrings, those with "tight" hamstrings, and those with low back pain.[112] Here's what they found:

- Those with low back pain had the lowest hip range of motion via the SLR test (even worse than those with just "tight" hamstrings). The researchers concluded that this decreased range of motion was due only to the hamstrings and did not have to do with any pelvic tilting or back mobility issues.

- The hamstrings in both the flexible group and the "tight" group showed a similar "defense reaction" as they were stretched. The farther the legs were stretched, the more electrical activity rose in all of the hamstring muscles. However, those with low back pain had an abnormal "defense reaction" and did not have simultaneous electrical activity in all of their hamstrings. Also, the electrical activity they did record did not increase at the same gradual pace as it did in those who were pain-free. This difference was attributed to a heightened arousal or sensitivity to movement that occurs in those with back pain.

- There was no difference in muscle stiffness between those with "tight" hamstrings and those in the low back pain group.

- Hamstring flexibility in those with low back pain was worse than in those with "tight" hamstrings, but this limited motion was not accompanied by an increase in muscular stiffness.

Here's what this means: low back pain coupled with limited hamstring flexibility is usually due to the nervous system going haywire. The hamstring muscles are reacting and behaving differently, which can affect a person's ability to tolerate a stretch.

The Treatment Plan

Armed with the information that limited hamstring flexibility is due to a neuro-muscular issue in individuals dealing with back pain, the solution is *not* passive stretching. So what should you do instead?

The three-step process for fixing back pain is as follows:

1. Wind down pain sensitivity by avoiding the motions, postures, and loads that trigger your pain. This will be different for each person and requires efficient screening.

2. Improve core stability and mobility of the joint complexes above and below the site of pain.

3. Improve movement quality: learn to move about the hips instead of the low back and reactivate the glutes.[113]

Viewing the Hamstrings in a New Light

Since we know that the hamstrings are not a cause of low back pain, we need to change our approach to how and when to improve hamstring *flexibility.* We must first discuss the difference between flexibility and mobility. We can test the flexibility or length of the hamstrings by performing the SLR test discussed on pages 104 and 105. *Mobility* is different; it has a movement component and describes the body's ability to use its flexibility, muscle tension/quality, and nervous system (aka motor control) to coordinate itself through a range.

Mobility should always be evaluated before flexibility. Let's take the example of Jim, a national-level Olympic weightlifter. Jim has great hip mobility and coordination of his core stability and posterior chain muscles. He shows great-looking technique during his barbell lifts of the clean and snatch. If you ask him to bend over and touch his toes, he will perform what looks like a barbell RDL without any weight in his hands because his body has been programmed to move correctly about the hips over and over again in the gym.

However, if you took Jim without looking at the quality of his movement and had him perform the SLR test, you might find that he has relatively "tight" hamstrings, as he is unable to lift his free leg straight past 80 degrees. Does this mean he should automatically be prescribed hamstring stretches?

What if I told you that the relatively "stiff" hamstrings of some athletes are an advantage and not a problem that needs to be stretched away? Think of your muscles as springs. When they are loaded with tension, they have the ability to explode with power and propel your body down a track.

Now, 20-plus years ago, long-duration stretching was all the rage because researchers believed that static stretches before a workout or an athletic completion could help reduce the risk of a muscular strain injury.[114] So, if Jim had gone to a physical therapist back then, he would have been prescribed some long-duration (1 minute–plus) static stretching for his hamstrings by lying on his back and pulling his foot to the sky.

Nowadays the tides are turning. A growing amount of new research is showing that this type of stretching before exercise can lead to decreases in strength, power, and speed, thereby limiting an athlete's performance.[115] This is part of the reason why both the American College of Sports Medicine and the European College of Sports Sciences have come out condemning long-duration static stretching as part of a warm-up routine![116]

Now, does this mean we should never stretch? Not at all. Some athletes would benefit from a certain amount of stretching to improve their flexibility, get into better technical positions, and move more efficiently during training and competition. If you want to stretch before a training session or competition, I recommend short-duration stretches (less than 30 seconds), which have been shown to have no harmful effects on muscular performance.[117] It's not until the stretch is held for *more than 45 seconds* that we see losses in strength, power, and speed. In fact, research has shown that the ability of a muscle to produce force when subjected to these long-duration stretches (which are still prescribed by many fitness trainers and coaches) is decreased for up to 30 minutes.[118]

Will there be athletes who need long-duration stretches? Sure. I wouldn't discontinue them completely, but their use must be individualized to the athlete who needs to improve flexibility in order to improve movement quality. If you are assigning a stretch just for the sake of stretching, you have already failed your client. I also recommend that, if you want to implement stretching into your own routine, you do it after a workout or on separate days/times from your training sessions.

On another note, if you have been stretching before your lifts for a long time and you have not seen any drops in performance, by all means continue with your routine. For instance, many gymnasts perform long-duration stretches before their sessions yet are capable of producing adequate power. I would not change that warm-up routine because stretching is deeply ingrained in the sport.

What may surprise you is that there is a way to improve flexibility without any stretching at all! Yes, you read that correctly. Research has shown that muscle stiffness can be decreased (and therefore muscle elasticity and flexibility can be increased) through a dynamic warm-up. By increasing the temperature of the muscle through activities like light jogging, fast walking, skipping, lunging, or doing bodyweight squats, we can make our muscles more supple and improve our ability to move freely.[119]

What you're feeling while you warm up is a thixotropic effect. *Thixotropy* is the ability of tissue (such as muscle) to become more pliable or liquid after motion and to return to a stiffer gel-like state when resting. Basically, movement decreases muscular stiffness. This is why your low back or legs feel stiff after you sit in a chair all day, but you feel much better after you get up and walk around for a few minutes.

Think about opening a container of yogurt. When you peel back the lid, the yogurt is sometimes clumped together. After you stick your spoon into the cup and stir the yogurt around, it becomes more gel-like. This is an example of a thixotropic effect. Just like the yogurt being stirred by the spoon, your muscles become less stiff and more responsive to movement.

A generalized warm-up that elevates the heart rate and improves blood flow to the muscles is recommended for all athletes before training or competition to promote this thixotropic effect. If you are a barbell athlete, your warm-up can include walking lunges, leg or arm swings, or even a fast-paced walk.

Following this general warm-up should be a sport-specific warm-up that includes movements tailored to your particular training/sport. For example, if your workout includes clean and jerks, you might start with an open bar and perform a number of shrugs and high pulls followed by some full-depth front squats before adding weight. The combination of a general and a specific warm-up is key for improving flexibility, mobility, and movement quality to perform at your best and be as safe as possible.

Final Thoughts on Hamstring Stretching

Every aspect of a training or rehab program has a purpose. At the end of the day, you have to ask yourself *why* you are implementing each exercise, including stretches. For years, we have been taught that if a muscle is tight, we need to stretch it to return it to what a textbook would tell us is "normal."

I hope you now understand that those who are in pain do not have "normal" hamstring flexibility. Their bodies are reacting differently due to pain/injury, which creates a facade of "muscle tightness."[120] For this reason, someone with back pain can't just stretch away the limited hamstring flexibility.

Also, just because someone has "tight" hamstrings does not mean they will develop back pain.[121] In fact, some athletes have short or stiff hamstrings for a reason. Remember, muscle length testing was developed years ago based on the idea that there is a "normal" or ideal range of muscle length for optimal movement and safety. Blindly prescribing long-duration stretching for an athlete's hamstring stiffness just because they appear "abnormal" on paper is not always a good idea. I'm going to share a little secret with you: *most elite athletes have abnormal traits that give them the ability to do things most of us "normal" people cannot.*

Instead, I urge you to address what you find in these athletes in a different manner than we have in the past. For those with back pain, treat the "why." Understand that the "tight" hamstrings are a reaction to the pain, and we need to learn how to stabilize the low back, turn the inactive glutes back on, and fix the movement pattern that led to the injury in the first place to find a lasting fix! For an athlete with "tight hamstrings," learn to incorporate a proper warm-up that includes dynamic movements and short-duration stretching (if warranted) that will improve mobility and movement quality without a decrease in performance. I hope this content empowers you to make more educated choices on *when* and *if* to include stretching in the future.

Notes

1. T. E. Dreisinger and B. Nelson, "Management of back pain in athletes," *Sports Medicine* 21, no. 4 (1996): 313–20.

2. G. B. Andersson, "Epidemiological features of chronic low-back pain," *Lancet* 354, no. 9178 (1999): 581–5.

3. T. J. Chandler and M. H. Stone, "The squat exercise in athletic conditioning: a review of the literature," *National Strength and Conditioning Association Journal* 13, no. 5 (1991): 51–8.

4. G. Calhoon and A. C. Fry, "Injury rates and profiles of elite competitive weightlifters," *Journal of Athletic Training* 34, no. 3 (1999): 232–8; E. W. Brown and R. G. Kimball, "Medical history associated with adolescent powerlifting," *Pediatrics* 72, no. 5 (1983): 636–44; J. Keogh, P. A. Hume, and S. Pearson, "Retrospective injury epidemiology of one hundred one competitive Oceania power lifters: the effects of age, body mass, competitive standard, and gender," *Journal of Strength and Conditioning Research* 20, no. 3 (2006): 672–81; Dreisinger and Nelson, "Management of back pain in athletes" (see note 1 above); J. W. Keogh and P. W. Winwood, "The epidemiology of injuries across the weight training sports: a systematic review," *Sports Medicine* 47, no. 3 (2016): 479–501.

5. A. Babińska, W. Wawrzynek, E. Czech, J. Skupiński, J. Szczygieł, and B. Łabuz-Roszak, "No association between MRI changes in the lumbar spine and intensity of pain, quality of life, depressive and anxiety symptoms in patients with low back pain," *Neurologia I Neurochirurgia Polska* 53, no. 1 (2019): 74–82.

6. W. Brinjikji, P. H. Luetmer, B. Comstock, B. W. Bresnahan, L. E. Chen, R. A. Deyo, S. Halabi, et al., "Systematic literature review of imaging features of spinal degeneration in asymptomatic populations," *American Journal of Neuroradiology* 36, no. 4 (2015): 811–6.

7. E. Carragee, T. Alamin, I. Cheng, T. Franklin, E. van den Haak, and E. L. Hurwitz, "Are first-time episodes of serious LBP associated with new MRI findings?" *Spine* 6, no. 6 (2006): 624–35.

8. M. C. Jensen, M. N. Brant-Zawadzki, N. Obuchowski, M. T. Modic, D. Malkasian, and J. S. Ross, "Magnetic resonance imaging of the lumbar spine in people without back pain," *New England Journal of Medicine* 331, no. 2 (1994): 69–73; Carragee, Alamin, Cheng, Franklin, van den Haak, and Hurwitz, "Are first-time episodes of serious LBP associated with new MRI findings?" (see note 7 above); K. Fukuda and G. Kawakami, "Proper use of MR imaging for evaluation of low back pain (radiologist's view)," *Seminars in Musculoskeletal Radiology* 5, no. 2 (2001): 133–6.

9. K. Singh, D. K. Park, J. Shah, and F. M. Phillips, "The biomechanics and biology of the spinal degenerative cascade," *Seminars in Spine Surgery* 17, no. 3 (2005): 128–36.

10. P. M. Ludewig, D. H. Kamonseki, J. L. Staker, R. L. Lawrence, P. R. Camargo, and J. P. Braman, "Changing our diagnostic paradigm: movement system diagnostic classification," *International Journal of Sports Physical Therapy* 12, no. 6 (2017): 884–93.

11. U. Aasa, V. Bengtsson, L. Berglund, and F. Öhberg, "Variability of lumbar spinal alignment among power- and weightlifters during the deadlift and barbell back squat," *Sports Biomechanics* 13 (2019): 1–17.

12. S. Sahrmann, D. C. Azevedo, and L. Van Dillen, "Diagnosis and treatment of movement system impairment syndromes," *Brazilian Journal of Physical Therapy* 21, no. 6 (2017): 391–9.

13. S. M. McGill, *Ultimate Back Fitness and Performance,* 4th Edition (Waterloo, Canada: Backfitpro Inc., 2009).

14. P. D'Ambrosia, K. King, B. Davidson, B. H. Zhou, Y. Lu, and M. Solomonow, "Pro-inflammatory cytokines expression increases following low- and high-magnitude cyclic loading of lumbar ligaments," *European Spine Journal* 19, no. 8 (2010): 1330–9.

15. S. M. McGill, "The biomechanics of low back injury: implications on current practice in industry and the clinic," *Journal of Biomechanics* 30, no. 5 (1997): 465–75; K. R. Wade, P. A. Robertson, A. Thambyah, and N. D. Broom, "How healthy discs herniate: a biomechanical and microstructural study investigating the combined effects of compression rate and flexion," *Spine* 39, no.

13 (2017): 1018–28; J. P. Callaghan and S. M. McGill, "Intervertebral disc herniation: studies on a porcine model exposed to highly repetitive flexion/extension motion with compressive force," *Clinical Biomechanics* 16, no. 1 (2001): 28–37.

16.   Wade, Robertson, Thambyah, and Broom, "How healthy discs herniate" (see note 15 above); Callaghan and McGill, "Intervertebral disc herniation" (see note 15 above); J. L. Gunning, J. P. Callaghan, and S. M. McGill, "Spinal posture and prior loading history modulate compressive strength and type of failure in the spine: a biomechanical study using a porcine cervical spine model," *Clinical Biomechanics* 16, no. 6 (2001): 471–80.

17.   Wade, Robertson, Thambyah, and Broom, "How healthy discs herniate" (see note 15 above); C. Tampier, J. D. Drake, J. P. Callaghan, and S. M. McGill, "Progressive disc herniation: an investigation of the mechanism using radiologic, histochemical, and microscopic dissection techniques on a porcine model," *Spine* 32, no. 25 (2007): 2869–74; L. W. Marshall and S. M. McGill, "The role of axial torque in disc herniation," *Clinical Biomechanics* 25, no. 1 (2010): 6–9; S. P. Veres, P. A. Robertson, and N. D. Broom, "The morphology of acute disc herniation: a clinically relevant model defining the role of flexion," *Spine* 34, no. 21 (2009): 2288–96.

18.   S. M. McGill, "Spine flexion exercise: myths, truths and issues affecting health and performance," Backfitpro, accessed March 10, 2018, https://www.backfitpro.com/documents/Spine-flexion-myths-truths-and-issues.pdf; A. G. Robling and C. H. Turner, "Mechanical signaling for bone modeling and remodeling," *Critical Reviews in Eukaryotic Gene Expression* 19, no. 4 (2009): 319–38.

19.   K. Spencer and M. Croiss, "The effect of increased loading on powerlifting movement form during the squat and deadlift," *Journal of Human Sport and Exercise* 10, no. 3 (2015): 764–74.

20.   J. Cholewicki, S. M. McGill, and R. W. Norman, "Lumbar spine loads during the lifting of extremely heavy weights," *Medicine & Science in Sports & Exercise* 23, no. 10 (1991): 1179–86.

21.   S. M. McGill, personal communication, March 28, 2019.

22.   Cholewicki, McGill, and Norman, "Lumbar spine loads during the lifting of extremely heavy weights" (see note 20 above); J. Cholewicki and S. M. McGill, "Lumbar posterior ligament involvement during extremely heavy lifts estimated from fluoroscopic measurements," *Journal of Biomechanics* 25, no. 2 (1992): 17–28.

23.   Cholewicki, McGill, and Norman, "Lumbar spine loads during the lifting of extremely heavy weights" (see note 20 above).

24.   R. Oftadeh, M. Perez-Viloria, J. C. Villa-Camacho, A. Vaziri, and A. Nazarian, "Biomechanics and mechanobiology of trabecular bone: a review," *Journal of Biomechanical Engineering* 137, no. 1 (2015): 0108021–215.

25.   J. H. van Dieën, H. Weinans, and H. M. Toussaint, "Fractures of the lumbar vertebral endplate in the etiology of low back pain: a hypothesis on the causative role of spinal compression in aspecific low back pain," *Medical Hypotheses* 53, no. 3 (1999): 246–52.

26.   Oftadeh, Perez-Viloria, Villa-Camacho, Vaziri, and Nazarian, "Biomechanics and mechanobiology of trabecular bone" (see note 24 above).

27.   R. D. Dickerman, R. Pertusi, and G. H. Smith, "The upper range of lumbar spine bone mineral density? An examination of the current world record holder in the squat lift," *International Journal of Sports Medicine* 21, no. 7 (2000): 469–70; H. Granhed, R. Jonson, and T. Hansson, "The loads on the lumbar spine during extreme weight lifting," *Spine* 12, no. 2 (1987): 146–9; P. H. Walters, J. J. Jezequel, and M. B. Grove, "Case study: bone mineral density of two elite senior female powerlifters," *Journal of Strength and Conditioning Research* 26, no. 3 (2012): 867–72; Cholewicki, McGill, and Norman, "Lumbar spine loads during the lifting of extremely heavy weights" (see note 20 above).

28.   Robling and Turner, "Mechanical signaling for bone modeling and remodeling" (see note 18 above).

29.   S. M. McGill and B. Carroll, *Gift of Injury* (Waterloo, Canada: Backfitpro Inc., 2017).

30.   J. C. Lotz, A. J. Fields, and E. C. Liebenberg, "The role of the vertebral end plate in low back pain," *Global Spine Journal* 3, no. 3 (2013): 153–64.

31. van Dieën, Weinans, and Toussaint, "Fractures of the lumbar vertebral endplate in the etiology of low back pain" (see note 25 above); Lotz, Fields, and Liebenberg, "The role of the vertebral end plate in low back pain" (see note 30 above).

32. L. Manchikanti, J. A. Hirsch, F. J. Falco, and M. V. Boswell, "Management of lumbar zygapophysial (facet) joint pain," *World Journal of Orthopedics* 7, no. 5 (2016): 315–37.

33. S. J. Dreyer and P. H. Dreyfuss, "Low back pain and the zygapophysial (facet) joints," *Archives of Physical Medicine and Rehabilitation* 77, no. 3 (1996): 290–300.

34. Dreyer and Dreyfuss, "Low back pain and the zygapophysial (facet) joints" (see note 33 above).

35. S. P. Cohen and S. N. Raja, "Pathogenesis, diagnosis, and treatment of lumbar zygapophysial (facet) joint pain," *Anesthesiology* 106 (2007): 591–614.

36. Dreyer and Dreyfuss, "Low back pain and the zygapophysial (facet) joints" (see note 33 above).

37. Cohen and Raja, "Pathogenesis, diagnosis, and treatment of lumbar zygapophysial (facet) joint pain" (see note 35 above).

38. P. T. Katani, N. Ichikawa, W. Wakabayashi, T. Yoshii, and M. Koshimune, "Studies of spondylolysis found among weightlifters," *British Journal of Sports Medicine* 6, no. 1 (1971): 4–8; C. J. Dangles and D. L. Spencer, "Spondylolysis in competitive weightlifters," *Journal of Sports Medicine* 15 (1987): 634–5.

39. Katani, Ichikawa, Wakabayashi, Yoshii, and Koshimune, "Studies of spondylolysis found among weightlifters" (see note 38 above).

40. Dangles and Spencer, "Spondylolysis in competitive weightlifters" (see note 38 above).

41. T. R. Yochum and L. J. Rowe, "The natural history of spondylolysis and spondylolysthesis," in *Essentials of Skeletal Radiology* (Philadelphia, PA: Lipincott, Williams & Wilkins, 2005): 433–84.

42. M. H. Stone, A. C. Fry, M. Ritchie, L. Stoessel-Ross, and J. L. Marsit, "Injury potential and safety aspects of weightlifting movements," *Strength and Conditioning* 15, no. 3 (1994): 15–21.

43. A. F. Reynolds, P. R. Weinstein, and R. D. Wachter, "Lumbar monoradiculopathy due to unilateral facet hypertrophy," *Neurosurgery* 10, no. 4 (1982): 480–6; G. P. Wilde, E. T. Szypryt, and R. C. Mulholland, "Unilateral lumbar facet hypertrophy causing nerve root irritation," *Annals of Royal College of Surgeons of England* 70, no. 5 (1988): 307–10.

44. S. M. McGill, *Back Mechanic: The Step by Step McGill Method to Fix Back Pain* (Waterloo, Canada: Backfitpro Inc., 2015); W. R. Frontera, J. K. Silver, and T. D. Rizzo, Jr., *Essentials of Physical Medicine and Rehabilitation: Musculoskeletal Disorders, Pain and Rehabilitation*, 3rd Edition (Philadelphia: Saunders, 2014).

45. A. Indahl, A. Kaigle, O. Reikeras, and S. Holm, "Electromyographic response of the porcine multifidus musculature after nerve stimulation," *Spine* 20, no. 24 (1995): 2652–8; Cohen and Raja, "Pathogenesis, diagnosis, and treatment of lumbar zygapophysial (facet) joint pain" (see note 35 above); M. W. Olson, L. Li, and M. Solomonow, "Flexion-relaxation response to cyclic lumbar flexion," *Clinical Biomechanics* (Bristol, Avon) 19, no. 8 (2004): 769–76.

46. McGill, *Back Mechanic* (see note 44 above); Frontera, Silver, and Rizzo, Jr., *Essentials of Physical Medicine and Rehabilitation* (see note 44 above).

47. McGill, "The biomechanics of low back injury" (see note 15 above).

48. Sahrmann, Azevedo, and Van Dillen, "Diagnosis and treatment of movement system impairment syndromes" (see note 12 above); L. R. Van Dillen, S. A. Sahrmann, B. J. Norton, C. A. Caldwell, M. K. McDonnell, and N. J. Bloom, "Movement system impairment-based categories for low back pain: stage 1 validation," *Journal of Orthopaedic & Sports Physical Therapy* 33, no. 3 (2003): 126–42.

49. Sahrmann, Azevedo, and Van Dillen, "Diagnosis and treatment of movement system impairment syndromes" (see note 12 above).

50. Sahrmann, Azevedo, and Van Dillen, "Diagnosis and treatment of movement system impairment syndromes" (see note 12 above).

51. Sahrmann, Azevedo, and Van Dillen, "Diagnosis and treatment of movement system impairment syndromes" (see note 12 above).

52. M. R. McKean, P. K. Dunn, and B. J. Burkett, "The lumbar and sacrum movement pattern during the back squat exercise," *Journal of Strength & Conditioning Research* 24, no. 10 (2010): 2731–41; R. List, T. Gülay, M. Stoop, and S. Lorenzetti, "Kinematics of the trunk and the lower extremities during restricted and unrestricted squats," *Journal of Strength & Conditioning Research* 27, no. 6 (2013): 1529–38; M. H. Campos, L. I. Furtado Aleman, A. A. Seffrin-Neto, C. A. Vieira, M. Costa de Paula, and C. A. Barbosa de Lira, "The geometric curvature of the lumbar spine during restricted and unrestricted squats," *Journal of Sports Medicine and Physical Fitness* 57, no. 6 (2017): 773–81.

53. K. Bennell, R. Talbot, H. Wajswelner, W. Techovanich, and D. Kelly, "Intra-rater and inter-rater reliability of a weight-bearing lunge measure of ankle dorsiflexion," *Australian Journal of Physiotherapy* 44, no. 3 (1998): 175–80.

54. McGill, *Back Mechanic* (see note 44 above).

55. McGill, *Back Mechanic* (see note 44 above); D. Hertling and R. M. Kessler, *Management of Common Musculoskeletal Disorders: Physical Therapy Principles and Methods* (Philadelphia: J. B. Lippincott, 1996); H. S. Robinson, J. I. Brox, R. Robinson, E. Bjelland, S. Solem, and T. Telje, "The reliability of selected motion- and pain provocation tests for the sacroiliac joint," *Manual Therapy* 12, no. 1 (2007): 72–9.

56. S. Freeman, A. Mascia, and S. M. McGill, "Arthrogenic neuromuscular inhibition: a foundational investigation of existence in the hip joint," *Clinical Biomechanics* 28, no. 2 (2013): 171–7; J. E. Bullock-Saxton, V. Janda, and M. I. Bullock, "Reflex activation of gluteal muscles in walking. An approach to restoration of muscle function for patients with low-back pain," *Spine* 18, no. 6 (1993): 704–8; V. Leinonen, M. Kankaanpaa, O. Airaksinen, and O. Hannien, "Back and hip extensor activities during trunk flexion/extension: effects of low back pain and rehabilitation," *Archives of Physical Medicine and Rehabilitation* 81, no. 1 (2008): 32–7; E. Nelson-Wong, B. Alex, D. Csepe, D. Lancaster, and J. P. Callaghan, "Altered muscle recruitment during extension from trunk flexion in low back pain developers," *Clinical Biomechanics* 27, no. 10 (2012): 994–8.

57. Freeman, Mascia, and McGill, "Arthrogenic neuromuscular inhibition" (see note 56 above).

58. McGill, *Ultimate Back Fitness and Performance* (see note 13 above).

59. M. Sadeghisani, F. D. Manshadi, K. K. Kalantari, A. Rahimi, N. Namnik, M. Taghi Karimi, and A. E. Oskouei, "Correlation between hip range-of-motion impairment and low back pain: a literature review," *Orthopedia, Traumatologia, Rehabilitacja* 17, no. 5 (2015): 455–62; G. P. Leão Almeida, V. L. da Souza, S. S. Sano, M. F. Saccol, and M. Cohen, "Comparison of hip rotation range of motion in judo athletes with and without history of low back pain," *Manual Therapy* 17, no. 3 (2012): 231–5.

60. K. D. Johnson, K. M. Kim, B. K. Yu, S. A. Saliba, and T. L. Grindstaff, "Reliability of thoracic spine rotation range-of-motion measurements in healthy adults," *Journal of Athletic Training* 47, no. 1 (2012): 52–60; K. D. Johnson and T. L. Grindstaff, "Thoracic rotation measurement techniques: clinical commentary," *North American Journal of Sports Physical Therapy* 5, no. 4 (2010): 252–6.

61. D. Ikeda and S. M. McGill, "Can altering motions, postures and loads provide immediate low back pain relief: a study of four cases investigating spine load, posture and stability," *Spine* 37, no. 23 (2012): E1469–75.

62. T. Giesecke, R. H. Gracely, M. A. B. Grant, A. Nachemson, F. Petzke, D. A. Williams, and D. J. Clauw, "Evidence of augmented central pain processing in idiopathic chronic low back pain," *Arthritis & Rheumatism* 50, no. 2 (2004): 613–23.

63. P. O'Sullivan, "Diagnosis and classification of chronic low back pain disorders: maladaptive movement motor control impairments as underlying mechanism," *Manual Therapeutics* 10, no. 4 (2005): 242–55.

64. Dreisinger and Nelson, "Management of back pain in athletes" (see note 1 above).

65. B. C. Lee and S. M. McGill, "Effect of long-term isometric training on core/torso stiffness," *Journal of Strength and Conditioning Research* 29, no. 6 (2015): 1515–26.

66. Lee and McGill, "Effect of long-term isometric training on core/torso stiffness" (see note 65 above).

67. S. G. Grenier and S. M. McGill, "Quantification of lumbar stability by using 2 different abdominal activation strategies," *Archives of Physical Medicine and Rehabilitation* 88, no. 1 (2007): 54–62.

68. S. M. McGill, "Stability: from biomechanical concept to chiropractic practice," *Journal of the Canadian Chiropractic Association* 43, no. 2 (1999): 75–88.

69. S. M. McGill, "The mechanics of torso flexion: sit-ups and standing dynamic flexion maneuvers," *Clinical Biomechanics* 10, no. 4 (1995): 184–92.

70. D. Juker, S. M. McGill, P. Kropf, and T. Steffen, "Quantitative intramuscular myoelectric activity of lumbar portions of psoas and the abdominal wall during a wide variety of tasks," *Medicine & Science in Sports & Exercise* 30, no. 2 (1998): 301–10.

71. McGill, *Back Mechanic* (see note 44 above).

72. S. M. McGill, "Core training: evidence translating to better performance and injury prevention," *Strength and Conditioning Journal* 32, no. 3 (2010): 33–46.

73. McGill, "Core training" (see note 72 above).

74. K. Boren, C. Conrey, J. Le Coguic, L. Paprocki, M. Voight, and T. K. Robinson, "Electromyographic analysis of gluteus medius and gluteus maximus during rehabilitation exercises," *International Journal of Sports Physical Therapy* 6, no. 3 (2011): 206–23.

75. T. M. Parkhurst and C. N. Burnett, "Injury and proprioception in the lower back," *Journal of Orthopaedic and Sports Physical Therapy* 19, no. 5 (1994): 282–95; K. P. Gill and M. J. Callaghan, "The measurement of lumbar proprioception in individuals with and without low back pain," *Spine* 23, no. 3 (1998): 371–7.

76. Indahl, Kaigle, Reikeras, and Holm, "Electromyographic response of the porcine multifidus musculature after nerve stimulation" (see note 45 above); Cohen and Raja, "Pathogenesis, diagnosis, and treatment of lumbar zygapophysial (facet) joint pain" (see note 35 above).

77. S. M. McGill, *Low Back Disorders: Evidence Based Prevention and Rehabilitation*, 2nd Edition (Champaign, IL: Human Kinetics Publishers, 2007).

78. McGill, *Ultimate Back Fitness and Performance* (see note 13 above).

79. M. Olfat, J. Perry, and H. Hislop, "Relationship between wire EMG activity, muscle length, and torque of the hamstrings," *Clinical Biomechanics* 17, no. 8 (2002): 569–79.

80. C. J. Durall, B. E. Udermann, D. R. Johansen, B. Gibson, D. M. Reineke, and P. Reuteman, "The effect of preseason trunk muscle training of low back pain occurrence in women collegiate gymnasts," *Journal of Strength and Conditioning Research* 23, no. 1 (2009): 86–92.

81. S. M. McGill, "Stability: from biomechanical concept to chiropractic practice," *Journal of the Canadian Chiropractic Association* 43, no. 2 (1999): 75–88.

82. McGill, *Back Mechanic* (see note 44 above).

83. E. Nelson-Wong, B. Alex, D. Csepe, D. Lancaster, and J. P. Callaghan, "Altered muscle recruitment during extension from trunk flexion in low back pain developers," *Clinical Biomechanics* 27, no. 10 (2012): 994–8.

84. McGill, *Ultimate Back Fitness and Performance* (see note 13 above).

85. D. Diggin, C. O'Regan, N. Whelan, S. Daly, V. McLoughlin, L. McNamara, and A. Reilly, "A biomechanical analysis of front versus back squat: injury implications," *Portuguese Journal of Sport Sciences* 11, Suppl 2 (2011): 643–6; H. Hartmann, K. Wirth, and M. Klusemann, "Analysis of the load on the knee joint and vertebral column with changes in squatting depth and weight load," *Sports Medicine* 43, no. 10 (2013): 993–1008.

86. D. A. Hackett and C. M. Chow, "The Valsalva maneuver: its effect on intra-abdominal pressure and safety issues during resistance exercise," *Journal of Strength and Conditioning Research* 27, no. 8 (2013): 2338–45.

87. Cholewicki, McGill, and Norman, "Lumbar spine loads during the lifting of extremely heavy weights" (see note 20 above).

88. R. M. Enoka, "The pull in Olympic weightlifting," *Medicine & Science in Sports & Exercise* 11, no. 2 (1979): 131–7.

89. C. M. Fenwick, S. H. Brown, and S. M. McGill, "Comparison of different rowing exercises: trunk muscular activation and lumbar spine motion, load, and stiffness," *Journal of Strength and Conditioning Research* 23, no. 2 (2009): 350–8.

90. S. M. McGill, L. Marshall, and J. Anderson, "Low back loads while walking and carrying: comparing the load carried in one hand or in both hands," *Ergonomics* 56, no. 2 (2013): 293–302.

91. S. Luoto, H. Aalto, S. Taimela, H. Hurri, I. Pyykkö, and H. Alaranta, "One-footed and externally disturbed two-footed postural control in patients with chronic low back pain and healthy control subjects. A controlled study with follow-up," *Spine* 23, no. 19 (1998): 2081–9; S. Taimela, M. Kankaanpää, and S. Luoto, "The effect of lumbar fatigue on the ability to sense a change in lumbar position: a controlled study," *Spine* 24, no. 13 (1999): 1322–7.

92. Fenwick, Brown, and McGill, "Comparison of different rowing exercises" (see note 89 above).

93. Dreisinger and Nelson, "Management of back pain in athletes" (see note 1 above).

94. J. Cholewicki, K. Juluru, A. Radebold, M. M. Panjabi, and S. M. McGill, "Lumbar spine stability can be augmented with an abdominal belt and/or increased intra-abdominal pressure," *European Spine Journal* 8, no. 5 (1999): 388–95.

95. J. E. Lander, J. R. Hundley, and R. L. Simonton, "The effectiveness of weight-belts during multiple repetitions of the squat exercise," *Medicine & Science in Sports & Exercise* 24, no. 5 (1992): 603–9; J. E. Lander, R. L. Simonton, and J. K. Giacobbe, "The effectiveness of weight-belts during the squat exercise," *Medicine & Science in Sports & Exercise* 22, no. 1 (1990): 117–26; S. M. McGill, R. W. Norman, and M. T. Sharratt, "The effect of an abdominal belt on trunk muscle activity and intra-abdominal pressure during squat lifts," *Ergonomics* 33, no. 2 (1990): 147–60; E. A. Harman, R. M. Rosenstein, P. N. Frykman, and G. A. Nigro, "Effects of a belt on intra-abdominal pressure during weight lifting," *Medicine & Science in Sports & Exercise* 21, no. 12 (1989): 186–90.

96. Lander, Hundley, and Simonton, "The effectiveness of weight-belts during multiple repetitions of the squat exercise" (see note 95 above); A. J. Zink, W. C. Whiting, W. J. Vincent, and A. J. McLaine, "The effect of a weight belt on trunk and leg muscle activity and joint kinematics during the squat exercise," *Journal of Strength and Conditioning Research* 15, no. 2 (2011): 235–40.

97. B. C. Clark, T. M. Manini, J. M. Mayer, L. L. Ploutz-Snyder, and J. E. Graves, "Electromyographic activity of the lumbar and hip extensors during dynamic trunk extension exercise," *Archives of Physical Medicine and Rehabilitation* 83, no. 11 (2002): 1547–52; J. P. Callaghan, J. L. Gunning, and S. M. McGill, "The relationship between lumbar spine load and muscle activity during extensor exercises," *Physical Therapy* 78, no. 1 (1998): 8–18.

98. E. Nelson-Wong, B. Alex, D. Csepe, D. Lancaster, and J. P. Callaghan, "Altered muscle recruitment during extension from trunk flexion in low back pain developers," *Clinical Biomechanics* 27, no. 10 (2012): 994–8.

99. Andersson, "Epidemiological features of chronic low-back pain" (see note 2 above).

100. P. W. McClure, M. Esola, R. Schreier, and S. Siegler, "Kinematic analysis of lumbar and hip motion while rising from a forward, flexed position in patients with and without a history of low back pain," *Spine* 22, no. 5 (1997): 552–8; M. A. Esola, P. W. McClure, G. K. Fitzgerald, and S. Siegler, "Analysis of lumbar spine and hip motion during forward bending in subjects with and without a history of low back pain," *Spine* 21, no. 1 (1996): 71–8.

101. W. Alston, K. E. Carlson, D. J. Feldman, Z. Grimm, and E. Gerontinos, "A quantitative study of muscle factors in the chronic low back syndrome," *Journal of the American Geriatrics Society* 14, no. 10 (1966): 1041–7; G. Hultman, H. Saraste, and H. Ohlsen, "Anthropometry, spinal canal width, and flexibility of the spine and hamstring muscles in 45–55-year-old men with and without low back pain," *Journal of Spinal Disorders* 5, no. 3 (1992): 245–53; G. Mellin,

"Correlations of hip mobility with degree of back pain and lumbar spinal mobility in chronic low-back pain patients," *Spine* 13, no. 6 (1988): 668–70; D. E. Feldman, I. Shrier, M. Rossignol, and L. Abenhaim, "Risk factors for the development of low back pain in adolescence," *American Journal of Epidemiology* 154, no. 1 (2001): 30–6.

102. J. P. Halbertsma and L. N. Göeken, "Stretching exercises: effect on passive extensibility and stiffness in short hamstrings of healthy subjects," *Archives of Physical Medicine and Rehabilitation* 75, no. 9 (1994): 976–81.

103. Halbertsma and Göeken, "Stretching exercises" (see note 102 above); B. S. Killen, K. L. Zelizney, and X. Ye, "Crossover effects of unilateral static stretching and foam rolling on contralateral hamstring flexibility and strength," *Journal of Sports Rehabilitation* 28, no. 6 (2018): 533–9; G. Hatano, S. Suzuki,
S. Matsuo, S. Kataura, K. Yokoi, T. Fukaya, M. Fujiwara, Y. Asai, and M. Iwata, "Hamstring stiffness returns more rapidly after static stretching than range of motion, stretch tolerance, and isometric peak torque," *Journal of Sports Rehabilitation* 28, no. 4 (2017): 325–31; T. Haab and G. Wydra, "The effect of age on hamstring passive properties after a 10-week stretch training," *Journal of Physical Therapy Science* 29, no. 6 (2017): 1048–53; N. Ichihashi, H. Umegaki, T. Ikezoe, M. Nakamura, S. Nishishita, K. Fujita, J. Umehara, S. Nakao, and S. Ibuki, "The effects of a 4-week static stretching programme on the individual muscles comprising the hamstrings," *Journal of Sports Sciences* 34, no. 23 (2016): 2155–9; S. R. Freitas, B. Mendes, G. Le Sant, and R. J. Andrade, "Can chronic stretching change the muscle–tendon mechanical properties? A review," *Scandinavian Journal of Medicine & Science in Sports* 28, no. 3 (2018): 794–806; M. P. McHugh and C. H. Cosgrave, "To stretch or not to stretch: the role of stretching in injury prevention and performance," *Scandinavian Journal of Medicine & Science in Sports* 20, no. 2 (2010): 169–81; A. D. Kay and A. J. Blazevich, "Effect of acute static stretch on maximal muscle performance: a systematic review," *Medicine & Science in Sports & Exercise* 44, no. 1 (2012): 154–64; American College of Sports Medicine, *ACSM's Resource Manual for Guidelines for Exercise Testing and Prescription,* 8th Edition (Philadelphia: Lippincott, Williams & Wilkins, 2010), 173; P. Magnusson and P. Renstrom, "The European College of Sports Sciences position statement: the role of stretching exercises in sports," *European Journal of Sport Science* 6, no. 2 (2006): 87–91; D. Kundson, P. Magnusson, and M. McHugh, "Current issues in flexibility fitness," *President's Council on Physical Fitness and Sports Research Digest* 3, no. 10 (2000): 1–8.

104. S. G. Spernoga, L. H. Timothy, B. L. Arnold, and B. M. Gansneder, "Duration of maintained hamstring flexibility after one-time, modified hold-relax stretching protocol," *Journal of Athletic Training* 36, no. 1 (2001): 44–8.

105. M. Moller, J. Ekstrand, B. Oberg, and J. Gillquist, "Duration of stretching effect on range of motion in lower extremities," *Archives of Physical Medicine and Rehabilitation* 66, no. 3 (1985): 171–3.

106. S. P. Magnusson, P. Aagaard, and J. J. Nielson, "Passive energy return after repeated stretches of the hamstring muscle-tendon unit," *Medicine & Science in Sports & Exercise* 32, no. 6 (2000): 1160–4.

107. C. H. Weppler and S. P. Maggnusson, "Increasing muscle extensibility: a matter of increasing length or modifying sensation?" *Physical Therapy* 90, no. 3 (2010): 438–49.

108. J. C. Tabary, C. Tabary, C. Tardieu, G. Tardieu, and G. Goldspink, "Physiological and structural changes in the cat's soleus muscle due to immobilization at different lengths by plaster casts," *Journal of Physiology* 224, no. 1 (1972): 231–44.

109. Tabary, Tabary, Tardieu, Tardieu, and Goldspink, "Physiological and structural changes in the cat's soleus muscle" (see note 108 above); M. R. Gossman, S. A. Sahrmann, and S. J. Rose, "Review of length-associated changes in muscle. Experimental evidence and clinical implications," *Physical Therapy* 62, no. 12 (1992): 1799–808.

110. K. Weimann and K. Hahn, "Influences of strength, stretching and circulatory exercises on flexibility parameters of the human hamstrings," *International Journal of Sports Medicine* 18, no. 5 (1997): 340–6; D. Knudson, "The biomechanics of stretching," *Journal of Exercise Science*

& *Physiotherapy* 2 (2006): 3–12; S. P. Magnussson, E. B. Simonsen, P. Aagaard, H. Sørensen, and M. Kjaer, "A mechanism for altered flexibility in human skeletal muscle," *Journal of Physiology* 497, Pt 1 (1996): 291–8; Weppler and Maggnusson, "Increasing muscle extensibility" (see note 107 above).

111. Magnussson, Simonsen, Aagaard, Sørensen, and Kjaer, "A mechanism for altered flexibility in human skeletal muscle" (see note 110 above).

112. J. P. Halbertsma, L. N. Göeken, A. L. Hof, J. W. Groothoff, and W. H. Eisma, "Extensibility and stiffness of the hamstrings in patients with nonspecific low back pain," *Archives of Physical Medicine and Rehabilitation* 82, no. 2 (2001): 232–8.

113. V. Leinonen, M. Kankaanpaa, O. Airaksinen, and O. Hannien, "Back and hip extensor activities during trunk flexion/extension: effects of low back pain and rehabilitation," *Archives of Physical Medicine and Rehabilitation* 81, no. 1 (2008): 32–7; M. Kankaanpää, S. Taimela, D. Laaksonen, O. Hänninen, O. Airaksinen, "Back and hip extensor fatigability in chronic low back pain patients and controls," *Archives of Physical Medicine and Rehabilitation* 79, no. 4 (1998): 312–7.

114. M. P. McHugh and C. H. Cosgrave, "To stretch or not to stretch: the role of stretching in injury prevention and performance," *Scandinavian Journal of Medicine & Science in Sports* 20, no. 2 (2010): 169–81.

115. Kay and Blazevich, "Effect of acute static stretch on maximal muscle performance" (see note 103 above); J. Kokkonen, A. G. Nelson, and A. Cornwell, "Acute muscle stretching inhibits maximal strength performance," *Research Quarterly for Exercise and Sport* 69, no. 4 (1998): 411–5.

116. American College of Sports Medicine, *ACSM's Resource Manual for Guidelines for Exercise Testing and Prescription*, 8th Edition; Magnusson and Renstrom, "The European College of Sports Sciences position statement: the role of stretching exercises in sports" (see note 103 above).

117. Kay and Blazevich, "Effect of acute static stretch on maximal muscle performance" (see note 103 above); W. D. Bandy, J. M. Irion, and M. Briggler, "The effect of time and frequency of static stretching on flexibility of the hamstring muscles," *Physical Therapy* 77, no. 10 (1997): 1090–6; A. D. Kay and A. J. Blazevich, "Moderate-duration static stretch reduces active and passive plantar flexor moment but not Achilles tendon stiffness or active muscle length," *Journal of Applied Physiology* 106, no. 4 (2009): 1249–56.

118. Hatano, Suzuki, Matsuo, Kataura, Yokoi, Fukaya, Fujiwara, Asai, and Iwata, "Hamstring stiffness returns more rapidly after static stretching" (see note 103 above).

119. Knudson, "The biomechanics of stretching" (see note 110 above).

120. J. P. van Wingerden, A. Vleeming, G. J. Kleinrensink, and R. Stoeckart, "The role of the hamstring in pelvic and spinal function," in *Movement Stability and Low Back Pain: The Essential Role of the Pelvis*, eds. A. Vleeming, V. Mooney, T. Dorman, C. Snijders, and R. Stoeckart (New York: Churchill Livingstone, 1997), 207–10; S. M. Raftry and P. W. M. Marshall, "Does a 'tight' hamstring predict low back pain reporting during prolonged standing?" *Journal of Electromyography and Kinesiology* 22, no. 3 (2012): 407–11; M. R. Nourbakhsh and A. M. Arab, "Relationship between mechanical factors and incidence of low back pain," *Journal of Orthopaedic & Sports Physical Therapy* 32, no. 9 (2002): 447–60.

121. A. L. Hellsing, "Tightness of hamstring and psoas major muscles. A prospective study of back pain in young men during their military service," *Upsala Journal of Medical Science* 93, no. 3 (1988): 267–76; F. Biering-Sorensen, "Physical measurements as risk indicators for low-back trouble over a one-year period," *Spine* 9, no. 2 (1984): 106–19.

CHAPTER 2

HIP PAIN

An injury to the hip is one of the most common problems for a strength athlete. Despite how prevalent this injury is, it can be one of the most complicated to diagnose and treat because pain can develop in any of several muscles that surround and attach to the femur or pelvis—hip flexor strains, groin pulls, piriformis syndrome, and so on.

To make matters even more difficult, hip pain can arise from the hip joint itself or even radiate down from an injury in the back! For this reason, performing a proper screening is imperative to uncovering why your symptoms are present, which will lead you to the right steps for fixing your pain.

Hip Anatomy

To understand how injury occurs at the hip, we need to start by discussing basic hip anatomy. The hip is a ball-and-socket joint. The end of the thigh bone (femur) is shaped like a small ball. It fits within the "socket" (acetabulum) of the hip and connects at a slight angle, allowing the foot to be positioned relatively straight forward when standing, walking, and squatting.

HIP/PELVIS BONY ANATOMY

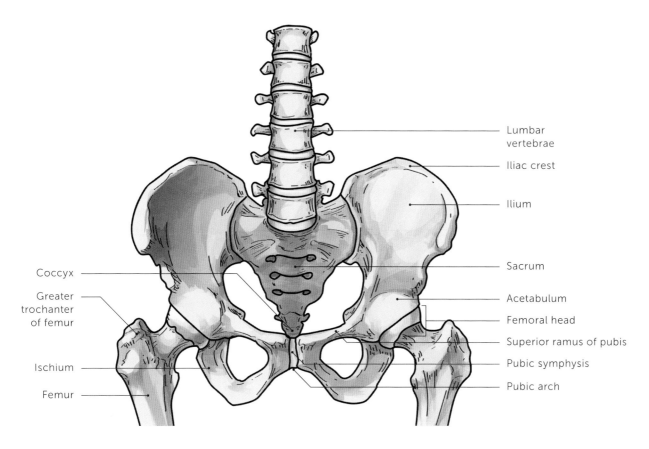

Coccyx

Greater trochanter of femur

Ischium

Femur

Lumbar vertebrae

Iliac crest

Ilium

Sacrum

Acetabulum

Femoral head

Superior ramus of pubis

Pubic symphysis

Pubic arch

However, not everyone fits this textbook bone structure. Variations in the ways our hips are shaped can impact how we move, especially the way we squat, deadlift, or catch a snatch in a deep receiving position. These anatomical differences must be assessed and uncovered during a proper evaluation, as they can play a large role in the development of hip pain.

So how prevalent are these variations? Well, in 2001, a group of researchers in Japan took a close look at the hip joint. While a majority of the subjects had "normal" hip sockets, close to 40 percent did not![1] Some people have hip sockets that open to the side, while others point more forward. A small change in how the hip socket opens can have a dramatic effect on how the body moves.

For example, as you squat, your femur rotates in the socket and your thigh moves toward your torso (the movement of hip flexion). If someone has a hip socket that opens laterally (called *acetabular retroversion*), their femur will come into contact with the front edge of the acetabulum sooner during a deep squat than if the socket opened more toward the front of the body.

ACETABULAR ALIGNMENT

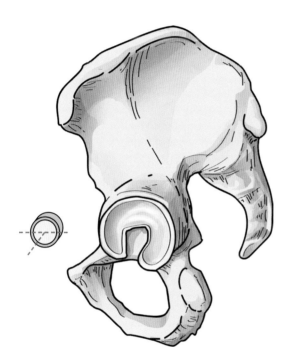
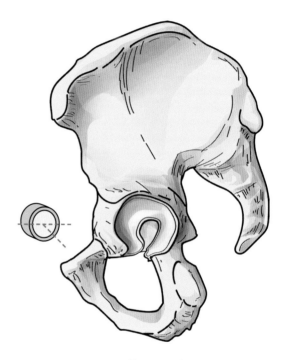

Normal acetabular position   Retroversion

A simple test can give you a better understanding of the alignment and shape of your hip sockets. Start by lying on your back. Bring your knee toward your chest in a straight line. See how far your thigh moves before you feel a "blocked" sensation. Next, perform the same movement but allow your thigh to move out to the side and your foot to rotate inward slightly (an abducted and externally rotated position of the hip).

What did you find? Research has shown that those with retroverted hip sockets are often able to bring their knee closer to their chest with the knee angled out to the side.[2]

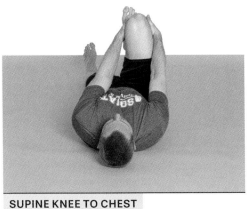

SUPINE KNEE TO CHEST

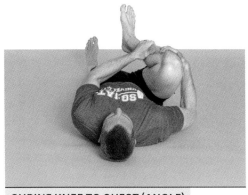

SUPINE KNEE TO CHEST (ANGLE)

This movement of bringing your knee to your chest also gives you insight into the depth of your hip socket. If you cannot bring your knee very close to your chest in either position (straight or angled away from your body) without feeling a blocked sensation in your hip, you may have a deep hip socket. Conversely, if you can bring your knee all the way to your chest without any pinching sensation (and without your lower back coming up off the ground), you likely have a shallower hip socket.

Think of the connection between your femur and hip socket like a small ball sitting on some dinnerware. If the ball (end of your femur) was sitting in a bowl, it could move around only so much before hitting the edge. But what would happen if you placed the ball on a plate? Clearly it would have more room to roll around than it would within the boundaries of a bowl. The same goes for how your femur moves within your hip socket.

HIP SOCKET DEPTH

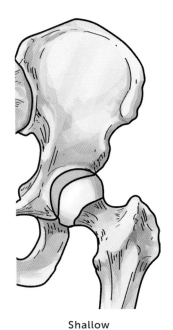

Shallow

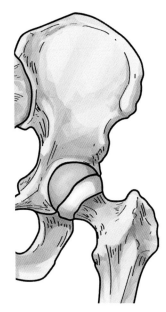

Deep

Now, the depth of your hip socket is based largely on your genetics—something you can thank or blame your parents for. For example, there is a higher rate of shallow hip sockets in people born in eastern Europe, such as Bulgaria and Poland. That is why this area of the world is found to have the highest incidence of hip dysplasia, a condition of extreme hypermobility due to a very shallow hip socket (an acetabulum shaped more like a plate).[3] Coincidentally—or perhaps not—this area of the world often produces the best weightlifters, in part because a shallow hip socket allows for more hip mobility and a deeper squat, giving a weightlifter more efficiency in the snatch and clean.

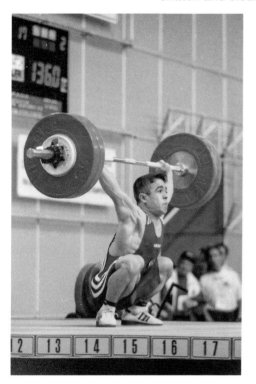

Deep receiving position in the snatch.
Halil Multu,
© Bruce Klemens

Conversely, someone with a very deep hip socket (an acetabulum shaped more like a bowl) will have a more difficult time squatting deeply. The deeper the hip socket, the less the femur can move and rotate. Research shows this anatomy to be more prevalent in western European countries, such as Scotland.[4] While this doesn't mean everyone born in Scotland has deep hip sockets and will be a poor squatter, it highlights the importance of assessing anatomy when it comes to understanding the relationship between barbell lifts and potential hip pain.

Some athletes are born with hips that make it easy for them to squat to great depths and deadlift with a wide sumo stance; others are not. Trying to make your lifting technique fit an "ideal" that is not right for your anatomy will not turn out well in the end.

Some people also have variations in the ways their femurs are shaped and connect with the pelvis. For example, some of us have femurs that are angled more forward or backward. This anatomy affects the alignment of the femur in the hip joint. A more forward-angled femur is called an anteverted hip, whereas a flatter angle gives us a retroverted hip.[5]

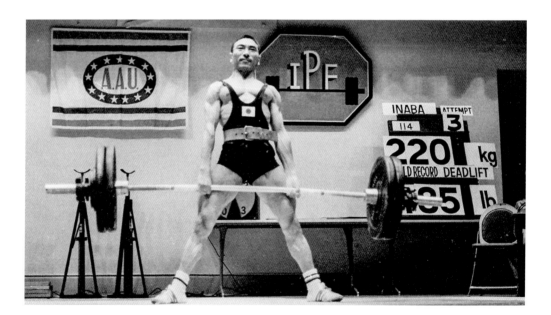

Sumo stance deadlift.
Hideaki Inaba,
© Bruce Klemens

FEMORAL ALIGNMENT

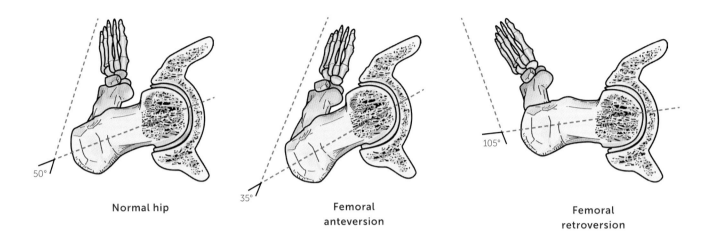

Normal hip

50°

Femoral
anteversion

35°

Femoral
retroversion

105°

If you preferred to sit in the W or "reverse tailor" position as a child, there's a good chance you have femoral anteversion. People with femoral anteversion tend to be pigeon-toed; however, there are always exceptions. To keep the toes from pointing inward, the lower leg bones (tibias) sometimes adapt and form an outward lateral twist to compensate for the inward medial twist of the femurs.

If you have the classic "duck walk," where your feet turn out excessively, you *may* have femoral retroversion. However, as before, the tibias can change shape as you grow and develop to "hide" this alignment so that you can walk with your toes pointing straight forward.

If your head is spinning, don't worry. Here's a simple way to think about hip anatomy: Someone with femoral anteversion will appear to have a *ton* of hip internal rotation (usually more than 50 degrees) and very limited hip external rotation (often less than 15 degrees) due to the way the bones of the pelvis and femur are aligned.[6] This asymmetry (excessive internal and limited external rotation) is apparent when sitting *and* when lying facedown. Meanwhile, someone with femoral retroversion will appear to have a ton of hip external rotation and very limited hip internal rotation both when sitting and when lying on their stomach.

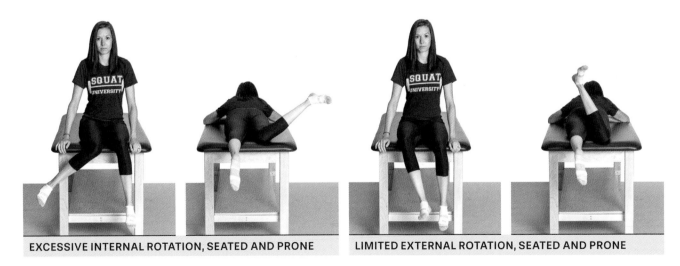

EXCESSIVE INTERNAL ROTATION, SEATED AND PRONE

LIMITED EXTERNAL ROTATION, SEATED AND PRONE

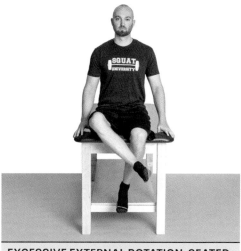

EXCESSIVE EXTERNAL ROTATION, SEATED

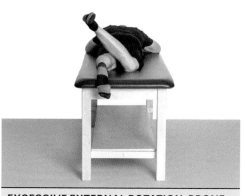

EXCESSIVE EXTERNAL ROTATION, PRONE

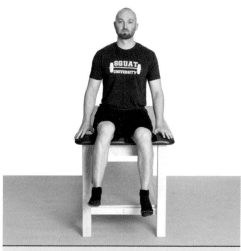

LIMITED INTERNAL ROTATION, SEATED

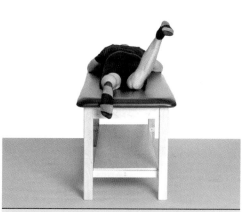

LIMITED INTERNAL ROTATION, PRONE

Forcing someone with hip anteversion to lift with a technique that requires a lot of external rotation (such as turning the toes out past 30 degrees during a sumo dead-lift) can place excessive pressure on the front of the hip joint and lead to the eventual development of pain. Similarly, forcing someone with hip retroversion to squat with a toes-forward technique (which requires a sufficient amount of hip internal rotation) will pull their femurs out of optimal alignment in the sockets and can eventually create anterior hip or groin pain. In short, having an athlete conform to a specific lifting technique without understanding their anatomy can be disastrous.

Another test that can give you insight into your hip anatomy is known as Craig's test. You'll need a friend for this screen.

Start by lying on your stomach on a bench or bed with one knee bent 90 degrees. Have a friend take their hand and feel for the notch of your femur (greater trochanter), which is located on the side of your upper thigh. With their other hand, they should rotate your lower leg toward and away from your body. As your leg moves, they'll notice the notch of the femur becoming more and less prominent against their hand. Have them stop moving your lower leg when they find this notch to be the most prominent.

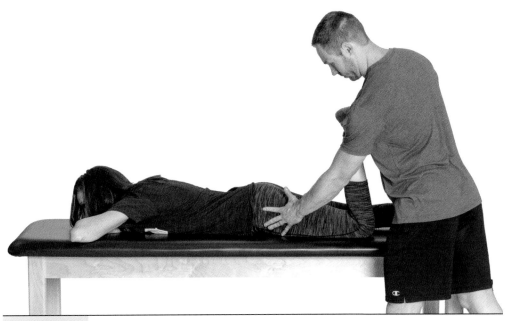

CRAIG'S TEST

"Normal" anatomy leaves the lower leg pointing only slightly away from the body (anywhere between 8 and 15 degrees from a vertical position). If your lower leg is positioned at a large angle to the side, it is a sign of an anteverted hip. If your lower leg is positioned vertically or even leaning back in toward the midline of your body, it is a sign of a retroverted hip. This method of assessing hip anatomy has been shown in research to be extremely reliable—even better than taking an X-ray.[7]

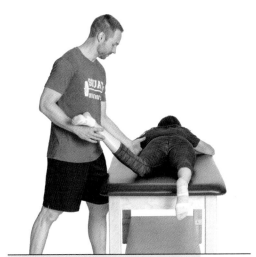

ANTEVERTED HIP
(EXCESSIVE INTERNAL ROTATION)

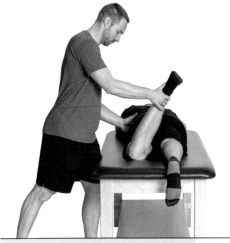

RETROVERTED HIP
(EXCESSIVE EXTERNAL ROTATION)

The results of Craig's test and the prior assessments are only small clues to understanding your hip anatomy. Don't hang your hat on what you find and dismiss the need for further screening! While you may have uncovered anteversion or retro-version, you may well have restrictions in mobility and/or flexibility that must also be addressed to find the ideal lifting technique for your body. Remember, bony anatomy gives us insight into how we move, but it does not tell the full story.

Hip Injury Anatomy 101

If in the past you decided to go the traditional medical route to address your hip pain and visited with your family practitioner or an orthopedic doctor, you likely received a diagnosis based on the particular anatomy the doctor believed was injured. Let's go over the most common diagnoses for strength athletes.

Groin Strain

Injuries to the groin can be difficult to diagnose and treat, primarily because pain can develop in this region for many reasons.[8] The anatomy in the groin region is very complex, and multiple injuries can occur at the same time and present with similar symptoms.

To simplify things, I am going to focus on an adductor strain when referring to a "groin strain." In fact, a strain (which describes small tears in the muscle fibers) in any of the adductor muscles is thought to be one of the most common forms of groin-related pain. Outside the weight room, injuries to this muscle group are most often seen in those who participate in ice hockey, a sport in which tremendous force is placed on the inner thigh muscles as they lengthen under tension during the push-off phase of skating.[9] A similar muscular action occurs during barbell lifts.

ADDUCTOR MUSCLES

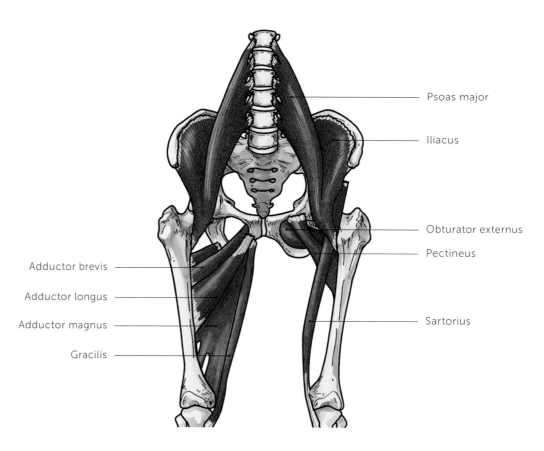

Psoas major

Iliacus

Obturator externus

Pectineus

Adductor brevis

Adductor longus

Adductor magnus

Sartorius

Gracilis

Anatomically, six muscles are considered "adductors":

- Adductor magnus, longus, and brevis
- Gracilis
- Obturator externus
- Pectineus

The adductor magnus, one of the largest muscles of the inner thigh, is the most commonly discussed of the adductor group when it comes to weight room movements, as the muscle is essential in extending the hip during the ascending phase of a squat or deadlift.[10] However, research has shown that the adductor longus, another large muscle of the inner thigh, is the most commonly injured of this group.[11]

Regardless of the specific anatomy that may be generating pain, most adductor strains cause tenderness in the upper inner thigh, close to where the muscles connect to the pubic bone.[12] Depending on the severity of the injury, it is common to see black or purple bruising in this area.

Hip Flexor Strain/Tendinopathy

When athletes have pain on the front side of the hip, they automatically label it a "hip flexor strain." However, I find that people are quick to give this diagnosis without really understanding what's going on.

HIP FLEXOR MUSCLES

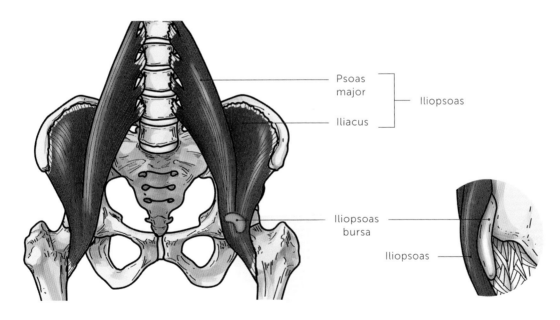

When most people say "hip flexor," they're referring to the iliopsoas. The iliopsoas is comprised of two muscles: the iliacus and psoas major. It may surprise you to learn that this is the only muscle group that directly connects the spine to the lower body. When the iliopsoas is activated, it helps flex and laterally rotate the hip or stabilize the core/pelvis and maintain posture. It can also be called upon to be a main mover in pulling the torso upward during a sit-up.

Pain can be created in this area in a few ways. The muscle group itself can be strained if placed under excessive tension. It can become excessively stiff and compress the underlying bursa sac, a fluid-filled bag that prevents friction. Its tendon can snap back and forth over a bony prominence during leg movement, creating a "popping" sensation in the front of the hip. An injury to the common hip flexor tendon (called *tendinopathy*) could even be present! While you may hear several medical diagnoses given to an injury in this area—hip flexor strain, iliopsoas syndrome, snapping hip syndrome, and so on—it is almost always due to overuse as opposed to a specific one-time tear, which is seen more often with adductor strains.[13]

However, we must not be too quick to label pain on the front side of the hip as a hip flexor strain. While pain in this region can be due to the iliopsoas muscle, it can also be generated by problems deeper in the joint itself, such as a labral tear or even a hip impingement. A proper screening process (which I will go over later) is imperative to figure out what you believe to be at fault so that you can take the right steps.

Hip Impingement (FAI)

Even if you feel pain when pushing into your hip flexor muscles, the reason for the tenderness may be coming from much deeper. A hip impingement, or femoral acetabular impingement (FAI), is one of the most common causes of hip joint–related groin pain. If the femur comes in contact with the front of the hip socket as you descend into a squat, it will cause pinching pain. If this contact happens repeatedly enough and under enough load, the tissues surrounding the joint can become irritated and generate pain.

HIP IMPINGEMENT

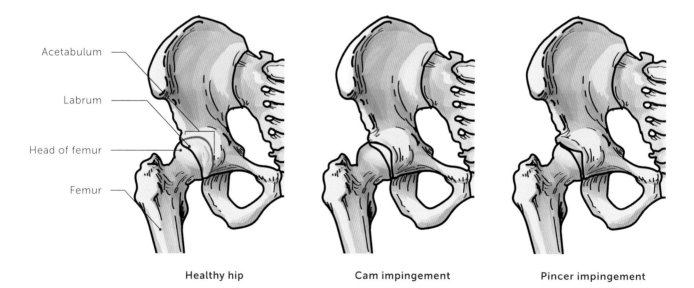

Acetabulum

Labrum

Head of femur

Femur

Healthy hip   Cam impingement   Pincer impingement

If you ignore this pain and push through your symptoms, new bone can form around the area as compensation (called a *cam* or *pincer deformity*). This excessive bone growth further narrows the available joint space, intensifies joint contact, and eventually leads to tearing of the labrum that surrounds the hip joint.

Sports Hernia

"Sports hernia" is a catchall term for several injuries that can occur around the inguinal canal, the area just above the ropelike ligament that creates the "V" in your lower abs. Despite the prevalence of this injury, the research on how to diagnose and treat a sports hernia is vague and contradictory. In fact, "sports hernia" doesn't even refer to an actual hernia, as there is no tear or deformity in the abdominal wall.[14] Technically, the term encompasses two groin injuries: inguinal disruption and athletic pubalgia, which have very similar symptoms.

Regardless of how accurate the name "sports hernia" is, it is still commonly used. The current consensus among experts in the field is that a sports hernia describes chronic pain (lasting many weeks to years) around the inner hip crease (inguinal area) or pubic region that is felt when exercising.[15]

The exact reason for sustaining a sports hernia is also unclear. Some of the possible causes are

- Excessive high-velocity cutting and twisting

- Imbalances in strength of the lower body compared to the rectus abdominus/core muscles

- A congenital abnormality (basically, your anatomy sets you up for this issue)

Diagnosing this injury is quite difficult, as there is no definitive test available. To make matters worse, many people with this injury have pain that mimics other forms of groin pain. For example, it's common to have pain that mimics a strained adductor.[16] To distinguish a sports hernia from an adductor strain, with a sports hernia, you'll sometimes notice pain when doing sit-ups, performing the Valsalva maneuver when lifting heavy (holding your breath and engaging your core/diaphragm to create intra-abdominal pressure), coughing, or sneezing.[17]

Researchers have outlined five signs that a sports hernia may be present:[18]

- Deep groin/lower abdominal pain

- Pain made worse with physical activity such as sprinting, cutting, and sit-ups; rest usually decreases pain

- Tenderness when the area around the pubic ramus (the front part of the pelvis near the inner groin) is poked

- Pain with resisted hip adduction (a test described later in this chapter)

- Pain with resisted abdominal sit-ups

This type of injury should be suspected if an athlete has complained of groin pain for months on end that does not get better with rest or traditional corrective exercises. If this is the case for you or someone you know, I highly recommend that you see an orthopedic specialist for a thorough examination.

Greater Trochanteric Bursitis/ Glute Medius Strain

If you have pain in the side(s) of your hip, chances are you've been given a diagnosis of greater trochanteric bursitis or glute medius strain. An injury to this area is commonly associated with a slow onset of dull, achy pain centered over the greater trochanter, the most prominent bone of the upper lateral thigh. You can typically pinpoint a painful area by pushing just under this bone.

GREATER TROCHANTER WITH GLUTE MEDIUS

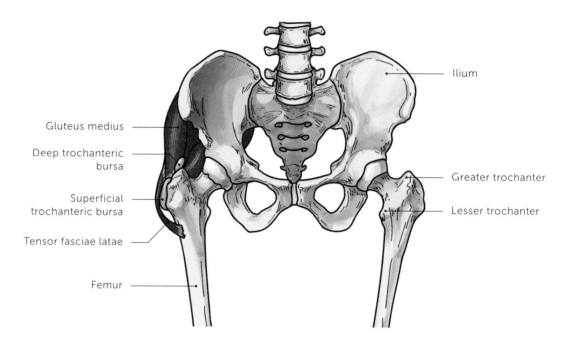

Gluteus medius

Deep trochanteric bursa

Superficial trochanteric bursa

Tensor fasciae latae

Femur

Ilium

Greater trochanter

Lesser trochanter

Lateral hip pain may present when lifting but is often most severe at night when trying to sleep on the affected hip.[19] Research shows that women, people with a history of low back pain, and individuals over the age of 40 are more likely to develop this kind of injury.[20]

Traditionally, many in the medical field have labeled this injury as trochanteric bursitis. *Bursitis* refers to inflammation of a bursa sac, a small fluid-filled "bumper pad" that provides cushioning and limits friction between bones and the muscles/ tissues that cover them. However, researchers have found that only a small proportion of lateral hip pain is due to an inflamed bursa sac—around 8 percent of cases, according to a 2001 study.[21] Nowadays, many believe that lateral hip pain is more often due to an overuse tendon injury of the two small muscles in the lateral hip, the gluteus minimus and medius; it is therefore referred to as a tendinopathy.[22]

Unfortunately, it's difficult for even the most knowledgeable medical practitioners to tell the difference between trochanteric bursitis and glute tendinopathy. In fact, these two problems can occur at the same time and are likely caused by the same issue![23] For this reason, you may see lateral hip pain described as greater trochanteric pain syndrome, or GTPS.[24]

Let's quickly go over the anatomy of the lateral hip to help you better understand how this injury occurs. The glute medius is a large fan-shaped muscle that runs from the lateral part of your pelvis (iliac crest) and connects with a single tendon to your femur.[25] The glute minimus is a smaller muscle that fits right behind the glute medius and also attaches to the femur.

In most anatomy classes, students are taught that these two muscles are the main abductors of the hip and that when activated, the medius/minimus muscles move the thigh away from the midline of the body. However, this isn't 100 percent accurate. It originated from research that dates back to the mid-1900s in which scientists used simplistic mathematical models to study how the body works.[26] These models fail to take into account the unique size, shape, and action of the lateral glute muscles.

LATERAL HIP ANATOMY

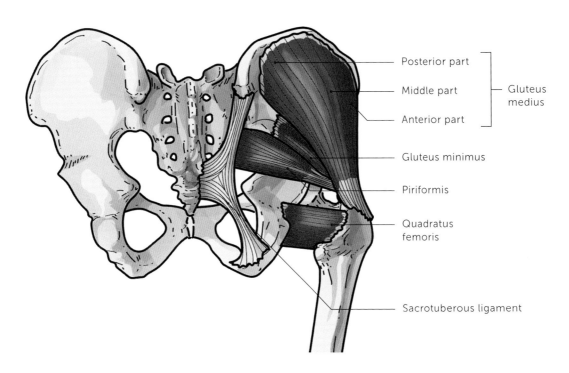

- Posterior part
- Middle part — Gluteus medius
- Anterior part
- Gluteus minimus
- Piriformis
- Quadratus femoris
- Sacrotuberous ligament

For example, while many people think the glute medius is one big muscle, research shows that it is composed of three distinct parts with unique actions.[27] The posterior muscle fibers act with the entire glute minimus muscle to pull the femur into the hip socket (acetabulum) to help stabilize the hip joint, basically keeping the ball in the middle of the socket. The middle and anterior portions work together to initiate lateral leg movement (abduction), which is then completed by the tensor fasciae latae (TFL). Along with beginning any lateral leg movement, the anterior fibers of the glute medius can create or limit pelvis rotation.

However, when you're on your feet, these muscles take on a slightly different role. When you run, lunge, or squat, the glute medius and minimus act together to steady the hip joint (limiting knee cave) and keep the pelvis from tipping, rotating, or shifting from side to side. This allows the larger muscles around the hip (TFL, glute max, hip flexors, hamstrings, and so on) to create movement. For this reason, the glute medius/minimus muscles are similar in function to the rotator cuff muscles of the shoulder. Both muscle groups act as stabilizers for their respective joints.

Contrary to what you may have learned in anatomy class, your lateral glute muscles are more of a movement stabilizer than a prime mover of the lower body. This understanding helps guide us in creating more efficient training and better corrective exercises for the hip joint.

As I explained earlier, most people with lateral hip pain have a gluteal tendinopathy injury. If you skip ahead to the Knee Pain chapter, specifically the section on patellar and quad tendinopathy (see pages 177 to 183), I explain there that tendon injuries occur due to relative overuse or overload of these tissues. They can occur in an untrained individual who starts a high-intensity program or even in an elite athlete who deconditions their body while on vacation and then jumps right back into "normal" training. If the body is not allowed to recover after a rapid increase in the intensity and/or frequency of training, the tendon becomes "reactive," and the injury process begins.

Gluteal tendinopathy occurs due to two main types of overloading: excessive stretching of the tendon fibers (much like stretching a rubber band) and/or too much compressive force (from the tendon being smashed into the tissues/bone underneath). These forces, called *tensile* and *transverse loads,* respectively, likely occur at the same time and reduce the overall strength of the tendons, making them susceptible to injury.[28]

One factor that can lead to overloaded tendons is individual anatomy. Some researchers believe that a wider-set and/or more angled alignment of the pelvis (often seen in women) can lead to greater compressive forces on the tendons of the lateral glute muscles and predispose them to injury.[29]

CHANGES IN GLUTE MEDIUS ANGLE OF PULL IN A WIDER-SET PELVIS

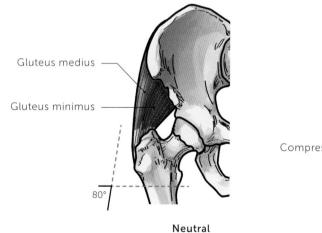

Gluteus medius

Gluteus minimus

80°

Neutral

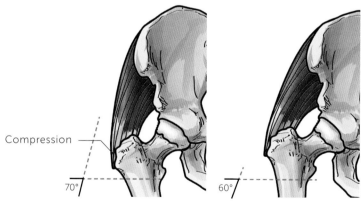

Lateral pelvic shift resulting in increased hip adduction

Compression

70°

60°

Wide

The second most common factor is movement or positional faults. I'll use the common technique fault of the hip shift on the squat as an example. If someone shifts to the right side on the way up from a squat, their right thigh shifts toward the midline of their body (the movement of hip adduction). This causes the right-side IT band to wrap more firmly around the lateral thigh in an effort to keep the pelvis stable, which compresses the underlying glute tendons and the associated bursae against the femur.[30]

Basically, anytime the thigh is pulled in toward the midline of the body (either with a hip shift or with the dreaded knee cave), the glute medius and minimus tendons are placed in poor positions and are exposed to a ton of compressive and tensile forces that can lead to injury.

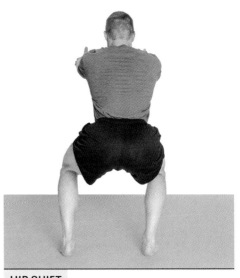

HIP SHIFT

Piriformis Syndrome

Let's turn our attention to the back side of the body. When it comes to pain deep in the glutes, the most common diagnosis is piriformis syndrome.

The piriformis is a small muscle that lies deep inside the hip underneath the larger glute muscles (glute max and medius). It is known mainly for lateral hip rotation. It also helps extend the thigh. The piriformis is responsible for preventing knee cave during squats. It can also function as a portion of the pelvic floor, helps stabilize the pelvis, and assists in controlling for anterior pelvic tilt.[31]

PIRIFORMIS MUSCLE

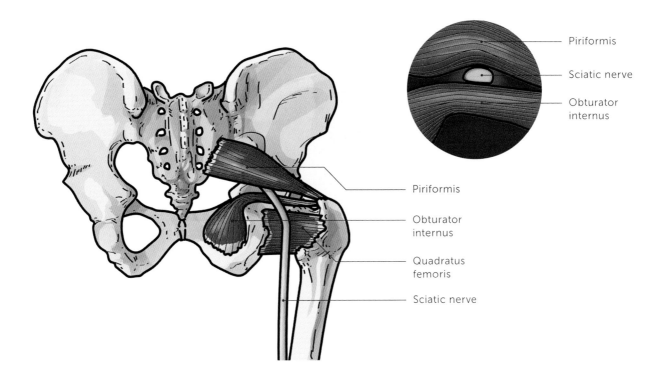

Piriformis

Sciatic nerve

Obturator internus

Piriformis

Obturator internus

Quadratus femoris

Sciatic nerve

Piriformis syndrome occurs when the piriformis muscle is compressed, which irritates the sciatic nerve. The sciatic nerve typically runs underneath the piriformis. For about 12 percent of the population, the nerve runs through the actual piriformis muscle.[32] This nerve runs from the low back (lumbar spine) down your thigh and extends to your feet. When irritated, it can cause pain deep in your glutes as well as symptoms like numbness and tingling that shoots down the back of your leg.

Historically, piriformis syndrome was thought to be caused by a muscle spasm or an excessively tight piriformis muscle. When shortened or in spasm, the piriformis can compress the sciatic nerve, creating pain that radiates down the leg. However, some experts now believe that this injury can also be caused when the piriformis is excessively stretched or elongated.[33]

With a lengthened piriformis, repetitive movements of the hip (such as knee collapse when squatting or lifting with an excessive anterior pelvic tilt) can strain the muscle and cause friction on the nearby sciatic nerve, resulting in inflammation and pain.[34]

Therefore, we actually have two possible causes of piriformis syndrome—long or short piriformis—that require two drastically different treatments to fix! The difficult part is distinguishing between the two, as they share some similar symptoms:

- **Short piriformis syndrome** is associated with pain when sitting for prolonged periods and limited hip internal rotation. This injury often responds well to stretching and soft tissue mobilization, while strengthening in a shortened muscular position (such as a side-lying clamshell) can re-create symptoms.

- **Long piriformis syndrome** is associated with pain that decreases with sitting and excessive internal rotation compared to the nonpainful hip. This injury is often due to poor technique (knee collapse and/or anterior pelvic tilt) when lifting and therefore responds well to strengthening and movement re-education.

I'll discuss later how to go about screening your body to understand which of these two syndromes you may be dealing with.

Hamstring Tendinopathy

Another common injury that can create pain deep in the glutes is a proximal hamstring tendinopathy. On the back side of the body under the larger glute max, the hamstring muscles all share a common tendon insertion point on a bony point of the pelvis called the *ischial tuberosity*. While a hamstring strain is common in sports such as soccer, hockey, and track and field, an injury to the tendon (tendinopathy) is more common in the strength sports of powerlifting, weightlifting, and CrossFit.

When the hip is flexed to a great degree, the hamstring tendon is tensioned and compressed against the bony pelvis. If this compression occurs often enough and with enough force, the tendon can become overloaded, leading to pain.[35]

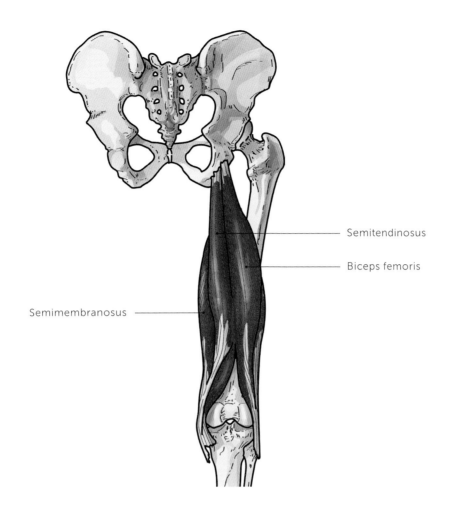

Semitendinosus

Biceps femoris

Semimembranosus

A tendinopathy injury can be sparked in a few ways. The first is acute overload in one specific workout or a group of training sessions that were much more intense than normal. In this scenario, the tendon experiences much higher load than it can currently tolerate. Tendinopathy can also occur upon returning to relatively normal training after taking an extended break (such as a weeklong vacation or time away to recover from a different injury). In this scenario, the time away from the gym leads to an adaptive lowering of the tendon's load capacity. Jumping quickly back into "normal training" causes a similar overload and sparks the exaggerated cellular response (called *reactive tendinopathy*).

For example, suddenly introducing high-volume sprinting, squatting, or hurdle exercises into an athlete's training may result in overload of a hamstring tendon and spark the injury process.[36] Because pain is generated when the tendon is loaded and compressed, this injury often brings out pain in a deep squat or when sitting on a hard surface, but rarely during activities like slow walking on a level surface, standing, or lying down. This injury does *not* create pain that radiates down the thigh (which would be seen with sciatic nerve irritation from the piriformis or an injury to the low back, such as a herniated disc).

Hamstring Strain

We always seem to be hearing about a professional football or soccer player with a pulled hammy on ESPN. Research shows that depending on the sport, hamstring strains account for 8 to 25 percent of all reported injuries.[37]

If you've ever had this injury, you know it can be stubborn. In fact, once you've had one hamstring strain, your chance of sustaining another is very high.[38] Research has shown that athletes are between two and six times more likely to suffer a recurrent strain within eight weeks of the first.[39] Strength and conditioning coach Eric Cressey compares the hamstring strain to an unpredictable mother-in-law: "Just when you think you've finally won her over, she brings you back down to Earth and reminds you how much more she liked your wife's old boyfriend."[40]

While hamstring strains are not nearly as prevalent in barbell training and competitive sports like weightlifting, powerlifting, and CrossFit as they are in football, soccer, and track and field, they still occur and require attention.

Most experts agree that hamstring strains happen while sprinting. If you want to get into the science, the muscle tear often occurs at the end of the swing phase of the running cycle, when you move or "swing" the leg from behind your body to the front.[41] During this time, the action of the hamstring is rapidly transitioning from slowing the forward-moving knee to preparing the body to propel itself forward as soon as the foot hits the ground. This quick change from an eccentric action (muscle lengthening under tension) to a concentric action (muscle shortening under tension) is thought to be when the muscle is most susceptible to injury. During this terminal swing phase, the hamstring lengthens quite a bit while experiencing a large amount of force.

As soon as this injury occurs, you'll know. It feels like a sharp pain in one specific part of the back of your thigh. You'll instantly have pinpoint tenderness and pain, usually where the muscle meets the tendon (the thicker ropelike part of your muscle).

Hamstring strains are graded into three degrees:

- **First degree:** Only a few muscle or tendon fibers are torn. There may be a small amount of swelling and discomfort. This is usually associated with minimal strength loss, and you'll likely be able to walk directly after the injury. Sprinting, however, will elicit pain.

- **Second degree:** A partial tear of the fibers. There will be a significant loss of strength and a good amount of pain. You'll likely feel some pain when walking.

- **Third degree:** A compete rupture of the muscle/tendon. This is associated with a huge loss of muscle function, often an inability to walk due to pain, and major bruising on the back of the thigh.

The five main risk factors people associate with hamstring strains are flexibility, strength, age, sport of choice, and previous history of the injury. Let's quickly cover these factors and whether or not each one has legitimacy:

- **Hamstring flexibility:** Hamstring flexibility has *not* been shown in research to be a significant risk factor for developing a muscle strain. Therefore, a program of endless hamstring stretches is unlikely to cut down your chances of sustaining this injury. However, there is evidence that the flexibility of your quad muscles can play a role.

- **Hamstring strength:** Isolated strength of the hamstrings is another factor that doesn't have a ton of research behind it. Some researchers say that weak hamstrings or muscle strength imbalances (hamstrings versus quads) can play a role. The thinking is that if the quads are extremely strong compared to the hamstrings, there will be a ton of force driving the leg forward during the swing phase of the running cycle, which would place increased demand on the relatively weak hamstrings to decelerate the fast-moving leg and possibly lead to injury. Unfortunately, there aren't many studies to back this up. It's never a bad idea to strengthen the hamstrings, though; most athletes overtrain their quads and have underdeveloped glutes/hamstrings. Overall, hamstring strength is a factor about which people have a lot of conflicting opinions.[42]

- **Age:** Age has been shown to be a significant risk factor for developing a hamstring strain.[43] Research has shown that athletes over the age of 25 are between 2.8 and 4.4 times more likely to suffer this injury.[44] Basically, the older you are, the higher your odds.

- **Sports involving sprinting:** As mentioned earlier, research has shown that an overwhelming majority of hamstring strains occur while running.[45] This is a big reason why athletes participating in the classic barbell sports of weight-lifting and powerlifting rarely sustain this injury. However, given the popularity of CrossFit, hamstring strains are not uncommon among CrossFitters due to the sprinting involved in training sessions and competition.

- **Prior hamstring strain:** As with most injuries, athletes with a previous hamstring strain have been shown to be between two and six times more likely to suffer another one in the future.[46] This is by far the biggest risk factor.

How to Screen Your Hip Pain

By now, you know that a *ton* of different injuries can occur at the hip. While the previous section was designed to help you understand the problems that can arise in this area, diagnosing the specific anatomical structure or tissue that is causing hip pain is no easy task. Doing so often requires expert assessment skills and expensive scans. To make matters even more difficult, it is not uncommon for more than one structure to be generating pain, such as a hip flexor tendinopathy and an irritated underlying bursa sac.

Instead of trying to diagnose the specific anatomy of the hip that may be injured, we need to uncover the movement problem associated with the pain. Identifying and classifying an injury by the specific motion or movement that generates symptoms rather than the specific anatomical tissue that is believed to be at fault helps us avoid tunnel vision in treatment by placing the emphasis on fixing problematic *movement*.

The framework for this theory has been called the *kinesiopathologic model*, or KPM.[47] This movement model approach does not dismiss or assume a specific anatomical problem as the cause of pain but instead treats any particular finding as a "piece of the pie" in the decision-making process. Treat the person, not the injury.

Here's a brief example of this concept at work. Brandon is a 36-year-old power-lifter who was referred to physical therapy with a diagnosis that read "right hip flexor strain." The hip flexor was the specific anatomical site of pain that the orthopedic doctor wanted to fix. Our examination uncovered poor glute coordination and strength along with a tight/stiff TFL muscle (the muscle that lies just lateral to the hip flexors on the front side of the hip). After performing soft tissue mobilization to the TFL with a foam roller along with some slow-tempo bodyweight squats with a resistance band around his knees to activate his glutes, he was able to squat and deadlift without pain.

Brandon did have pain in the front of his hip where his hip flexors are located. However, the *cause* of his pain was not a faulty hip flexor! Instead, his pain was due to a movement issue associated with a stiff TFL and weak/poorly coordinated glutes. These factors led to an overload of the hip flexor muscles and the eventual development of pain. For this reason, no amount of hip flexor stretching or other treatments (like dry needling or electrical stimulation) directed to the site of pain would have truly fixed the problem.

As you go through the screening process outlined in the next portion of the chapter, I want you to think about which of the following categories best fits your hip pain:

- Limited mobility/flexibility
- Strength imbalance/weakness
- Poor movement/technique

It could be a combination of problems. Each test can give you clues on how to piece together a plan of action to fix your injury.

Movement Screening

Every evaluation I perform on an athlete in pain starts with assessing the athlete's movement. I want you to begin by grabbing a friend or videorecording yourself performing the following tests so you can analyze how you're moving. You're going to begin by performing a squat.

In your normal squat stance, do a slow squat to full depth and hold the bottom position for a few seconds. Slowly return to the start position and then perform five more repetitions. What did you notice? Did you feel any pain? If so, write down which part of the squat brought out the pain and where the pain was located.

For example, an athlete dealing with a hip impingement may not report pain until they get into the bottom of a deep squat. Not until the athlete moves into a deep flexed position does the femur run into the front of the hip socket, generating pain. An issue like this could be due to a flexibility problem in the surrounding muscles of the joint, poor joint mobility, or even a strength imbalance. (You'll find more on how to screen for these problems soon.)

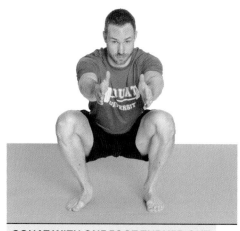

SQUAT WITH ONE FOOT TURNED OUT

As you analyze your squat, also notice the position of your feet. Is one foot angled outward more than the other? If you try to keep your feet firmly planted, does one foot spin out to the side as you descend? Do your hips shift to one side or the other as you move into a deep squat? These movement problems are clues to possible weaknesses/flexibility limitations.

If you passed the bodyweight squat test easily, let's make things a little more challenging. Videorecord yourself lifting, taking footage from different angles for the most efficient assessment. Start with light weight, but make sure to evaluate how you're moving when lifting heavy as well. Load is an incredible teacher, and it can expose many movement problems commonly missed in a traditional bodyweight-only screen.

Did you notice any movement problems after adding weight to the equation? The more load is placed on the body, the clearer and more obvious movement problems become.

Next, stand on one foot and try to balance for 30 seconds. Did you notice any pain? For some people, standing on one leg for an extended period re-creates their lateral hip pain (such as greater trochanteric bursitis or glute medius tendinopathy).[48] To maintain balance in a single-leg stance, your stance leg naturally shifts slightly inward toward the midline of your body (a motion called *adduction*). This motion can compress the lateral hip tissues, re-creating pain.

Lastly, perform a single-leg squat, going as deep as you can without falling over or using anything to assist your balance. What happened? If you found it difficult to balance and squat on one leg without the knee of your stance leg caving in and your hip shifting, you've uncovered a problem in stability that you may not have noticed in your double-leg squat! This movement problem is often due to weak/poorly coordinated lateral hip muscles (such as the glute medius).

Mobility Assessment

Restrictions in mobility limit optimal movement. While significant differences from side to side (such as limited hip internal rotation on the right hip compared to the left) are a common adaptation in certain sports, such as baseball, they can be very problematic for strength athletes. When you squat, deadlift, press, or lift an Atlas Stone from the ground, you want to have symmetrical mobility in your lower body. Significant asymmetries in mobility can both be a cause and an effect of injury. Try some of the following tests to see if you may be dealing with a mobility restriction.

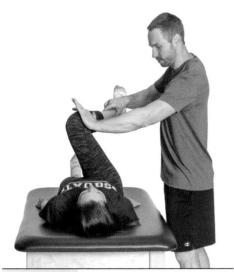

FADIR TEST

Lie on your back, pull your knees together, and bring them toward your chest. Completely relax your lower body during this motion. What did you notice?

Those who have hip impingement often experience pain in the front of the hip when the hip is fully flexed (knee to chest). This is because the femur is moving incorrectly in the hip socket, smashing into the front side of the capsule and creating inflammation in the tissues surrounding the joint.

If you have a friend available, try the FADIR test, which stands for flexion-adduction-internal rotation.[49] Start by lying on your back. Have your friend push your thigh toward your chest while pushing your knee toward your opposite shoulder and pulling your foot away from the midline of your body. This is another common test to determine whether someone has a hip impingement due to faulty joint issues.

If you noticed a pinching pain in the front of your hip with either of these tests, try the banded joint mobilizations discussed later in this chapter. After performing them, immediately retest using this screen and see if you notice a difference. This test-retest method is a simple tool that you can use to ensure you're performing corrective exercises that are efficient and effective for your body.

Make sure to continue along with the rest of the lower body screens. Pain in the front of the hip can occur by itself or at the same time as a hip flexor tendinopathy/bursitis. This means other movement problems (such as a weak hip flexor, excessively stiff TFL, and/or weak glutes) may also be contributing to your pain. If you skip ahead and perform only banded joint mobilizations without uncovering all of your weak links, you may not fully resolve your pain!

Next, you're going to perform the FABER test, which stands for flexion-abduction-external rotation.[50] Again, start by lying on your back. Cross one leg over the other and rest your ankle just above your opposite-side knee. Relax your body and allow your knee to drop slowly toward the ground. Make sure to keep your pelvis level as you do; don't let your opposite hip rise as your knee drops. Test both sides and see what you find.

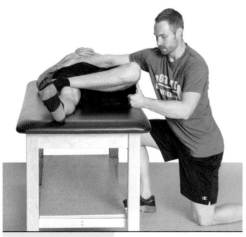

FABER TEST: GOOD

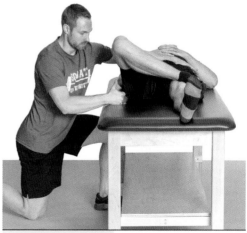

FABER TEST: POOR

Your knee should drop to a width of two fists from the floor. If you found a big asymmetry or if one side was painful, consider it a positive test. If you tested positive, you probably have a difficult time extending or externally rotating your hip. This mobility issue could be due to restricted joint mechanics (something that requires mobility exercises like the assisted hip airplane to correct; see page 151).

Next, you're going to assess hip internal rotation. While lying on your back, have a friend grab your leg, bend your knee, and lift your thigh to a 60-degree angle to the ground. From this position, rotate your lower leg away from the midline of your body to assess the amount of medial or internal rotation you have. Perform the same movement on both legs.

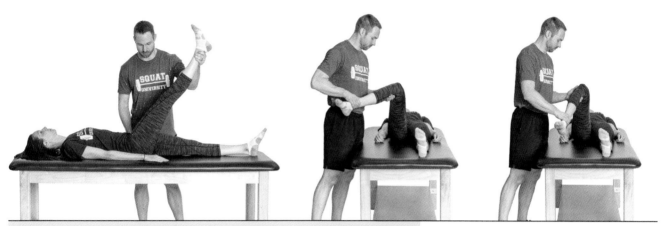

HIP INTERNAL ROTATION AT 60-DEGREE HIP ELEVATION: GOOD AND POOR

Did you find limited internal rotation on one leg? This restriction could be due to a problem at the joint or to limited muscular flexibility (such as the piriformis muscle). If your pain was located on the front or side of the hip, chances are your restriction is due to the way your femur is moving in the hip joint. I recommend trying the banded joint mobilizations and the assisted hip airplane presented later in the chapter.

If your pain was on the back of your hip (deep in your glute), however, the results of this test can help you differentiate between forms of injury to the piriformis muscle. One of the easiest ways to differentiate between short and long piriformis syndrome is to evaluate the amount of rotation you have at the hip. If you have short piriformis syndrome, you will show less internal rotation on the painful side. At this angle of the thigh (around 60 degrees of hip elevation), the piriformis performs the movement of external rotation. If it is short or in spasm, it won't allow your leg to move internally. If you have long piriformis syndrome, you will show excessive internal rotation on the painful side. This is because the piriformis has become elongated due to the excessive strain placed on it while you move, usually as a result of allowing your knee to cave in during squatting.

In the past, one of the most common treatments for piriformis syndrome was to stretch the muscle. However, we now know that this treatment isn't appropriate for everyone! You should stretch your piriformis only if you have *short* piriformis syndrome. Stretching a muscle that is already lengthened would only exacerbate the injury. I'll talk about other forms of treatment for this problem later in the chapter.

Flexibility Assessment

Many hip injuries can be caused not only by joint capsule restrictions but also by stiffness in the surrounding muscles on the front of the thigh, like the TFL. This muscle has a tendency to become overused and stiff. A flexibility screen that can help you assess the length of these muscles is the modified Thomas Test.[51]

Stand at the end of a bench or bed, with your hips in contact with the edge. As you gently fall backward onto the bench, grab both knees and pull them toward your chest. While lying on your back, allow one leg at a time to relax completely and drop toward the bench.

In what position did your body end up? Having a friend take a photo or video of your end position can be extremely helpful. After you screen one leg, perform the same test on the other side and see what you find. Was there a difference from side to side?

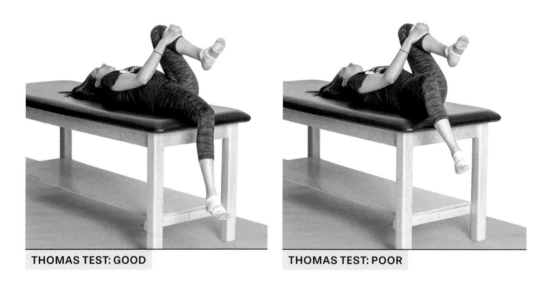

THOMAS TEST: GOOD　　　**THOMAS TEST: POOR**

If your free leg was unable to come to rest completely on the bench in a straight line with the rest of your body and instead wanted to hang out to the side slightly, your TFL muscle is stiff/short. If your knee was unable to hang at a 90-degree angle, your rectus femoris (one of your quad muscles) is stiff/short. If you found either of these problems, you'll need to do soft tissue mobilization of these muscles with a foam roller or small ball and/or stretch. I'll go over these exercises later in the chapter.

Strength and Load Assessments

Every time you perform a squat, climb a staircase, or jump from a small height, a force called *load* is placed upon your body. Depending on how you've trained over the years, every muscle and tendon in your body has a set point of load tolerance. If a particular day of training or a longer period of training exceeds this tolerance level, injury can occur and pain can set in. Load tolerance testing allows you to get an idea of how your body is tolerating these forces.

If you have pain in the front of your hip, try this test. Sit on the edge of a bench and raise your thigh a few inches. Do you feel pain? If not, attempt to hold this position while a friend tries to push your knee back down toward the bench. What did you notice?

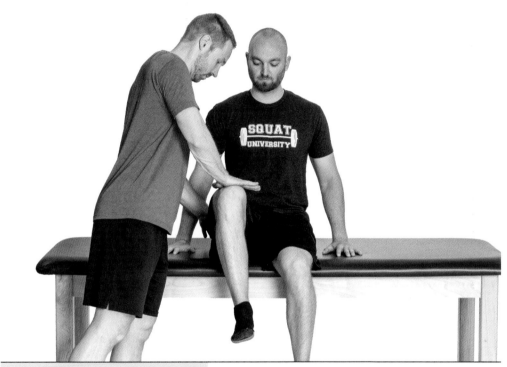

HIP FLEXION MANUAL MUSCLE TEST

Those who are dealing with a hip flexor injury (such as iliopsoas tendinopathy) often experience pain during this test. The forceful push on your thigh places excessive load on the injured tissue. If you fall into this group, the last thing you want to do at this time is stretch your hip flexors. Instead, you want to start hip flexor isometrics as a part of your rehab plan—which I'll address later.

An injury to the adductor muscle/tendon often creates pain with the resisted adductor test. To perform this test, start by lying on your side. Straighten your bottom leg and lift it about 12 inches. Hold this position and try to keep the leg from moving as a friend attempts to push it down by applying force with their hand around your ankle.[52] If this added force reproduces your pain, one of your first steps will be adductor isometrics to gradually improve load tolerance in this part of your body.

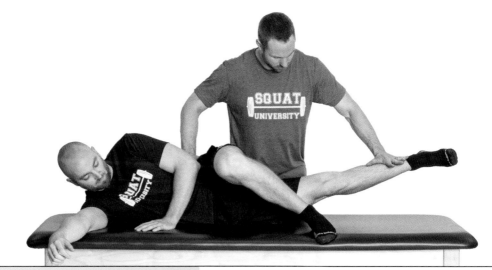

ADDUCTOR MANUAL MUSCLE TEST

If an athlete has lateral hip pain, I like to use the external derotation test to determine if the issue is a glute medius tendinopathy. Lie on your back and raise one thigh to 90 degrees. Have a friend externally rotate your hip by pushing your foot toward the midline of your body. (Don't push the leg too far into this position; doing so may create pain.) Next, try to rotate your lower leg back to a straight position as your friend applies light resistance to the outside of your foot. This test is positive if this motion (resisted external rotation) re-creates pain in your lateral hip.[53]

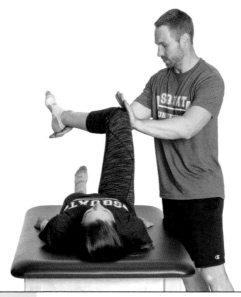

EXTERNAL DEROTATION TEST

Lastly, you will perform a single-leg bridge test. The goal is twofold. First, you want to assess the load tolerance of your hamstrings. Start by performing a single-leg bridge with your foot elevated on a bench or box and your knee bent to 90 degrees. Hold your hips in the air for 10 seconds and notice if this movement brings out any pain.

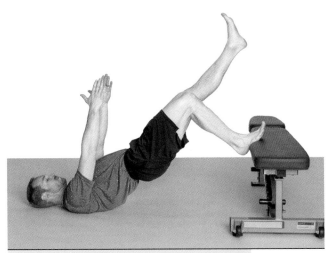

SINGLE-LEG BRIDGE TEST, FOOT ELEVATED

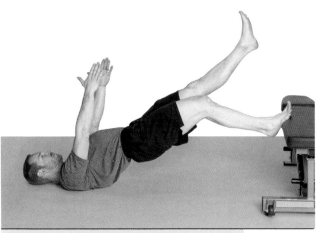

SINGLE-LEG BRIDGE TEST, FOOT ELEVATED, KNEE STRAIGHTER

If the single-leg bridge reproduced pain in the back of your hips (where the hamstrings attach), perform the same test with your knee a little more extended but not fully straight. Did this position make the pain worse? Straightening the knee slightly elongates the hamstring muscles and increases the load placed on the tendon.[54] If you felt pain, you are potentially dealing with a hamstring tendinopathy. The intensity and/or volume of your recent training has exceeded the strength of your tendon (your load tolerance level) and sparked this injury. Hamstring isometrics and bent-knee bridges will be a part of your early rehab plan, followed by single-leg RDLs (Romanian deadlifts).

The second reason I use the single-leg bridge test is to look for the level of glute involvement from side to side. As you perform the bridge and hold your hips in the air for 10 seconds, I want you to feel for which muscles are working hard to keep you up. I often find that those who have a hip injury fail the single-leg bridge and have a hard time activating their glutes. If this is you, performing exercises that improve the strength and coordination of the glute max will be key to a successful rehab plan.

Looking Outside the Hip

As I mentioned at the start of this chapter, hip pain is sometimes created by a problem in the low back. For this reason, I highly recommend going through the testing portion of the Back Pain chapter as well to ensure that you're uncovering all of the weak links that could be contributing to your hip pain.

When Is It Time to See a Doctor?

If you have any of the following symptoms, you should seek help from a medical professional:

- Catching, locking, or clicking in your hip
- Shooting pain down your thigh
- A sensation of your leg giving out

These symptoms may be indicative of a neurological issue or a serious hip issue (labral tear). Also, if your symptoms are associated with any type of bladder or bowel problem, it is important to seek medical attention.

The Rebuilding Process

Now that you have made your way through the screening process, you should have a better understanding for the "weak links" associated with your pain/injury. With this newfound knowledge, you can craft a treatment plan targeted specifically at addressing each problem area.

Soft Tissue Mobilization: Foam Rolling

If you failed the modified Thomas test (see page 144) due to a stiff TFL/rectus femoris, your first go-to should be soft tissue mobilization. A foam roller or even a small ball can decrease tension in stiff muscles and release myofascial trigger points that limit flexibility and cause pain.[55]

Lie on your stomach and position the foam roller or ball on the front of your hip. Putting pressure on this area is often a little painful. Slowly roll around until you find the tender area of muscle. Apply direct pressure for one to two minutes before slowly moving forward and back over this area in a wavelike motion.

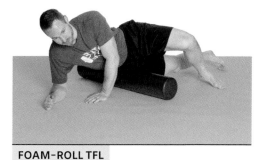

FOAM-ROLL TFL

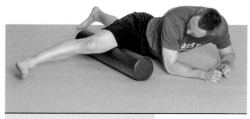

FOAM-ROLL ADDUCTORS

Mobilizing the tissues of the inner thigh (adductors) can be another great way to relieve pain and promote healing of an injured groin. Lie on your stomach with your injured leg positioned as close to 90 degrees to your torso as possible. Place the foam roller close to your groin, running perpendicular to your injured thigh. Roll slowly on this section of your thigh for two minutes, pausing for a few seconds on areas of tenderness when you find them. If you can't tolerate a hard form roller, you can switch to a softer roller or hold off for now.

If you found yourself to have a shortened piriformis with flexibility testing, soft tissue work with a small ball works great. Sustained pressure to this short or spasmed muscle can help it relax and decrease tension. Cross one leg over the other to help expose the piriformis muscle. Place the ball in the middle of your glute max muscle and roll slowly on it until you find a painful spot. Sit on the tender area for a minute before rolling off. If this treatment is right for your body, you should notice a decrease in symptoms after standing back up.

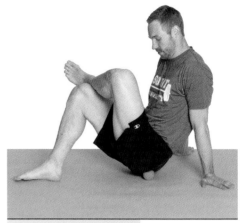

BALL INTO PIRIFORMIS

Joint Mobility

After performing soft tissue mobilization, you want to clear up any joint restrictions that may be hindering your mobility and creating hip pain.

Banded Joint Mobilizations

The first exercise that I want to discuss is the lateral banded joint mobilization.[56] The goal is to address restrictions in the lateral and posterior portions of the hip capsule fibers.

As shown in the photos on the next page, place a long resistance band around your thigh, getting it as high as you can toward your hip. Put a ton of pressure on the band as you assume a kneeling lunge with the hip you want to work on in the forward position. Once in the lunge, use your hand to pull your forward knee across your body and push it back to the start position.

This movement, along with the pull from the band, will help stretch the lateral and posterior fibers that surround the hip. If the band is pulling hard enough, the inward knee movement should not bring out any pinching pain in the front of your hip. Instead, it will bring out a light stretch to the side of your hip.

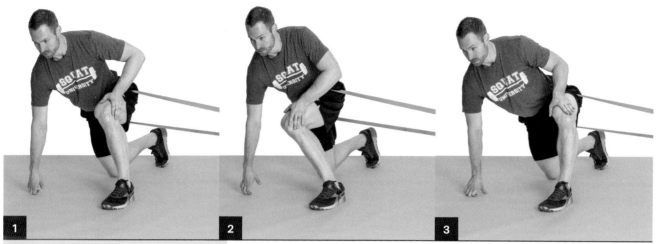

LATERAL BANDED JOINT MOBILIZATION

Next, you can perform a mobilization in an all-fours (quadruped) position. With the band still around your upper thigh and your hips flexed to around 90 degrees, rock your hips back and forth, toward and away from the pull of the band. This posterior–lateral motion will bring out a stretch to the back and side of your hip. Hold each part of the rocking motion for about five seconds before returning to the start position.

If you need to work on improving internal rotation motion, kick your foot out to the side slightly. In this position, you can also externally rotate your hip by moving your foot toward your stomach. This may increase the stretch to the lateral hip.

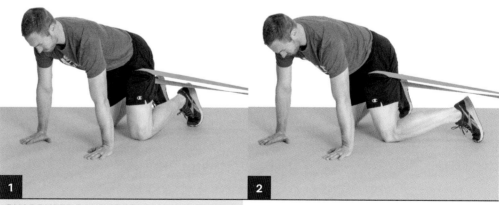

QUADRUPED BANDED JOINT MOBILIZATION

Assisted Hip Airplane/Tippy Bird

Another great exercise that helps improve full joint mobility is the assisted hip airplane, also known as the "tippy bird." If you failed the FADIR or FABER test (see page 142), I recommend trying this exercise and then retesting your mobility afterward.

Assume a single-leg stance. Lock your rib cage down by bracing your core. With your hands in front of you holding onto a rig or racked barbell for balance, rotate your torso forward over your stance leg while kicking your back leg behind you. Keep your trail leg completely straight and your stance-leg knee locked in a slightly bent position. Imagine that your body is a seesaw. This first part of the movement mimics a single-leg RDL.

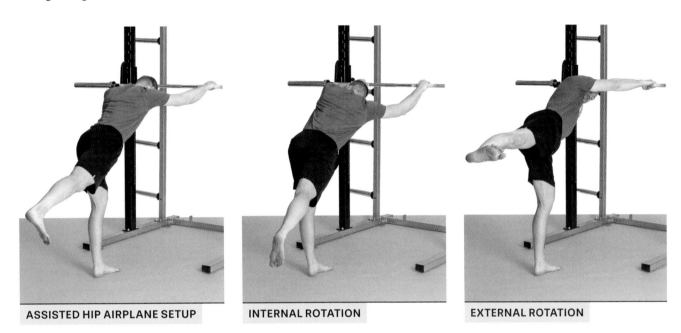

ASSISTED HIP AIRPLANE SETUP   INTERNAL ROTATION   EXTERNAL ROTATION

When your torso is parallel to the floor, rotate your pelvis as far up toward the sky as possible. This motion of hip external rotation may bring out a slight stretching sensation deep in your hip joint. Go as far as you can and hold for five seconds before rotating in the opposite direction. Drop your pelvis as far toward your stance leg as you can. This motion of hip internal rotation may bring out a slight stretch in the lateral hip muscles of your stance leg. Again, hold this position for five seconds before returning to the start position and repeating on the other side.

Recommended sets/reps: 10 reps of a 5-second hold in each end position

Stretching

Piriformis Stretch

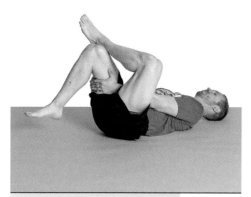

SUPINE PIRIFORMIS STRETCH

As discussed earlier in this chapter, stretching the piriformis should be performed only for cases of *short* piriformis syndrome.

The figure-four stretch is an easy-to-perform treatment for short piriformis syndrome. If you have long piriformis syndrome (as indicated by excessive internal rotation compared to your pain-free side), a stretch like this could aggravate your symptoms.

For the supine version of this stretch, lie on your back with your knees bent. Cross the ankle of your affected leg over your opposite thigh. From this position, grab your pain-free thigh and pull it toward your chest until you feel a stretch deep in your hip.

Because of how your piriformis is aligned in your hips, it becomes a medial rotator when you flex your hip past 90 degrees. This is why this stretch helps elongate the muscle when your hip is in a laterally rotated position close to your chest.

You can also perform the piriformis stretch while seated. Cross your legs by placing the ankle of your painful leg on your opposite thigh. With your back flat, lean your chest forward until you feel a stretch deep in your hip. I recommend doing the figure-four stretch on your back *or* in the seated position—whichever version gives you the better stretch.

Recommended sets/reps: 3 sets of 30-second stretches

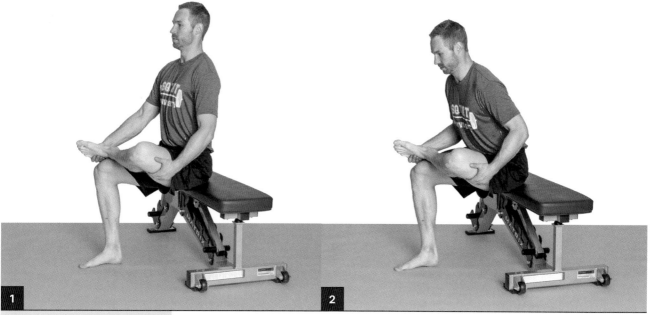

SEATED PIRIFORMIS STRETCH

Pigeon Stretch

The pigeon stretch is a progression of the piriformis stretch. Find a tall box, bench, or bed and place your painful leg on top in an externally rotated position.

With your lower leg completely flat on the box, lean your torso forward until you feel a light stretch in your hip. Make sure to keep your back from rounding. You can play around with this movement and lean your torso at different angles (toward your foot or your knee, for example) to maximize the stretch in the back of your hip. You can also perform this stretch on the ground if you don't have access to a box or bench.

Recommended sets/reps: 3 sets of 30-second stretches

After performing any of the prior stretches, retest your hip internal rotation (with the hip flexed to 60 degrees) to see if you were effective at clearing up this restriction. If you do not see any improvements, I suggest performing the banded joint mobilization next.

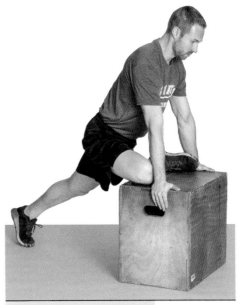

PIGEON STRETCH ON BOX

Kettlebell Weight Shift

Start in a half-kneeling position (one knee on the ground) with your front leg pointing laterally away from your body. Your back-leg hip should be in an externally rotated position, with your foot pointed toward the midline of your body. With an upright posture, hold a kettlebell in front of you below your hips.

Next, shift your weight toward your forward leg, trying to drive your knee over the middle of your foot. Your back hip will remain in an extended position during the entire movement.

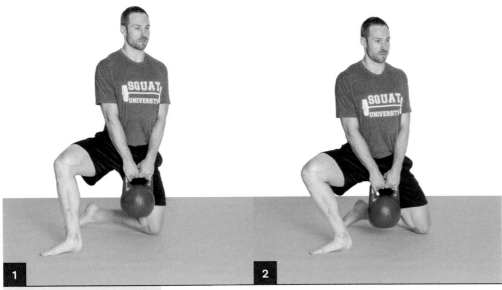

KETTLEBELL WEIGHT SHIFT

This shift may bring out a good stretch to both hips, depending on your restrictions. Because a stretch to the back-leg hip flexor and adductor muscles as you shift toward your forward leg is common, use of this stretch in the early days following a hip flexor or adductor muscle strain should be avoided, as the tension may re-create pain. However, as long as the stretch feels good in both hips, feel free to continue using it.

Recommended sets/reps: 2 sets of 10 reps of 5-second stretches

Rebuilding Strength

After addressing your soft tissue and/or joint mobility restrictions, you need to address your strength. A rehab progression for safely rebuilding strength looks like this:

- Isometrics to decrease pain and improve muscular control
- Strength exercises (called *isotonics*) to improve muscle/tendon capacity to handle load
- Movement re-education and technique fixes for barbell training

Early Strengthening with Isometrics

While taking a step back from lifting big weights is an important first step when you experience pain, it can't be the only thing you do to fix the injury. After a day or two of rest, you need to do something to facilitate healing.

Initially following an injury, aggressive strengthening (especially for a tendinopathy) can make symptoms worse. For this reason, if you had pain with any of the isolated strength tests, you want to start by performing a low-level strength exercise called an *isometric*. Activating the muscle without movement (called an *isometric contraction*) can be a great way to kick-start healing.

ADDUCTOR ISOMETRIC

For the adductors, lie on your back with your knees bent and place a small ball (or a pillow if you're at home) between your knees. Squeeze your knees together like you're trying to pop the ball. When you start doing these exercises, think about contracting 50 to 75 percent of maximum effort, and don't push through pain! Hold the contraction for five seconds before relaxing. As it becomes easier, start squeezing with more intensity or increase the hold time to 10 to 15 seconds. You can eventually progress to having your legs straight once the exercise becomes more tolerable.

Recommended sets/reps: 2 sets of 20 reps for a 5-second hold

ADDUCTOR SQUEEZE WITH BALL

When you eventually reach a point where you no longer have pain with the isometric adductor squeeze (in either the bent-leg or the straight-leg position), it's time to progress strengthening of the inner groin tissues. A great way to increase load on these tissues is with the Copenhagen side plank.

To start, assume a side-lying position perpendicular to a bench or box with an open frame. Your entire torso should be in line with your legs as if performing a classic side plank. Next, push yourself into a side plank, supported only by your affected leg positioned on top of the bench. You can have the down arm either bent or straight, depending on the height of the bench.

The bent-knee position is easier for most people to perform, but you can progress to the straight-leg version as long as it doesn't create knee pain. As with the earlier isometrics, hold this position for 10 seconds before dropping back to the start position. If this exercise is right for your body, you should not feel pain during the exercise or directly after performing it.

Recommended sets/reps: 2 sets of 10 reps for a 5-second hold

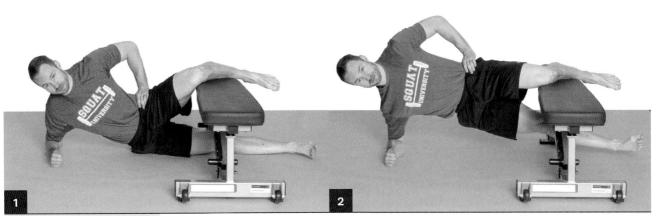

COPENHAGEN SIDE PLANK

HIP FLEXOR ISOMETRIC

For the hip flexors, lie on your back with your knees bent and your feet up at a 90-degree angle. Loop a small resistance band around your feet.

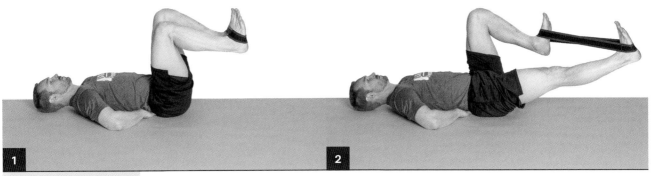

HIP FLEXOR ISOMETRIC

Brace your core and then straighten one leg. Make sure your other leg remains bent. Hold the extended leg for five seconds before returning to the start position. This exercise requires an isometric contraction of the hip flexors to prevent the bent leg from moving.

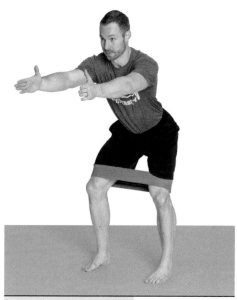

BANDED SQUAT HOLD

GLUTE MEDIUS ISOMETRIC

There are two simple ways to perform an isometric for the glute medius. The first is to assume the same stance you would take during a squat with a resistance band around your knees. Perform a mini squat and hold that position. While keeping your feet glued to the ground, drive your knees out to the sides against the band to turn on your lateral glutes (don't lose your tripod foot). Hold this position until your lateral glutes start burning!

This contraction does not need to be intense. In fact, research has shown that low-intensity isometrics (around 25 percent of your maximum ability to contract the muscle) can be more efficient at decreasing pain than high-intensity isometrics (around 80 percent).[57]

Recommended sets/reps: 5 reps of a 10- to 30-second hold

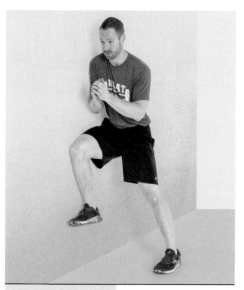

LATERAL WALL SIT

You can also perform a wall sit while pushing laterally into a wall. Stand next to a wall with your outer foot at least 12 inches from the wall (which gives you some room to lean into it). Bring your inner thigh up to 90 degrees and lean your body into the wall.

Push with your outer leg and jam your hip into the wall. This action should turn on the lateral glute muscles of your pushing leg. Make sure that the knee of the leg you're pushing with is in line with your foot and not caving inward.

Recommended sets/reps: 5 reps of a 10- to 30-second hold

Progressing Strength

Eventually, you must progress past simple isometric exercises and move to more dynamic movements to address strength and stability imbalances in your lower body. None of the following exercises should create pain or worsen your pain symptoms. If these exercises exacerbate your pain, I recommend seeing a medical doctor or physical therapist for assistance with your recovery.

BRIDGE

Regardless of which type of hip injury you may be experiencing, the bridge is often a part of a comprehensive rehab program.[58] If you did not feel your glutes working hard when performing the single-leg bridge test on page 147, this exercise will help.

Lie on your back with your knees bent. Squeeze your butt muscles and then lift your hips. Squeeze your glutes as hard as you can for five seconds before coming back down. Work your way up to a 10-second hold.

If your hamstrings start cramping, two modifications can help. First, bring your heels closer to your hips, which shortens the hamstrings and puts them at a disadvantage to contribute to the movement (a concept called *active insufficiency*).[59] You can also jam your toes into the ground and think about pushing your feet away from your hips. This turns on your quads slightly, which decreases hamstring activity (a concept called *reciprocal inhibition*). The only muscles left to create hip extension with the hamstrings out of the picture are—you guessed it—the glutes!

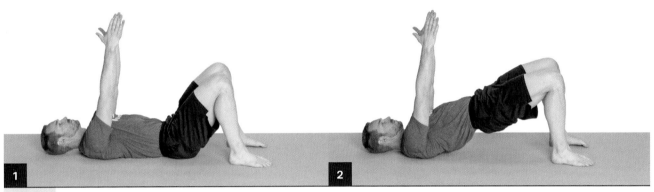

BRIDGE

Recommended sets/reps: 2 sets of 20 reps for a 5- to 10-second hold

To increase the difficulty of this exercise, you can perform it with your back against a bench and a barbell across your hips (not shown). This variation is called a *hip thrust*.

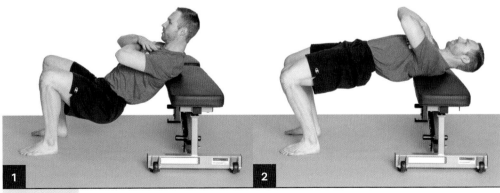

HIP THRUST

Recommended sets/reps: 3 sets of 10 reps for a 5-second hold

MARCHING RESISTED BRIDGE

This exercise is great for hip flexor, core, and posterior chain strength and stability. I recommend it for those who are recovering from any hip flexor injury, as confirmed by a positive load tolerance test from earlier in this chapter.

Lie on your back with your legs extended and your heels resting on a bench. Loop a resistance band around your feet. Brace your core and raise your hips in a bridging movement. Squeeze your glutes hard in this position. Next, pull one knee to your chest while keeping the other on the bench. Keep your core braced during the entire movement. Repeat with the other knee.

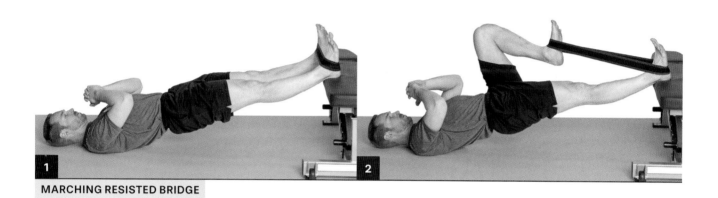

MARCHING RESISTED BRIDGE

Recommended sets/reps: 2 or 3 sets of 10 alternating reps

SIDE PLANK CLAMSHELL

The next area you want to concentrate on is lateral hip strength and stability. The side plank clamshell is a helpful exercise for those dealing with a hip impingement or hip flexor injury, both of which are related to weak hip rotation strength and coordination.[60]

Lie on your right side with your legs bent and a resistance band around your knees. Keep your right elbow and right knee in contact with the ground as you raise your hips and hold them in a side plank position.

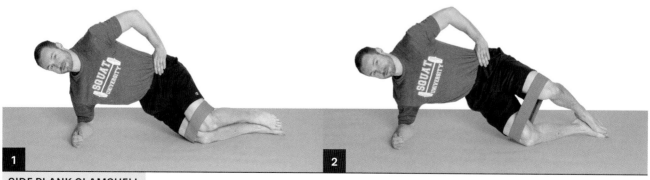

SIDE PLANK CLAMSHELL

While maintaining this side plank, rotate your left leg against the band resistance. Hold for five seconds before lowering it back down. I often cue my patients to imagine that their legs are the mouth of a clamshell opening and closing.

Recommended sets/reps: 2 sets of 10 reps for a 5-second hold on each side

Movement Re-education

The last step in the rehab process is to retrain any faulty coordination, balance, and stability with movements that resemble the lifts we perform in the gym. This is an essential aspect of rehab that is often missed.

Hip Airplane/Tippy Bird Progression

Let's start by progressing the assisted airplane (or "tippy bird"; see page 151). This version was designed by Stuart McGill as an active flexibility exercise for the glute muscles, and it is an essential part of a comprehensive warm-up for those who lift weights![61] To adequately prepare your body to hoist massive weights in training or competition—and do so pain-free—you must first enhance your sense of control and balance. This exercise does just that.

But why would someone who can easily squat 600 pounds need to work on their balance and sense of control? Because a majority of the injuries we develop as athletes don't arise due to strength deficits but instead are due to poor control of the strength we do have. This lack of balance and control leads to an accumulation of microtrauma that develops into the aches and pains of injury.

I want to share with you not only the hip airplane but also the progression I use to teach the exercise, which I call the Superman. To perform the full airplane movement, you must first show the necessary stability and coordination to balance on one leg. Perform this exercise barefoot so you can feel your toes gripping the floor and your body weight spread evenly across the tripod foot. This will help you activate the smaller muscles of your feet that are essential in creating a stable body from the ground up.

Assume a single-leg stance. Lock your rib cage down by bracing your core. Spread your arms out to the sides and rotate your torso forward over your stance leg while kicking your back leg behind you. Keep your trail leg completely straight and the knee of your stance leg locked in a slightly bent position. Imagine that your body is a seesaw. Draw a line from your shoulder through your hip down to your knee/ankle. Keep this line straight throughout the exercise. This is similar to a single-leg RDL.

Once you have gone as far forward as you can without losing your balance, hold that position for 10 seconds before returning to a standing position. Make sure to jam your heel into the ground and grip the ground with your toes. The end goal of this movement is to be able to balance with your chest completely parallel to the floor for the full 10 seconds. If you are doing this exercise correctly, you should feel some tension in your upper hamstrings and the glutes of your stance leg.

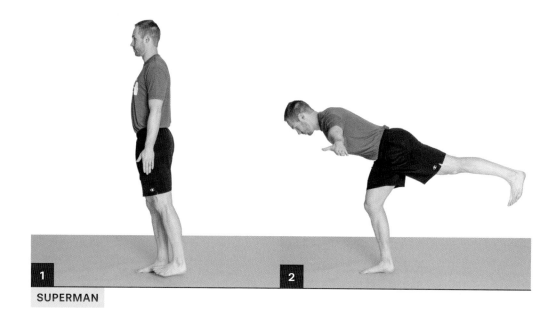

SUPERMAN

Recommended sets/reps: 1 or 2 sets of 10 reps for a minimum 10-second hold

The airplane is performed exactly like the Superman exercise, except it introduces rotation. The addition of rotation not only increases the difficulty of maintaining balance (as you'll soon find out) but also teaches your body to actively control your glute muscles through a full range of motion. Dr. McGill refers to this concept as "steering" your strength.[62]

Assume a single-leg stance. Lock your rib cage down by bracing your core. Rotate your body forward over your stance leg to a point where you can hold the position without losing your balance. (Your chest does not need to be parallel to the ground to start.)

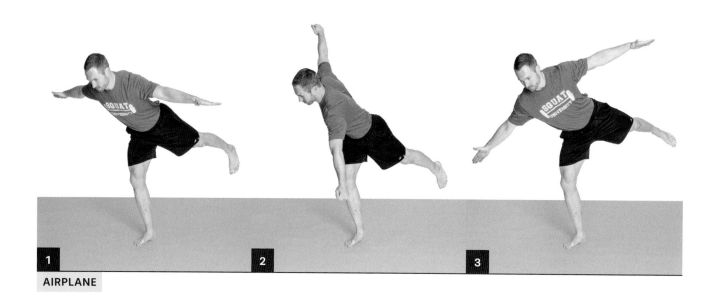

AIRPLANE

Instead of holding this position for 10 seconds, rotate your torso toward your stance leg (hip internal rotation) and then away from your stance leg (hip external rotation). A helpful cue is to imagine moving your belly button toward your stance leg and then rotating it away to the side. Perform three to five rotations before standing up again. You should feel this exercise working the glutes of your stance leg.

Recommended sets/reps: 1 or 2 sets of 10 to 20 reps

I find this exercise extremely helpful for those who have been dealing with anterior hip pain, especially a hip joint impingement. As you gain better control over your balance and steering ability during the rotational part of the movement, you can increase the difficulty by assuming a more inclined trunk position.

Single-Leg RDL

Being able to perform the prior exercise progression without falling over means that you now have the ability to sufficiently control a hip hinge motion on one leg. You can begin to load this pattern with the single-leg RDL. Hold a kettlebell or dumbbell in the hand opposite your stance leg. Perform the same movement as you did with the unweighted Superman. Go as far forward as you can without losing the straight line from your shoulder through your torso and free leg to your heel. If you are doing this exercise correctly, you should feel tension building in your hamstrings and glutes. You don't need to hold the bottom position, but make sure to perform the entire exercise in a slow, controlled manner.

This exercise is excellent for rebuilding strength in the posterior chain (glutes and hamstrings). If you found a hamstring load intolerance with the testing at the beginning of this chapter (a notable increase in pain with a single-leg bridge performed with a semistraight leg compared to a bent-knee bridge), slowly building your hamstring strength with this exercise will be key to your recovery. You should not have any pain while performing the reps or the day after. If you find that your pain increases during this exercise or over the next 24 hours, you used too much weight; decrease the load next time.

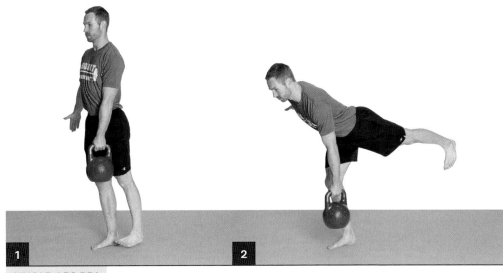

SINGLE-LEG RDL

If you have a problem maintaining balance and coordination while performing the single-leg RDL (for example, your chest drops quicker than your free leg rises), place a resistance band around your foot and shoulder. Maintaining tension on the band throughout the entire RDL will improve your stability and help you move entirely about your hip joint.

Recommended sets/reps: 2 or 3 sets of 10 to 15 reps

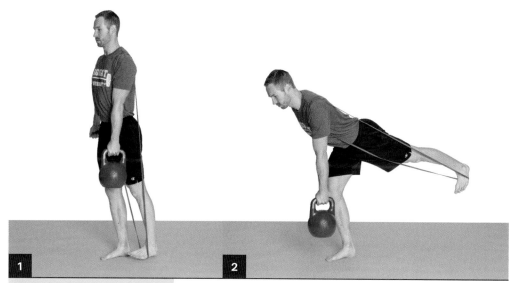

SINGLE-LEG RDL WITH BAND

RNT Progression

First introduced by physical therapists Michael Voight and Gray Cook, reactive neuromuscular training (RNT) exercises are designed to improve movement quality by teaching athletes to feel for how they are moving (known as *proprioception*).[63]

To perform these exercises, you use a resistance band to pull your body into an exaggerated movement fault (knee cave or hip shift). When you "feed" the movement problem, your body should reflexively realize the error and learn how to correct itself by pushing in the opposite direction.

RNT SQUAT

Assume your normal squat stance with a small resistance band around your knees. As you squat, keep your knees in alignment with your feet. Your lateral glutes must kick on to stabilize your femurs and pelvis to keep the tension of the band from pulling your knees together. As you drive your knees wide against the resistance band, make sure your feet stay glued to the ground. A good cue to prevent your feet from rolling to the side is to keep your big toes jammed into the ground.

Recommended sets/reps: 2 sets of 20 reps

As your movement quality improves and your pain lessens, you can start performing this banded squat as part of your warm-ups with light weight before attempting heavier lifts.

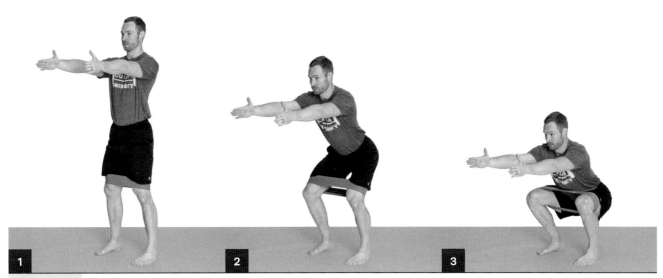

1 **2** **3**

RNT SQUAT

RNT SPLIT SQUAT

Assume a lunge position (one leg in front of the other) with the heel of your back foot elevated off the ground. Place a resistance band around your forward leg and have your friend pull the band inward toward the midline of your body in an effort to collapse your knee.

As you perform the split squat, work to maintain your knee in alignment with your foot. The resistance from the band should stimulate your lateral glutes to kick on at the appropriate time and keep your knee in a good, stable position.

Recommended sets/reps: 2 sets of 20 reps

Again, as the quality of your movement progresses and your pain decreases, you can start using a loaded barbell on your back or holding dumbbells in your hands to increase the challenge of this exercise and ease back into your normal training routine.

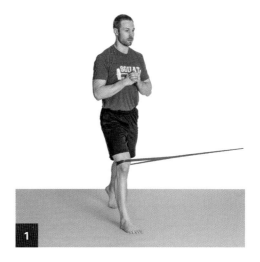

1

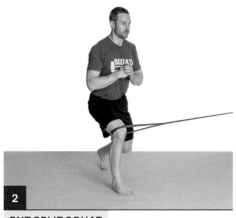

2

RNT SPLIT SQUAT

TOUCHDOWN

No matter the type of hip injury you are dealing with, I recommend working on your single-leg squat with the touchdown. Flip to pages 206 and 207 in the Knee Pain chapter for a full explanation of this exercise.

Early in the rehab process of a lateral hip injury (such as a glute medius tendinopathy or greater trochanteric bursitis), you don't want to perform a ton of single-leg squats, as the injured leg naturally moves into slight adduction in order to stay balanced (meaning a small amount of tendon compression cannot be avoided). This normal increase in compression with the single-leg stance is why the position is used as a provocation test for this injury in the first place. If you have lateral hip pain in a single-leg stance and/or pain with the external derotation test, hold off on touchdown squats until those tests are symptom-free.

LOAD CONSIDERATIONS

Within 24 hours of performing any of the prior strength exercises, assess whether your symptoms are getting better or worse.[64] If your pain is worse, your corrective exercises or training program may be too intense and may need to be adjusted. Eventually, you can progress back to your regular barbell lifts and other strength training exercises as long as you are pain-free.

Technique Considerations Based on Anatomy

SQUAT WITH TOES RELATIVELY FORWARD

The squat is a movement first and an exercise second. When I screen a new athlete, I want to see their ability to squat with shoes off and toes facing forward. My goal is to assess their *movement*. This method allows me to identify any weak links. Squatting with your feet relatively straight forward (5- to 7-degree toe-out angle) is more difficult than squatting with the toes pointed slightly outward. However, that is the point of the screen.

To squat to full depth with your toes straight forward, you must have adequate ankle and hip mobility and sufficient pelvic/core control. You also must have acceptable coordination and balance. Turning the toes out allows most people to achieve a full-depth squat with a more upright chest position. There will always be a few individuals who are simply unable to get into a deep squat due to abnormal anatomy. With that said, *most* athletes should be able to achieve a full-depth bodyweight squat.

The bodyweight squat sets the movement foundation for other athletic actions, such as jumping and landing. Many knee injuries occur when you land with your foot pointing out and your knee caving in. Players who have to jump and cut tear their ACL when the knee caves in and rotates. My goal is for athletes to land and jump with good mechanics, thereby decreasing their chance of season-ending injuries.

If you suspect that you have femoral or acetabular retroversion based on the prior testing, it may be "normal" for your body to have a more exaggerated toe-out angle (around 30 degrees) when you squat, catch a clean/snatch, or deadlift. This is especially true for Olympic lifters trying to receive a clean or snatch in the deepest possible positions.

If you found a possible retroverted hip socket or femur, try this test. Assume a bodyweight squat stance with your toes relatively straight. Squat as deeply as you can. Next, point your toes out a little and perform the same deep squat. Athletes with retroverted hips often feel an uncomfortable and painful sensation in the fronts of their hips that limits depth during the toes-forward squat.[65]

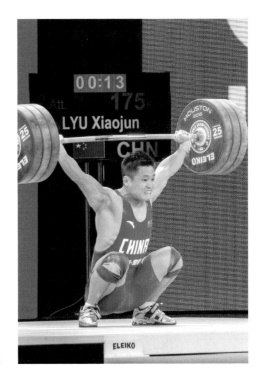

Weightlifter with toes turned out during reception of lift.
Liu Xiaojun snatch,
© Bruce Klemens

If this describes you, it means you have a bone structure that does not allow for a deep squat with your feet straight. It is normal and natural for your body to squat with your toes angled out slightly, and no amount of mobility work will bring about *significant* change.

Now, this does *not* mean you should stop performing all hip mobility work! Quite the opposite. I still want you to perform mobility and flexibility exercises based on the restrictions you have uncovered with the tests in this chapter. Rarely do I find an athlete who has maxed out their mobility potential. That being said, understand that not everyone has a "textbook" bone structure, and trying to conform to a squat stance that isn't right for your body (regardless of the amount of mobility work you do) can be disastrous. If you have a hard blocking sensation or pinching pain in your hips when lifting that isn't relieved by doing any of these corrective exercises *and* your anatomy screening exposed potential retroversion, your body is telling you to move differently. Listen to it.

Just because you didn't hit the genetic lottery with perfect hip anatomy doesn't mean you should hang up your weightlifting shoes and quit training altogether. You simply need to understand the potential technique adjustments and mobility modifications your body requires to reach your potential and stay pain-free. If your pain persists or worsens despite these interventions and the prior exercises, I highly recommend seeking out a medical doctor or other rehabilitation professional, like a physical therapist.

Notes

1. M. Maruyama, J. R. Feinberg, W. N. Capello, and J. A. D'Antonio, "The Frank Stinchfield award: morphologic features of the acetabulum and femur: anteversion angle and implant positioning," *Clinical Orthopaedics and Related Research* 393 (2001): 52–65.

2. D. Reynolds, J. Lucas, and K. Klaue, "Retroversion of the acetabulum: a cause of hip pain," *Journal of Bone & Joint Surgery,* British Volume 81, no. 2 (1999): 281–8.

3. R. T. Loder and E. N. Skopelja, "The epidemiology and demographics of hip dysplasia," *ISRN Orthopedics* (2011): 238607.

4. Loder and Skopelja, "The epidemiology and demographics of hip dysplasia" (see note 3 above).

5. M. T. Cibulka, "Determination and significance of femoral neck anteversion," *Physical Therapy* 84, no. 6 (2004): 550–8.

6. R. H. Gelberman, M. S. Cohen, S. S. Desai, P. P. Griffin, P. B. Salamon, and T. M. O'Brien, "Femoral anteversion: a clinical assessment of idiopathic intoeing gait in children," *Journal of Bone & Joint Surgery,* British Volume 69, no. 1 (1987): 75–9.

7. P. A. Ruwe, J. R. Gage, M. B. Ozonoff, and P. A. DeLuca, "Clinical determination of femoral anteversion: a comparison with established techniques," *Journal of Bone & Joint Surgery* 74, no. 6 (1992): 820–30.

8. A. Weir, P. Brunker, E. Delahunt, J. Ekstrand, D. Griffin, K. M. Khan, G. Lovell, et al., "Doha agreement meeting on terminology and definitions in groin pain in athletes," *British Journal of Sports Medicine* 49, no. 12 (2015): 768–74.

9. T. F. Tyler, H. J. Silvers, M. B. Gerhardt, and S. J. Nicholas, "Groin injuries in sports medicine," *Sports Health* 2, no. 3 (2010): 231–6.

10. A. D. Vigotsky and M. A. Bryanton, "Relative muscle contributions to net joint movements in the barbell back squat," 40th Annual Meeting of the American Society of Biomechanics, Raleigh, NC, August 2–5, 2016; M. L. Benn, T. Pizzari, L. Rath, K. Tucker, and A. I. Semciw, "Adductor magnus: an EMG investigation into proximal and distal portions and direction specific action," *Clinical Anatomy* 31, no. 4 (2018): 535–43.

11. P. Renstrom and L. Peterson, "Groin injuries in athletes," *British Journal of Sports Medicine* 14, no. 1 (1980): 30–6.

12. Renstrom and Peterson, "Groin injuries in athletes" (see note 11 above).

13. T. F. Tyler, T. Fukunaga, and J. Gellert, "Rehabilitation of soft tissue injuries of the hip and pelvis: invited clinical commentary," *International Journal of Sports Physical Therapy* 9, no. 6 (2014): 785–97.

14. A. A. Ellsworth, M. P. Zoland, and T. F. Tyler, "Athletic pubalgia and associated rehabilitation: invited clinical commentary," *International Journal of Sports Physical Therapy* 9, no. 6 (2014): 774–84.

15. C. A. Unverzagt, T. Schuemann, and J. Mathisen, "Differential diagnosis of a sports hernia in a high-school athlete," *Journal of Orthopaedic & Sports Physical Therapy* 38, no. 2 (2008): 63–70.

16. Ellsworth, Zoland, and Tyler, "Athletic pubalgia and associated rehabilitation" (see note 14 above).

17. Weir et al., "Doha agreement meeting on terminology and definitions in groin pain in athletes" (see note 8 above).

18. A. F. Kachingwe and S. Grech, "Proposed algorithm for the management of athletes with athletic pubalgia (sports hernia): a case series," *Journal of Orthopaedic & Sports Physical Therapy* 38, no. 12 (2008): 768–81.

19. A. Grimaldi and A. Rearon, "Gluteal tendinopathy: integrating pathomechanics and clinical features in its management," *Journal of Orthopaedic & Sports Physical Therapy* 45, no. 11 (2015): 910–22.

20. Grimaldi and Rearon, "Gluteal tendinopathy" (see note 19 above); G. Collee, B. A. C. Dijkmans, J. P. Vandenbroucke, and A. Cats, "Greater trochanteric pain syndrome (trochanteric bursitis) in low back pain," *Scandinavian Journal of Rheumatology* 20, no. 4 (1991): 262–6; P. J. Tortolani, J. J. Carbone, and L. G. Quartararo, "Greater trochanteric pain syndrome in patients referred to orthopedic spine specialists," *Spine Journal* 2, no. 4 (2002): 251–4; N. A. Segal, D. T. Felson, J. C. Torner, Y. Zhu, J. R. Crutis, J. Niu, M. C. Nevitt, et al., "Greater trochanteric pain syndrome: epidemiology and associated factors," *Archives of Physical Medicine and Rehabilitation* 88, no. 8 (2007): 988–92.

21. P. A. Bird, S. P. Oakley, R. Shnier, and B. W. Kirkham, "Prospective evaluation of magnetic resonance imaging and physical examination findings in patients with greater trochanteric pain syndrome," *Arthritis & Rheumatology* 44, no. 9 (2001): 2138–45.

22. A. S. Klauser, C. Martinoli, A. Tagliafico, R. Bellmann-Weiler, G. M. Feuchtner, M. Wick, and W. R. Jaschke, "Greater trochanteric pain syndrome," *Seminars in Musculoskeletal Radiology* 17, no. 1 (2013): 43–8.

23. Grimaldi and Rearon, "Gluteal tendinopathy" (see note 19 above); Klauser et al., "Greater trochanteric pain syndrome" (see note 22 above).

24. B. S. Williams and S. P. Cohen, "Greater trochanteric pain syndrome: a review of anatomy, diagnosis and treatment," *Anesthesia & Analgesia* 108, no. 5 (2009): 1662–70.

25. G. Gottschalk, S. Kourosh, and B. Leveau, "The functional anatomy of the tensor fasciae latae and gluteus medius and minimus," *Journal of Anatomy* 166 (1989): 179–89.

26. Gottschalk, Kourosh, and Leveau, "The functional anatomy of the tensor fasciae latae and gluteus medius and minimus" (see note 25 above).

27. Gottschalk, Kourosh, and Leveau, "The functional anatomy of the tensor fasciae latae and gluteus medius and minimus" (see note 25 above).

28. Grimaldi and Rearon, "Gluteal tendinopathy" (see note 19 above).

29. Grimaldi and Rearon, "Gluteal tendinopathy" (see note 19 above); N. K. Viradia, A. A. Berger, and L. E. Dahners, "Relationship between width of greater trochanters and width of iliac wings in trochanteric bursitis," *American Journal of Orthopedics* 40, no. 9 (2011): E159–62; D. Woyski, A. Olinger, and B. Wright, "Smaller insertion area and inefficient mechanics of the gluteus medius in females," *Surgical and Radiologic Anatomy* 35, no. 8 (2013): 713–9.

30. Grimaldi and Rearon, "Gluteal tendinopathy" (see note 19 above).

31. D. Hertling and M. K. Randolph, *Management of Common Musculoskeletal Disorders: Physical Therapy Principles and Methods* (Philadelphia: J. B. Lippincott, 1996).

32. D. J. Magee, *Orthopedic Physical Assessment* (Philadelphia: Saunders, 2002).

33. F. P. Kendall, E. K. McCreary, and P. G. Provance, *Muscles: Testing and Function*, 4th Edition (Baltimore: Williams & Wilkins, 1993); S. A. Sahrmann, *Diagnosis and Treatment of Movement Impairment Syndromes* (St. Louis: Mosby, 2002).

34. C. M. Hall and L. T. Brody, *Therapeutic Exercise: Moving Toward Function*, 2nd Edition (Philadelphia: Lippincott Williams & Wilkins, 2005).

35. J. L. Cook and C. Purdam, "Is compressive load a factor in the development of tendinopathy?" *British Journal of Sports Medicine* 46, no. 3 (2012): 163–8.

36. T. S. Goom, P. Malliaras, M. P. Reiman, and C. R. Purdam, "Proximal hamstring tendinopathy: clinical aspects of assessment and management," *Journal of Orthopaedic & Sports Physical Therapy* 46, no. 6 (2016): 483–93; L. Lempainen, K. Johansson, I. J. Banke, J. Ranne, K. Mäkelä, J. Sarimo, P. Niemi, and S. Orava, "Expert opinion: diagnosis and treatment of proximal hamstring tendinopathy," *Muscles, Ligaments and Tendons Journal* 5, no. 1 (2015): 23–8.

37. M. Prior, M. Guerin, and K. Grimmer, "An evidence-based approach to hamstring strain injury: a systematic review of the literature," *Athletic Training* 1, no. 2 (2009): 154–64.

38. Maruyama, Feinberg, Capello, and D'Antonio, "The Frank Stinchfield award" (see note 1 above).

39. A. Arnason, S. B. Sigurdsson, A. Gudmundsson, I. Holme, L. Engebretsen, and R. Bahr, "Risk factors for injuries in football," *American Journal of Sports Medicine* 32, 1 Suppl (2004): 5S–16S; K. Bennell, H. Wajswelner, P. Lew, A. Schall-Riaucour, S. Leslie, D. Plant, and J. Cirone, "Isokinetic strength testing does not predict hamstring injury in Australian Rules footballers," *British Journal of Sports Medicine* 32, no. 4 (1998): 309–14; B. J. Gabbe, K. L. Bennell, C. F. Finch, H. Wajswelner, and J. W. Orchard, "Predictors of hamstring injury at the elite level of Australian football," *Scandinavian Journal of Medicine & Science in Sports* 16, no. 1 (2006): 7–13; M. Hagglund, M. Walden, and J. Ekstrand, "Previous injury as a risk factor for injury in elite football: a prospective study over 2 consecutive seasons," *British Journal of Sports Medicine* 40, no. 9 (2006): 767–72.

40. E. Cressey, "5 reasons you have tight hamstrings," June 12, 2012, https://ericcressey.com/5-reasons-tight-hamstrings-strain.

41. G. Verrall, J. Slavatinek, P. Barnes, G. Fon, and A. Spriggins, "Clinical risk factors for hamstring muscle strain injury: a prospective study with correlation of injury by magnetic resonance imaging," *British Journal of Sports Medicine* 35, no. 6 (2001): 435–40.

42. Prior, Guerin, and Grimmer, "An evidence-based approach to hamstring strain injury" (see note 37 above); Bennell et al., "Isokinetic strength testing does not predict hamstring injury in Australian Rules footballers" (see note 39 above); J. Orchard, J. Marsden, S. Lord, and D. Garlick, "Preseason hamstring muscle weakness associated with hamstring muscle injury in Australian footballers," *American Journal of Sports Medicine* 25, no. 1 (1997): 81–5; T. Yamamoto, "Relationship between hamstring strains and leg muscle strength," *Journal of Sports Medicine and Physical Fitness* 33, no. 2 (1993): 194–9.

43. Prior, Guerin, and Grimmer, "An evidence-based approach to hamstring strain injury" (see note 37 above).

44. B. J. Gabbe, K. L. Bennell, C. F. Finch, H. Wajswelner, and J. W. Orchard, "Predictors of hamstring injury at the elite level of Australian football," *Scandinavian Journal of Medicine & Science in Sports* 16, no. 1 (2006): 7–13; B. J. Gabbe, K. L. Bennell, and C. F. Finch, "Why are older Australian football players at greater risk of hamstring injury?" *Journal of Science and Medicine in Sport* 9, no. 4 (2006): 327–33.

45. C. Woods, R. D. Hawkins, S. Maltby, M. Hulse, and A. Thomas, "The Football Association Medical Research Programme: an audit of injuries in professional football—analysis of hamstring injuries," *British Journal of Sports Medicine* 38, no. 1 (2004): 36–41.

46. Prior, Guerin, and Grimmer, "An evidence-based approach to hamstring strain injury" (see note 37 above).

47. S. Sahrmann, D. C. Azevedo, and L. Van Dillen, "Diagnosis and treatment of movement system impairment syndromes," *Brazilian Journal of Physical Therapy* 21, no. 6 (2017): 391–9.

48. M. Lequesne, P. Mathieu, V. Vuillemin-Bodaghi, H. Bard, and P. Djian, "Gluteal tendinopathy in refractory greater trochanter pain syndrome: diagnostic value of two clinical tests," *Arthritis & Rheumatism* 59, no. 2 (2008): 241–6.

49. M. Tijssen, R. van Cingel, L. Willemsen, and E. de Visser, "Diagnostics of femoroacetabular impingement and labral pathology of the hip: a systematic review of the accuracy and validity of physical tests," *Arthroscopy* 28, no. 6 (2012): 860–71.

50. J. J. Bagwell, L. Bauer, M. Gradoz, and T. L. Grindstaff, "The reliability of FABER test hip range of motion measurements," *International Journal of Sports Physical Therapy* 11, no. 7 (2016): 1101–5.

51. D. Harvey, "Assessment of the flexibility of elite athletes using the modified Thomas test," *British Journal of Sports Medicine* 32, no. 1 (1998): 68–70.

52. T. F. Tyler, S. J. Nicholas, R. J. Campbell, S. Donellan, and M. P. McHugh, "The effectiveness of a preseason exercise program to prevent adductor muscle strains in professional ice hockey players," *American Journal of Sports Medicine* 30, no. 5 (2002): 680–3; T. F. Tyler, S. J. Nicholas, R. J. Campbell, and M. P. McHugh, "The association of hip strength and flexibility with the incidence of adductor muscle strains in professional ice hockey players," *American Journal of Sports Medicine* 29, no. 2 (2001): 124–8.

53. M. Lequesne, P. Mathieu, V. Vuillemin-Bodaghi, H. Bard, and P. Djian, "Gluteal tendinopathy in refractory greater trochanter pain syndrome: diagnostic value of two clinical tests," *Arthritis & Rheumatism* 59, no. 2 (2008): 241–6.

54. Goom, Malliaras, Reiman, and Purdam, "Proximal hamstring tendinopathy" (see note 36 above).

55. J. Paolini, "Review of myofascial release as an effective massage therapy technique," *Athletic Therapy Today* 14, no. 5 (2009): 30–4.

56. M. P. Reiman and J. W. Matheson, "Restricted hip mobility: clinical suggestions for self-mobilization and muscle re-education," *International Journal of Sports Physical Therapy* 8, no. 5 (2013): 729–40.

57. M. K. Hoeger Bement, J. Dicapo, R. Rasiarmos, and S. K. Hunter, "Dose response of isometric contractions on pain perception in healthy adults," *Medicine & Science in Sports & Exercise* 40, no. 11 (2008): 1880–9.

58. J. C. Tonley, S. M. Yun, R. J. Kochevar, J. A. Dye, S. Farrokhi, and C. M. Powers, "Treatment of an individual with piriformis syndrome focusing on hip muscle strengthening and movement reeducation: a case report," *Journal of Orthopaedic & Sports Physical Therapy* 40, no. 2 (2010): 103–11.

59. M. Olfat, J. Perry, and H. Hislop, "Relationship between wire EMG activity, muscle length, and torque of the hamstrings," *Clinical Biomechanics* 17, no. 8 (2002): 569–79.

60. C. A. Johnston, D. M. Lindsay, and J. P. Wiley, "Treatment of iliopsoas syndrome with a hip rotation strengthening program: a retrospective case series," *Journal of Orthopaedic & Sports Physical Therapy* 29, no. 4 (1999): 218–24; N. C. Casartelli, N. A. Maffiuletti, J. F. Item-Glatthorn, S. Staehli, M. Bizzini, F. M. Impellizzeri, and M. Leunig, "Hip muscle weakness in patients with symptomatic femoroacetabular impingement," *Osteoarthritis Cartilage* 19, no. 7 (2008): 816–21.

61. S. McGill, *Ultimate Back Fitness and Performance*, 6th Edition (Waterloo, Canada: Backfitpro Inc., 2014); C. Liebenson, "Training the hip: a progressive approach," *Journal of Bodywork and Movement Therapies* 17, no. 2 (2013): 266–8.

62. McGill, *Ultimate Back Fitness and Performance* (see note 61 above).

63. G. Cook, L. Burton, and K. Fields, "Reactive neuromuscular training for the anterior cruciate ligament-deficient knee: a case report," *Journal of Athletic Training* 34, no. 2 (1999): 194–201.

64. Loder and Skopelja, "The epidemiology and demographics of hip dysplasia" (see note 3 above).

65. Sahrmann, *Diagnosis and Treatment of Movement Impairment Syndromes* (see note 33 above).

CHAPTER 3

KNEE PAIN

If you're reading this chapter, chances are you've dealt with knee pain at one time or another. Of all the joints in the human body, the knee is one of the most commonly injured.[1] To keep it simple, the types of injuries that can be sustained at this joint can be broken down into two main categories: traumatic and nontraumatic.

A traumatic knee injury, as you can probably imagine, happens in one violent incident. For example, while you're playing basketball, you land from a jump and your knee collapses inward, tearing your anterior cruciate ligament (ACL). These types of injuries are serious and often season-ending for athletes who participate in sports like basketball, football, and soccer.

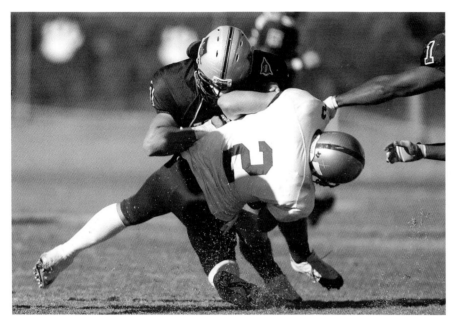 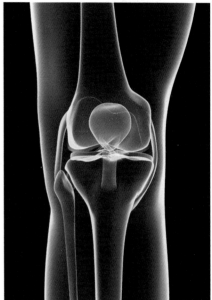

When it comes to barbell training, however, it is rare for someone to sustain a traumatic knee injury. I'm not saying these horrible injuries don't happen; they're just not very prevalent during weight training or in weightlifting/powerlifting competition.[2]

Research shows that knee pain associated with barbell training is often due to overuse injuries.[3] These nontraumatic injuries can become nagging and often lead to further issues down the road. Over time, this type of injury could affect your training and your quality of life.

After following a group of elite Olympic weightlifters for over six years, researchers Gregg Calhoon and Andrew Fry found that 51 percent of the athletes reported chronic knee pain (lasting many weeks), yet 95 percent of the time, they didn't miss more than a day of training.[4] This goes to show how common it is for athletes to push through nontraumatic but irritating knee pain.

These numbers also speak to the power of the "no pain, no gain" mantra that many athletes live by. Often, aggressive-minded coaches push their clients/athletes to train through pain in order to compete. Today, athletes do their best to mask pain by wearing knee sleeves, taking painkillers, or using topical creams. Trust me, I've been there, and I know what you're going through.

If you flipped to this chapter to address knee pain, it's likely because your performance is suffering. Most athletes don't seek help when they start to feel pain. It's not until their lifting is compromised that they finally turn to a professional.

Knee Injury Anatomy 101

If you decide to go the traditional medical route, which is to see your primary care physician or an orthopedic specialist, you'll likely receive a diagnosis that is anatomy based. Usually, the diagnosis is based on where the pain is and not on why you have knee pain. While there are many anatomical sources of pain surrounding the knee joint, here are some of the most common:

- Patellofemoral pain syndrome
- IT band syndrome
- Patellar or quad tendinopathy

Patellofemoral Pain Syndrome (PFPS)

If you have pain around your kneecap (patella), you'll likely be given a diagnosis of patellofemoral pain syndrome (PFPS). Unfortunately, PFPS is a blanket term and will never reveal how or why pain is present at the kneecap. Using such an ambiguous term only leads to confusion. For example, pain around the kneecap could be traced to degrading cartilage under the patella, to a bone bruise, or even to irritation of nearby tissues like the superior fat pad or the retinaculum (sections of the tough, fibrous capsule that surrounds the joint). Fortunately, you don't need to know with 100 percent certainty which specific anatomical tissue is at fault to take the first steps toward becoming pain-free!

Let's talk briefly about the mechanics of the knee joint. As you move your knee, your kneecap travels within a small notch in your femur called the *patellar groove*. This bony connection (called the *patellofemoral joint*) is placed under tremendous stress during a deep squat. Fortunately, the human body is uniquely designed for such movements! If you were to look closely at this joint, you would find that the kneecap and femur are lined with some of the thickest cartilage in the entire body. This dense layer of tissue distributes the load and keeps the joint healthy.

PATELLA IN PATELLAR GROOVE

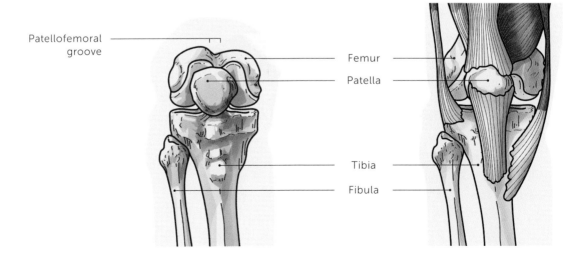

Patellofemoral groove · Femur · Patella · Tibia · Fibula

As your knee bends and straightens, the tissues (muscles, fascia, ligaments, and retinaculum) that surround the joint keep the patella in a stable position. If you perform a squat or catch a snatch in a deep receiving position and maintain your knees in alignment with your feet, the load is evenly distributed across the patellofemoral joint. If the knee does not track in this ideal manner and begins to wobble from side to side, however, problems can eventually arise.

The most common reason strength athletes develop pain around the kneecap is a lack of ability to control for rotation at the knee (i.e., demonstrating poor knee stability when lifting). If your knee wobbles as you squat, catch a clean, or stand up in a deadlift, the patella shifts and tilts off-axis in the patellar groove.[5] This wobbling not only creates uneven pressure on the underside of the bone but also places excessive strain on the surrounding tissues that connect to the kneecap.

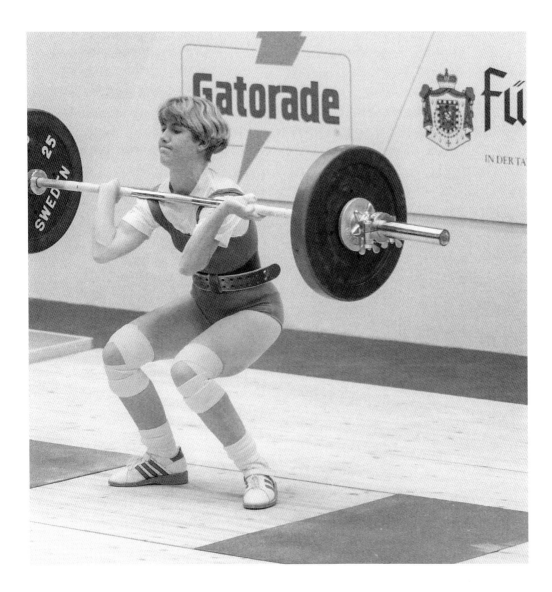

Knee cave squat.
Victoria Futch,
© Bruce Klemens

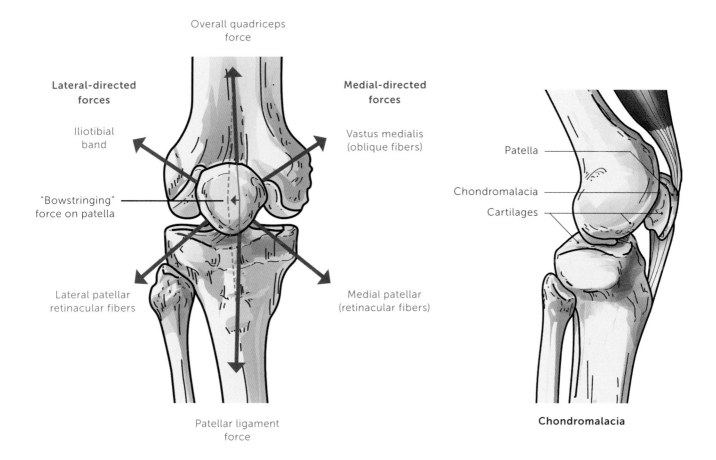

Overall quadriceps force

Lateral-directed forces

Medial-directed forces

Iliotibial band

Vastus medialis (oblique fibers)

"Bowstringing" force on patella

Lateral patellar retinacular fibers

Medial patellar (retinacular fibers)

Patellar ligament force

Patella

Chondromalacia

Cartilages

Chondromalacia

Think of this problem like a train being pulled off the tracks. If the pressure pulling the joint off-axis occurs often enough and under enough load, problems can ensue. This uneven tracking of the joint can also create popping and grinding noises in the knee, called *crepitus*. If left untreated, this friction between the kneecap and femur can lead to erosion of the smooth cartilage on the underside of the bone, an injury called *chondromalacia*.

IT Band Syndrome (ITBS)

The iliotibial (IT) band is a thick piece of fascia (dense connective tissue) that runs from the top of the hip all the way to the outside (lateral) part of the knee. It encloses the tensor fasciae latae (TFL) and has connections to the gluteus maximus (the largest butt muscle), lateral hamstrings, and lateral quads. The TFL and IT band work together to move the leg, one of those motions being internal or medial rotation of the femur.

ILIOTIBIAL (IT) BAND

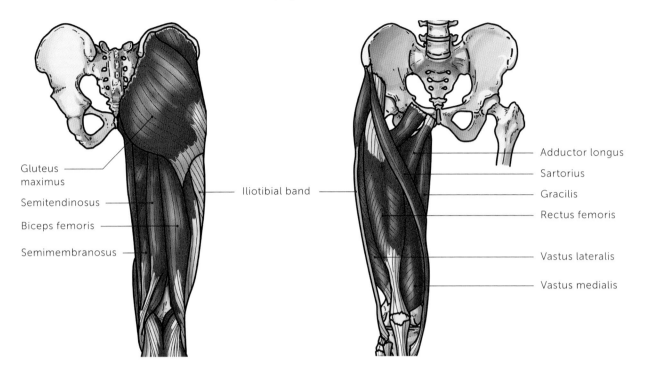

Gluteus maximus

Semitendinosus

Biceps femoris

Semimembranosus

Iliotibial band

Adductor longus

Sartorius

Gracilis

Rectus femoris

Vastus lateralis

Vastus medialis

The diagnosis of IT band syndrome (ITBS) is usually given when someone experiences pain on the lateral part of the knee, often over the prominent bony part of the femur called the *lateral femoral condyle*. Symptoms usually get worse over time and are not linked to one specific incident or trauma (like getting hit on the side of the leg). While this pain can start off dull and achy, it often progresses to a sharp pain that can be pinpointed to one specific area on the lateral surface of the knee where the band inserts. Some people even complain of a painful popping or snapping sensation at times.

Historically, ITBS has been thought to be a repetitive overuse injury typically found in runners. An athlete suffering from this injury commonly experiences more pain when they run for longer periods. In fact, ITBS has been found to encompass upwards of 12 percent of all running-related injuries.[6] However, it also appears in those participating in weight training. The exact reason for the development of this pain is debated; some people blame it on excessive friction, while others believe it is a compression issue. Let me explain.

The initial thinking was that when the IT band is excessively tight, it shifts forward and backward repetitively over the lateral femoral condyle as the knee bends and straightens.[7] This shifting causes friction underneath the IT band that eventually results in inflammation and pain.

However, recent research has shown that the IT band is, in fact, firmly attached to the distal femur by strong fibrous strands, preventing it from rolling over the condyle as previously thought. In fact, the rolling movement that many see when the knee is flexed and straightened is not a true movement but instead is a shifting in the tension of the IT band. As the knee bends, tension shifts from the anterior to the posterior fibers of the IT band.

For this reason, most experts now believe that the symptoms of pain are not due to friction underneath the band but instead to compression of a layer of highly innervated fat (fat that contains a lot of nerve endings).[8] Thus, it is not the IT band itself but the tissue underneath that is generating pain at the lateral knee. Medically, this is classified as a form of enthesopathy.

ILIOTIBIAL BAND CONNECTION

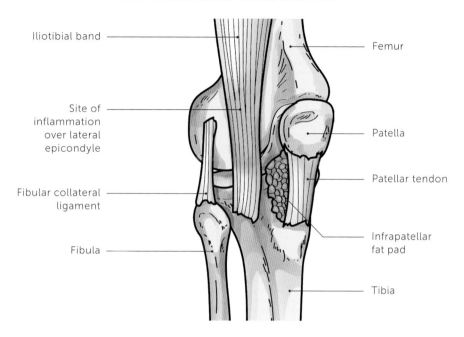

Iliotibial band

Femur

Site of inflammation over lateral epicondyle

Patella

Fibular collateral ligament

Patellar tendon

Fibula

Infrapatellar fat pad

Tibia

So now you know that compression is the main anatomical cause of IT band pain. How does this compression start? It all comes down to the way you move. Just like patellofemoral pain syndrome, research has linked problems in controlling rotational force at the knee with ITBS. In fact, studies have shown that athletes with IT band pain showed more knee internal rotation (knee cave) when their foot hit the ground compared to those without pain.[9] By now, you may be noticing a trend in how injuries occur at the knee.

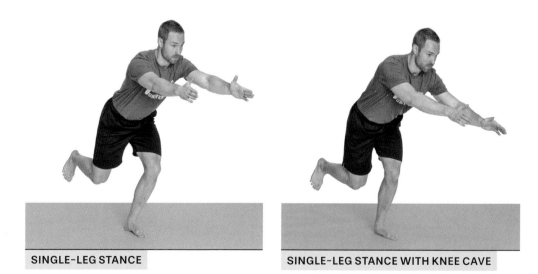

SINGLE-LEG STANCE

SINGLE-LEG STANCE WITH KNEE CAVE

Patellar/Quad Tendinopathy

When it comes to understanding patellar and quad tendon pain, things are a bit more complicated. Let's start by discussing a little anatomy.

A tendon is essentially a fibrous band of tissue that connects muscle to bone. The patellar tendon runs from the kneecap (patella) to the tibial tuberosity (the prominent bony part of your shin bone). Above the kneecap is another band of fibrous tissue, the quad tendon, which attaches to the large and strong quadriceps muscles. These two tendons work together to absorb and release tremendous power for movements such as jumping, much like a spring.

PATELLAR AND QUAD TENDON

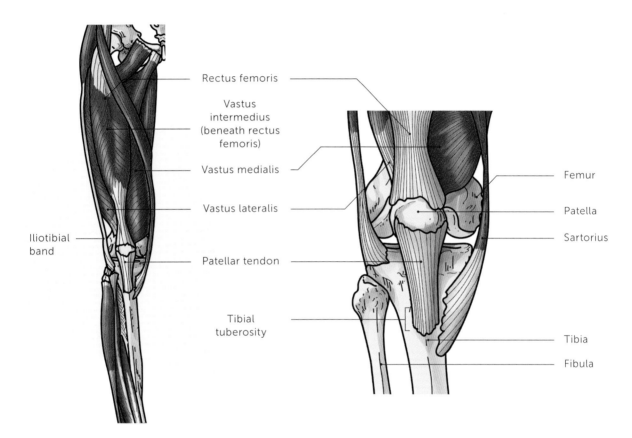

Every day, the tissues of your body—muscles, tendons, and even bones—are in a constant state of fluctuation. Every time you place stress on your body (such as when working out), tissue is broken down and then regenerated. Over time, this natural replenishing process is how strength is built.

In your tendons, this process is largely controlled by small cells called *tenocytes* that are dispersed among aligned fibers called *collagen*—type 1 collagen, to be exact. Tenocytes react to the forces and loads placed on the tendon and adapt the cellular makeup of the tissue (called the *extracellular matrix*) accordingly. Depending on several factors, such as how intensely you have trained over your years as an athlete, which medications you take, and whether you have diabetes, your body will have adapted your tendon to a certain set point of strength, known as its *load tolerance level*.

Training loads placed on the tendon that do not severely exceed this set point create a cellular response in the tendon that will return to normal in two to three days given proper recovery. This response can be seen through ultrasound imaging. The two- to three-day recovery is the normal time frame for the adaptation "replenishment" process.[10] However, if the load placed on the tendon is too extreme or the athlete's training program does not allow for adequate recovery, this balance is disrupted, and the process tips from being adaptive to pathological. A spark is lit, and the injury process begins.

Young athletes (under the age of 30) who are involved in sports that require sudden explosive and repetitive movements of the knee are the most susceptible to developing an injury at the quad or patellar tendon. Movements that use the tendons of the knee as a spring, such as a jump, place significantly more load on those tendons than a slower movement, like a squat. This is why sports such as basketball and volleyball that involve a lot of jumping have such a high incidence of this injury, hence the term "jumper's knee."

Interestingly, long-distance runners usually don't get diagnosed with patellar tendinopathy because there isn't a high enough load on the tendon to generate pain. In contrast, jumping (double and single leg) places a lot of stress on the patellar tendon.[11]

Of the two tendons at the knee, the patellar tendon is the more commonly injured. However, patellar and quad tendon pain are both prevalent in sports such as weightlifting and CrossFit due to the high forces that are sustained during the repetitive ballistic movements of the snatch and clean, as well as nonweighted repetitive movements like box jumps.

Historically, tendon injuries have been separated into two categories: tendinitis and tendinosis.[12] The *-itis* ending refers to an acute injury caused by inflammation. The *-osis* ending traditionally means that the problem is due to the tendon degrading and becoming weak. Medical practitioners often throw out the word *tendinitis* when referring to a recently painful injury and *tendinosis* when referring to more chronic tendon injuries.

However, recent research has challenged the idea that the inflammation commonly seen with tendon pain is a main driver of the injury and the pain.[13] Furthermore, leading researchers in the field of tendon injuries now believe that tendonitis and tendinosis are not mutually exclusive but are different parts of the same injury process. Therefore, when we speak about tendon injuries, it is advised to use the term *tendinopathy* rather than *tendonitis* or *tendinosis*.

The most practical way to understand how tendon injuries occur comes from the Continuum of Tendon Pathology by renowned expert Jill Cook.[14] This model describes a sequence with three overlapping stages of injury:

1. Reactive tendinopathy

2. Tendon disrepair

3. Degenerative tendinopathy

Progression from one stage to the next is met with a decreasing ability to recover to the prior healthy state.

THE CONTINUUM MODEL

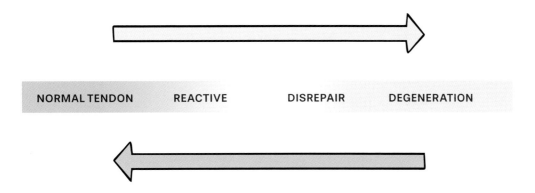

As mentioned before, when exposed to an overload of any nature, there is a short-term exaggerated response of the cells that make up the tendon. Specifically, small proteins called *proteoglycans* flood the extracellular matrix, causing the tendon to become swollen and painful. Again, this swelling is not caused by inflammation—a big reason why ice and rest alone won't fix the injury![15]

So how exactly does this overload occur? If preventing tendon injuries was as simple as not lifting more than a certain amount of weight or not lifting too frequently, how is an elite weightlifter able to pull two-a-day training sessions multiple times per week without developing pain while a novice athlete might develop this injury after training for only a few weeks? It all comes down to the individual and the relative load capacity of their tendons. Let me explain.

The human body does an amazing job of adapting to the stresses applied to it. Depending on the kind and amount of stress, the cells in our tendons can respond positively or negatively. In response to acceptable training loads, our tendons become stronger by increasing in stiffness.[16] An elite athlete who performs explosive and heavy barbell training every day with minimal rest can do so because they have deliberately conditioned their tendons over years to withstand high levels of stress. By routinely subjecting their tendons to high levels of load through proper training programs, elite athletes are able to raise the load tolerance level of their tendons.

If a relatively untrained athlete tries to perform the same higher-level training of an elite athlete, they can spark a "reactive" phase of injury—the short-term exaggerated response of the cells due to the unexpected overload. This common scenario takes place when athletes have one extremely difficult training session or jump from a three-days-a-week program to daily lifting.

The spark that sets off the reactive phase for a novice can also occur in an elite athlete. If an athlete who is able to tolerate a lot of load day in and day out took a long break from training (two or more weeks, for example) and all of a sudden jumped right back into a relatively normal training program ("normal" being relative to what they were used to), they would subject their tendons to a significant amount of unexpected stress. This is because their tendons would have become somewhat deconditioned over the extended break, adapting their tissues to a lower load capacity level.

There is no set amount of weight or number of reps of any drill that will automatically trigger this injury response; it comes down purely to whether an individual's tendon load capacity has been exceeded. Basically, any unexpected loading on the tendon can trigger a reaction, and the tendon can subsequently thicken in an attempt to handle the stress.[17] At this time, an athlete may experience pain as well as a small amount of swelling around the tendon.

Now, here's the good thing: this process is reversible if properly managed. Researchers believe that reactive tendons have the potential to return to their normal healthy state within a few weeks if the initial training load is significantly reduced and proper rehabilitation steps are taken.[18] However, if someone continues to train past this point of reactivity, the tendon will enter the disrepair stage as it continues to thicken in an attempt to heal itself. In fact, researchers have found this exaggerated repair process can cause the patellar tendon to double in thickness (from around 4 to 8 millimeters) as a protective response.[19] In reaction to the continued overload, more and more proteoglycans flood the extracellular matrix, drawing in water, which eventually starts to disrupt the architectural struts (collagen) that make up the tendon. At this point, we also see new blood vessels and nerves growing in the tendon, which may play a part in creating pain.[20]

If the proper steps are not taken to address the injury at this time, the disorganized collagen starts to break down even further and die off as the injury enters the third stage, degeneration. Unfortunately, it is very hard to distinguish whether a tendon is in disrepair. To make matters worse, you may not even know that your tendon has slipped into the third stage because the degenerated part of the tendon doesn't elicit pain.

So how do we figure out which stage of injury a tendon is in?

What researchers like Cook have found is that tendon pain is primarily a symptom of the reactive stage. For this reason, if you are currently experiencing patellar or quad tendon pain, you can stage your injury into an even simpler two-phase model of either "reactive" or "reactive on disrepair/degeneration" tendinopathy.[21]

Let's say this is the first time you've experienced patellar tendon pain. The day after a really difficult training session, your tendon hurt so badly that you were forced to limp around. Because this is an acute (brand-new) episode of tendon pain, you're likely experiencing the first stage of reactive tendinopathy.

However, let's say this is *not* the first time you've experienced patellar tendon pain. You had a small flare-up last year and another a few months ago. You took a few weeks off, and the pain eventually went away, but it keeps coming back. Due to the chronic nature of these symptoms, you are likely experiencing a case of reactive on disrepair/degeneration tendinopathy.

NORMAL, REACTIVE, AND REACTIVE ON DISREPAIR

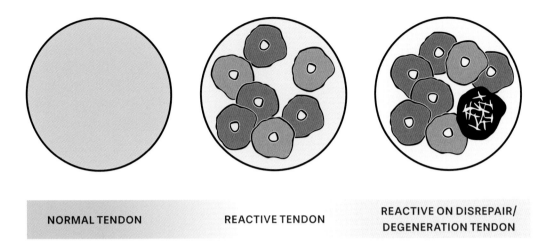

| NORMAL TENDON | REACTIVE TENDON | REACTIVE ON DISREPAIR/ DEGENERATION TENDON |

When a tendon experiences continued episodes of overload, degradation can begin, but the entire tendon doesn't just die off. If you looked deep into the tendon, you'd notice small "islands" of degenerated collagen tissue dispersed among healthy tendon tissue. These islands are unable to bear load. They usually lose tensile strength and springlike capacity, which renders them "mechanically deaf," as Cook says.[22]

Think of these islands of degenerated patellar or quad tendon fibers as holes in donuts. The holes are surrounded by healthy tissue. However, research has shown that the body will adapt and "grow" more normal tendon tissue around these dead spots in an effort to recover lost strength.[23]

NORMAL TENDON WITH DEGENERATION ISLAND

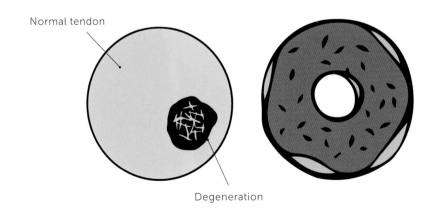

Normal tendon

Degeneration

As noted earlier, these degenerated "holes" in the tendon do not create pain.[24] It is not until the surrounding portion of healthy tissue becomes overloaded and slips into the reactive phase (in the exact same way a perfectly healthy tendon would) that pain can develop in a degenerated tendon. This is why someone could have a very degenerated tendon without experiencing any pain symptoms.[25]

Good ways to differentiate between reactive tendon pain and reactive on disrepair/degeneration tendon pain (other than a history of symptoms) are how intense the pain is, which exact mechanism set off the injury, and how long it takes to recover. For example, a truly reactive tendon is very painful and swollen. It is sparked by a severe overload, such as an extremely difficult training session filled with plyometric exercises like box jumps.

On the other hand, a reactive on disrepair/degeneration tendon can be sparked by much less dramatic activity overload and often isn't accompanied by much swelling. Pain from this particular tendinopathy can resolve in as little as a few days with proper rest, whereas truly reactive tendons can take four to eight weeks to heal.[26] Understanding which stage you're in will dramatically affect how you manage the injury.

Those with patellar tendinopathy typically complain of tenderness and pain at the connection point of the kneecap and patellar tendon, called the *inferior pole of the patella.* You might even experience pain where the patellar tendon attaches to the tibia (a small bump on the front of your shin called the *tibial tuberosity*).[27] You won't usually have pain in the center of your patellar tendon unless you've sustained a direct blow to the knee (like hitting your knee on a corner of a desk). Those with quadriceps tendinopathy will have pain and tenderness at the connection point of the kneecap and the quad tendon, called the *superior pole of the patella.*

PATELLAR TENDON

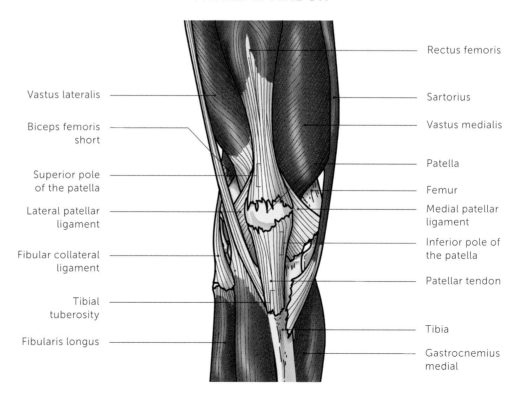

- Rectus femoris
- Vastus lateralis
- Sartorius
- Biceps femoris short
- Vastus medialis
- Superior pole of the patella
- Patella
- Lateral patellar ligament
- Femur
- Medial patellar ligament
- Fibular collateral ligament
- Inferior pole of the patella
- Tibial tuberosity
- Patellar tendon
- Fibularis longus
- Tibia
- Gastrocnemius medial

Initially, most people report feeling a dull ache in the front of the knee after an intense workout. People who have this injury typically experience pain that worsens as the load to the knee increases (for example, a repetitive tuck jump brings out more pain than a slow bodyweight squat). This is called *load-related pain*. Remember this term; it will be an important part of how we fix this injury.

Interestingly enough, the patellar and quad tendons are also placed under considerably more load in a very deep squat where the knee must move forward over the toes. For this reason, someone with either type of tendon injury may complain of pain during a loaded squat, but only at the very bottom portion of the lift.

The Mechanism of Injury

The prior sources of pain are only a few of the common anatomy-based diagnoses you may receive from a medical doctor; others include a bone bruise, meniscus tear, fat pad irritation, and plica or even bursa irritation. Unfortunately, it can be difficult for even the best clinicians to diagnose the exact anatomical structure that is causing knee pain with 100 percent certainty. Doing so requires expert assessment skills and often expensive scans of the knee joint. Luckily, you don't need to spend hundreds or even thousands of dollars to take the first steps toward understanding and addressing your pain.

What causes knee pain? The simplest answer is that the pain is the result of cumulative microtrauma on the structures of the knee caused by two things:

- Specific movements
- Excessive training loads

Every part of your body, from the small bones and joints to the large muscles that span them, has a set amount of force or load that it can tolerate before it fails and breaks. Athletes who push themselves to the brink of this tipping point without going overboard often find massive success in improving their strength and performance. If they exceed that threshold, however, injury occurs and pain sets in.

Sometimes the mechanism that triggers an injury is blatant. Take, for instance, a powerlifter who is going for a heavy PR during a competition. One of their knees collapses into extreme valgus, and they tear every ligament in their knee. Other times the trauma is slowly applied over months or years through micromovements that cannot be seen with the naked eye. For example, I have worked with many athletes who developed knee pain due to a side-to-side imbalance in hip rotation. Even to a seasoned coach, their lifting technique looked sufficient. What the coach couldn't see, however, was that limited hip internal rotation in one leg was creating microtrauma at the knee joint that eventually led to the development of pain.

While pain may strike at a specific moment, nontraumatic knee pain is usually the result of something that has been building for some time. The signs of injury are often present even before symptoms appear. For example, numerous research studies have found a connection between knee problems (like patellofemoral pain syndrome, iliotibial band syndrome, and even the development of osteoarthritis) and movement problems such as excessive hip adduction (thigh moving toward the midline of the body) and internal rotation.[28]

This means that while you may have experienced pain for the first time after a heavy squat workout last week, the cause of the injury may have been building up for a while. Therefore, the quality of your technique and how you load your body during training will always be the most important factors in whether you get stronger and find success or you fail to progress because of an injury.

If you've been told that you have one of the above injuries, don't hang your head. There is hope! Step one of fixing your injury is diving into how to screen your knee pain, which starts with evaluating the way you move.

How to Screen Your Knee Pain

The idea that flawed movement or technique leads to the development of pain has been called the *kinesiopathologic* model, or KPM.[29] While the model has a pretty fancy name that most of you will never have to remember, the theory behind it is key to fixing your pain: start by finding out which movement problems led to the development of the injury in the first place.

For hundreds of years, the traditional medical field has attempted to address pain by diagnosing the specific tissue or body part that may be injured, such as patellofemoral pain syndrome or IT band syndrome. Rather than take a medical approach to analyzing the body, we are going to go through a movement-based screening process to uncover the cause of your pain. You don't need an MRI or other expensive scans. Instead, we're going to take a step back and view how the body moves from head to toe. This way, we treat the person, not the injury.

Here's a brief example of this concept at work. Selena is an 18-year-old avid weightlifter. She has competed for 8 years and is on the cusp of qualifying for her first international team. In the weeks leading up to an important national competition, she begins to feel pain in her right knee—a dull ache around the inside of her kneecap. At first, she felt it only when lifting heavy, but it has progressed to the point where she feels it on almost every lift. Despite endless foam rolling, the pain never seems to go away, so she decides to see her family doctor. After listening to Selena's story, the doctor gives her a diagnosis of patellofemoral pain syndrome, gives her a prescription for anti-inflammatories, and tells her to cut back on lifting for a few weeks.

Does this story sound familiar to you?

While rest and medication often decrease symptoms, they do nothing to address *why* the pain started in the first place. This is the reason many who find themselves in this situation see their pain return when they go back to lifting.

When Selena came to see me for an examination, I started the screening process by having her perform some basic movements. During her bodyweight squat, everything looked great. She began with a sufficient hip hinge and controlled her body to full depth and back to the standing position with optimal technique.

However, when I asked her to perform a simple single-leg squat, things started to break down. While she had good control of her left knee, her right knee collapsed inward, and her pain was re-created. However, with some proper cuing, she was able to control her knee a little better and reported feeling less pain.

Further screening revealed that she had great mobility in her lower body (ankles and hips) but limited strength in her lateral right hip muscles compared to her left. Therefore, her movement problem was due to a stability deficit—weakness/coordination problem of these muscles turning on at the appropriate time and intensity.

Screening and classifying based on movement problems that cause pain (an issue with knee control or a "biomechanical dysfunction") is more useful for driving the treatment process than the pathoanatomical diagnosis. If we concentrate on the fact that Selena has an injury to the patellofemoral joint (PFPS), then we miss the big picture. Knowing that she has a patellofemoral joint injury doesn't necessarily tell me *why* she has pain or *what* needs to be corrected.

Therefore, instead of labeling Selena as a person with a patellofemoral joint injury, I would classify her injury as "right knee pain due to a biomechanical dysfunction with a stability deficit." By switching the focus to a movement diagnosis, we can then address her deficits and correct the technique/movement problem.

During the screening process, I want you to think about which of the following categories best describes your knee pain. While physical therapists use other movement diagnoses to categorize injuries, I find the following to be the most common among strength athletes:

- Biomechanical dysfunction
  - Mobility deficiency
  - Stability deficiency
- Load intolerance

Gather clues from each of the screens and tests that follow to help you figure out what type of movement or load triggers your knee pain. The understanding you receive from this self-assessment will empower you to take control of your injury and become your own best advocate for alleviating your pain.

Movement Screening

Grab a friend or videorecord yourself performing the following tests so you can analyze how you're moving.

Bodyweight Squat

You're going to start by performing a squat. Make sure to take off your socks and shoes to expose any problems that occur at the foot/ankle.

In your normal squat stance, perform a slow squat to full depth and hold the bottom position for a few seconds. Slowly return to the start position and then perform five more repetitions. What did you notice? Did you feel any pain? If you did, take note of where the pain was located and how intense it was on a scale of 0 to 10,

0 being no pain and 10 being the worst pain you could imagine. Both of these factors will come in handy later in the screening process.

As you analyze your movement, notice the position of your feet. Is one foot more angled out than the other? If you try to keep your feet firmly planted, does one foot spin out to the side as you descend into the squat? If so, make a mental note, because this may be due to a mobility imbalance between your right and left hip and/or ankle (something we'll screen for soon).

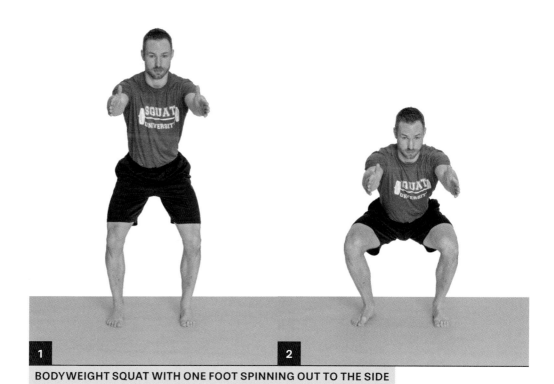

BODYWEIGHT SQUAT WITH ONE FOOT SPINNING OUT TO THE SIDE

Also observe the position of your hips. Did your hips shift to one side or the other? If you videorecord your squat from behind, does your pelvis seem uneven in the bottom position, with one side higher than the other?

Single-Leg Squat

If you easily passed the bodyweight squat, let's make things a little harder. Stand on one leg and perform a single-leg squat, going as deep as you can without falling over or using anything to assist your balance. What happened?

If you found it difficult to balance and squat on one leg without the arch of your foot collapsing (excessive pronation) and your knee waving around like crazy, you've uncovered a stability problem that you may not have noticed in your double-leg squat. In my experience, many strong athletes can "hide" problems with stability when they perform a bodyweight squat. However, some of these athletes fail a single-leg squat on one side but pass on the other side! You can uncover a laundry list of stability/mobility issues with a single-leg squat screen.

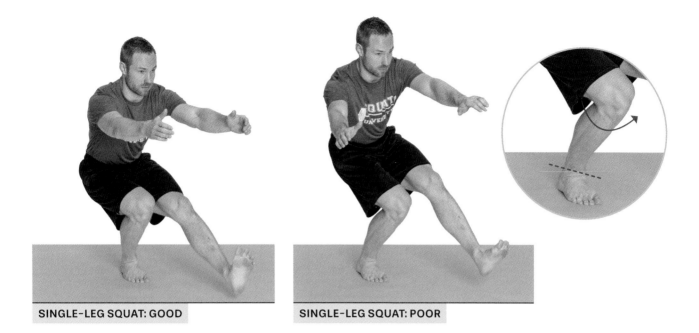

SINGLE-LEG SQUAT: GOOD

SINGLE-LEG SQUAT: POOR

Understanding the importance of stability when it comes to keeping your knees healthy starts with focusing attention on the foot. You see, the foot is like your body's house of cards. Good foot stability sets the foundation for the rest of your body to move. When the foot collapses (excessive pronation), it leads to rotation in the tibia that forces the patella to move off-axis.[30]

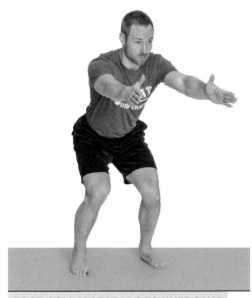
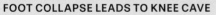

FOOT COLLAPSE LEADS TO KNEE CAVE

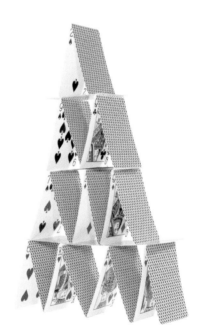

The hip also plays a crucial role in providing stability to the knee joint. Observe what happens to your thigh as you perform a single-leg squat. Does it shift inward (a motion called *adduction*) or even rotate inward toward your other leg (internal rotation)? These problems are often due to poor hip coordination. If the muscles on the side and back of your hip (glute medius and glute max) don't turn on at the right time and maintain sufficient activation during a motion like the squat, your knee will collapse inward toward the midline of your body. This motion increases contact pressure on the back side of your patella against the femur *and* increases compression of the IT band against the lateral knee.

Think about opening and closing a door. The movement of the metal hinge that connects the door to its frame operates similarly to your knee joint. When you pull on the door handle, the door opens smoothly. However, what would happen if you simultaneously pulled upward while pulling the handle toward you? The door obviously wouldn't open nearly as smoothly. This is because the hinge is being pulled off-axis. These same uneven forces are placed on the knee joint when it moves out of ideal alignment during a squat.

If you videorecorded and viewed your single-leg squat from the side, what did you notice? While knee cave is the most obvious movement fault during a squat, we must also consider how the body is moving in a forward-and-back plane of motion (called the *sagittal plane*). I find that many athletes with knee pain have a difficult time engaging their posterior chain muscles and don't hinge at the hips optimally when initiating a double-leg or single-leg squat. While the knee and hip joint should flex at the same time as you descend, jamming the knee forward excessively at the very start can increase compressive forces on the patella. As you can see, there are many factors to consider when breaking down and analyzing movement.

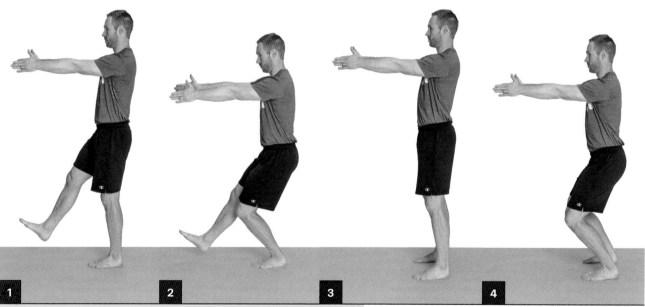

1 **2** **3** **4**

SINGLE- AND DOUBLE-LEG SQUATS WITH FORWARD KNEE TRAVEL

If you noticed knee pain with the single-leg squat, see if you can modify it by changing the way you move. Using a mirror will give you helpful feedback on what your foot, knee, or hip is doing.

Start by creating a stable foot with your big toe jammed into the floor. Attempt to grab the ground with your foot to create sufficient stability. Next, initiate a small single-leg squat by pushing your hips back and bringing your chest forward in a hinging action. Your knee will bend slightly during this hinge, but your shin will not shift forward. If you do this correctly, your foot should not move whatsoever, and your body weight should be centered directly over the middle of your foot. As you continue to squat, try to keep your knee from wobbling. Your kneecap should point directly toward your second to fourth toes.

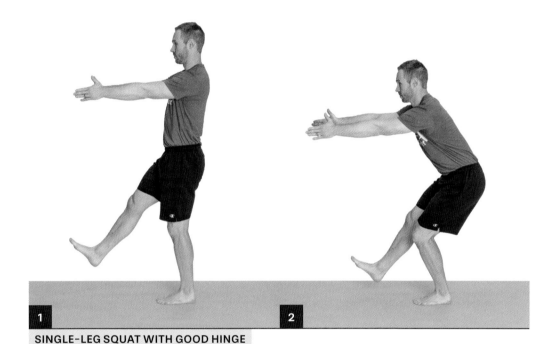

SINGLE-LEG SQUAT WITH GOOD HINGE

What did you notice? If retesting your single-leg squat with cues to create a proper hip hinge and maintain better knee control decreases your symptoms, you're likely dealing with a biomechanical dysfunction due to a stability deficit. Prioritizing a movement diagnosis over a pathoanatomical diagnosis will make your treatment more focused and efficient. Your recovery time should be shorter since you are less obsessed about the painful site and more driven to fix mobility or stability deficits—which are two things that an athlete actually has control over.

Mobility Screening

While it is sometimes easy to identify a biomechanical dysfunction due to a stability deficit with movements like the single-leg squat, mobility deficits are often a little less noticeable. I have worked with many patients who failed to make significant progress in fixing their knee pain because they addressed only strength/stability problems. They were never screened for underlying mobility deficits! No matter how much strength and stability work you perform to improve knee control, pain often persists until a mobility problem is also addressed. The two most common mobility deficits that can lead to biomechanical dysfunction are found at the joints directly above and below the knee: the hip and ankle.

Hip Mobility

To assess hip mobility, I like to use the supine hip rotation screen. The goal of this screen is to uncover any side-to-side differences in hip internal or external rotation. Lacking hip rotation in either direction will cause the patella to sit and move awkwardly against the femur. Over time, this abnormal tracking—much like a train being pulled off the tracks—can lead to pain on the front of the knee.[31] Flip to pages 52 and 53 in the Back Pain chapter to go through this assessment and see what you find.

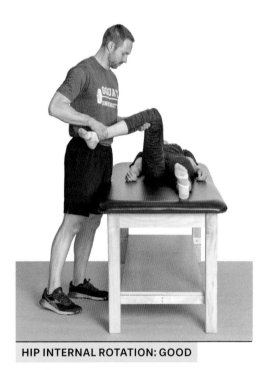

HIP INTERNAL ROTATION: GOOD

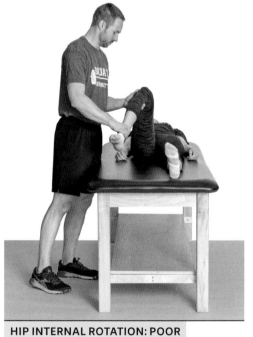

HIP INTERNAL ROTATION: POOR

While asymmetries are normal in most people, if you find a significant difference in hip rotation between your painful and nonpainful side (larger than 10 degrees, for example), you have uncovered a weak link in hip mobility that needs to be addressed. Flip to the Hip Pain chapter for some of my favorite mobility exercises for the hip to clear up rotation problems.

I recommend a simple test-retest method to see if the mobility exercise you choose is right for your body. Videorecord the supine hip rotation screen and then perform the suggested hip mobility exercises in the Hip Pain chapter (see pages 149 to 151). Immediately retest and see if you made any significant changes. If so, also retest your double- and single-leg squats and notice if you have less pain. If so, you just confirmed that your knee pain can be classified as "biomechanical dysfunction with a mobility deficit."

Ankle Mobility

Testing ankle mobility should also be a part of the screening process when dealing with a knee injury. If the gastroc and/or soleus muscles are stiff or short, there is less range of motion to absorb load during activities such as landing from a jump. For example, research shows that between 37 and 50 percent of the total force absorbed by the body when landing from a jump occurs at the ankle joint.[32] Ankle stiffness reduces the body's capacity to absorb energy in this manner, which means that higher loads are transferred upward to the knee. Therefore, structures like the patellar tendon are placed under greater strain as the tendon must take more load more quickly when landing from a jump or receiving a clean or snatch, increasing the risk of injuries like tendinopathy.[33]

Limited ankle mobility can also play a part in changing your ability to stabilize the knee when lifting.[34] In his book *Anatomy for Runners,* physical therapist Jay Dicharry uses a perfect metaphor to describe how these types of restrictions alter movement patterns.[35]

An ankle with full mobility allows the tibia to move freely on the foot. Think of it like a car being able to travel straight through an intersection. A restriction in ankle mobility is like a European-style roundabout in the middle of the road. When the car enters the intersection, it must go around the island before proceeding along its route. Essentially, the lower leg spins off its normal route and collapses inward. As the lower leg goes around the restriction, the knee is pulled inward. Movement breaks down. Therefore, limited ankle mobility is a potential factor in the development of a biomechanical dysfunction.

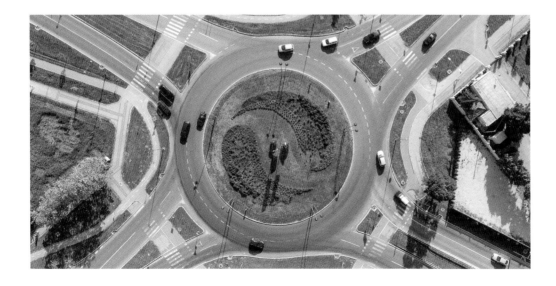

The 5-inch wall test is a simple screen that you can perform on your own.[36] Kneel down facing a wall and place your toes 5 inches from its base. Drive your knee straight forward over your toes, attempting to touch the wall without letting your heel pop up off the ground.

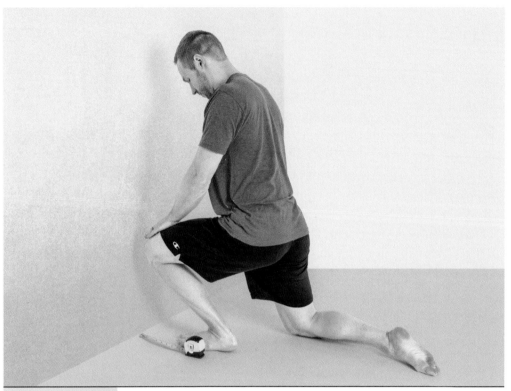

5-INCH WALL TEST

Were you able to touch the wall with your knee, or did your heel pull up off the ground first? If you failed the 5-inch wall test, you have uncovered a weak link in ankle mobility that needs to be addressed. Make sure to check out the ankle mobility exercises (foam rolling/stretching of the calf and joint mobilizations) discussed in the Ankle Pain chapter. Working every day to improve this mobility should be a priority if you wish to return to lifting pain-free!

As with the hip, make sure to perform the test-retest method with the ankle. Record your 5-inch wall test by measuring the distance from your knee to the wall. Perform the recommended ankle mobility exercises and then immediately retest to see if you have made any significant progress. Also retest your double- and single-leg squats to see if you notice improvements.

Load Screening

If you have pain when performing a bodyweight squat, it is important to figure out if it is due to a biomechanical dysfunction or if you are dealing with a tendinopathy. First, ask yourself, "Do I have pain when resting or only when moving?" Tendinopathies *rarely* hurt when you are completely at rest.[37] This is because sitting or lying down removes the load on the tendon.

If you have pain only when moving, you should perform more testing to confirm the idea that you may be dealing with a tendinopathy. Perform 10 double-leg tuck jumps in a row, jumping as high off the ground as you can, without resting between jumps. Did the intensity of your pain increase from the rating you gave your symptoms when performing the bodyweight squat at the start of the screening process?

If you can, perform 10 single-leg tuck jumps in a row. Did your knee pain increase again? If so, we can say that your pain is load intolerant. The bodyweight squat puts very little load through the knee compared to the springlike forces generated at the tendons during multiple tuck jumps. Performing single-leg tuck jumps places even *more* load on your patellar and quad tendons than the double-leg version.

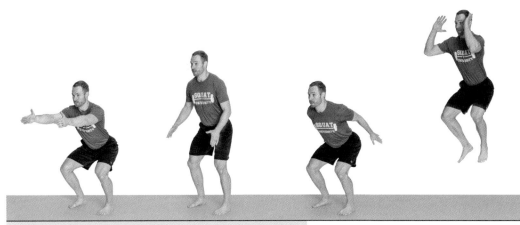

LOAD TOLERANCE TESTING: DOUBLE-LEG TUCK JUMP

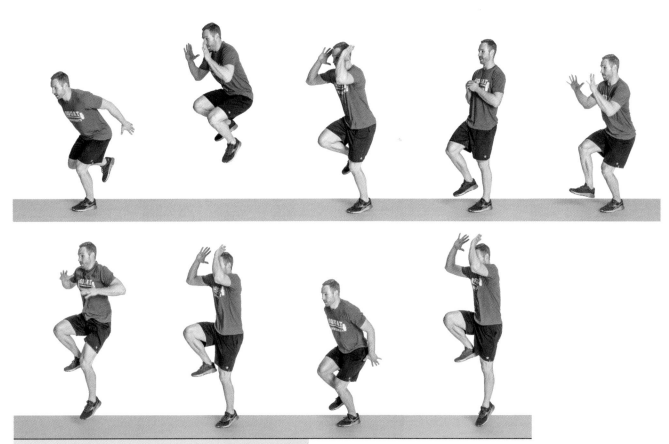

LOAD TOLERANCE TESTING: SINGLE-LEG TUCK JUMP

If your pain did increase in each of the prior steps, did the pain remain localized to the inferior pole (bottom tip) of the kneecap, or did it begin to spread to other parts of the knee joint over time? Pain that moves around the knee, sometimes on the inside and sometimes on the bottom by the patellar tendon, is often a symptom of a biomechanical dysfunction. On the other hand, pain that remains pinpointed to one specific area during these tests is a sign of a tendinopathy. A biomechanical dysfunction rarely coexists with a load intolerance problem like that seen with patellar or quad tendinopathy, so make sure you can clearly answer each of the prior questions to decipher which type of injury you're dealing with.[38]

Single-Leg Bridge Screen

It is common to see strength deficits and coordination issues in how the muscles are activated at the hip in athletes dealing with knee pain. In my experience, these athletes often have weak glutes, or their glutes have timing/coordination issues. A simple screen to expose this weakness is the single-leg bridge.

Lie on your back with one leg bent and the other straight. Elevate your hips and hold the highest position for 10 seconds. Which muscles did you feel working hard after holding this bridge?

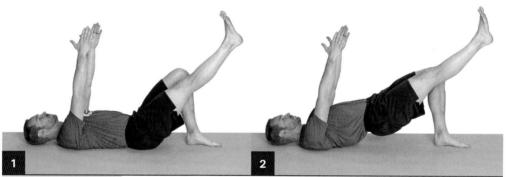

SINGLE-LEG BRIDGE

The goal of this screen is to identify your go-to muscles for hip extension (the movement that drives you out of the bottom of a squat, clean, snatch, and so on). If you felt anything other than your glutes working hard, you have a coordination and/ or strength problem to work on.

When Is It Time to See a Doctor?

Locking or clicking of your knee, significant swelling, tingling, numbness, or throbbing in the back of your knee likely indicates a more significant problem that requires an evaluation by a medical professional, such as a sports physical therapist or an orthopedic medical doctor.

The Rebuilding Process

There is no one-size-fits-all approach to fixing knee pain. Everyone responds differently based on their individual cause for pain. What may help decrease pain in one person may increase pain in another. The screening process outlined in the preceding section should highlight whether you have a stability issue or a mobility issue. You may also discover that you have a load intolerance problem at the patellar or quad tendon. Classifying your pain into one of these categories should help you take the next step toward finding a real fix.

Mobility First

A mobility restriction at the hip and/or ankle can lead to movement compensations at the knee. For this reason, if you perform only stability exercises and never address mobility restrictions at the hip or ankle, your pain will probably persist despite your best efforts.

Hip and ankle mobility exercises can be found in the Hip Pain and Ankle Pain chapters of this book. To make sure you have found the right exercise (or combination of exercises) for your body, use the test–retest method. The screen that uncovers your imbalance/restriction will serve as your baseline measurement. Next, perform a mobility exercise that targets that specific problem area. Immediately retest and see if you notice any significant changes. If you do, you have succeeded in finding a helpful exercise to address your restriction. I recommend performing 5 to 10 minutes of mobility work specific to what your body requires every day.

After performing mobility exercises for the hip and/or ankle joints, you can address any possible stiffness in the tissues that lie directly above the knee. If the tissues of the lateral leg (such as the vastus lateralis of the quads) become stiff, they can pull excessively on the kneecap, tilting it on its side and causing it to track laterally in the groove. Using a foam roller to perform soft tissue mobilization is a great way to address stiffness in your quads.

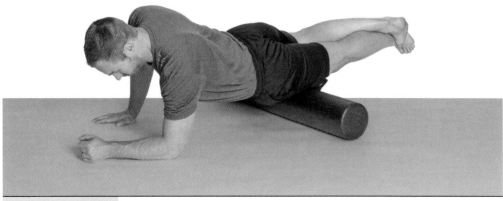

FOAM ROLL QUADS

Start by lying prone and place the foam roller under your quad, just above the kneecap. Slowly roll up and down to identify tender spots. Make sure to pause when you find a trigger point to allow that muscle to downregulate/release. You can also move to the inner thigh, the lateral leg, and up to the hip (TFL muscle). Go slowly when rolling, and spend some extra time on areas that feel stiff or painful, holding pressure on these tender areas for 30 to 60 seconds at a time.[39]

Many people ask whether they should foam-roll the IT band. When I was in physical therapy school, we dissected cadavers and physically cut into the IT band in the anatomy lab. Let me tell you, the IT band is an *extremely thick* piece of tissue. For this reason, deep tissue work like foam-rolling isn't likely to make a ton of change in tension. However, the IT band also has fascial connections to many other muscles of the lower leg, which are like a spider web of connective tissue that encapsulates and connects all the muscles of the body.

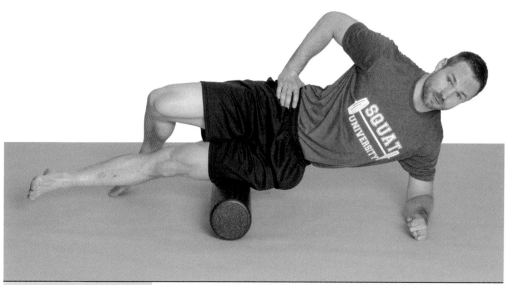

FOAM-ROLL LATERAL LEG

When foam-rolling your lateral leg, you're not *only* hitting your IT band. You're also rolling over tissues that connect to the IT band, such as the vastus lateralis (lateral quad), biceps femoris (lateral hamstrings), glutes, and TFL. Restrictions in these muscles can contribute to excessive tension on the IT band.[40] Trigger points in these muscles can even refer pain to the lateral part of the knee, mimicking the symptoms of IT band syndrome. For this reason, foam-rolling the lateral thigh to address restrictions in these connections can be extremely beneficial for decreasing lateral knee pain. That being said, I wouldn't roll over a painful spot on the outside of your knee! Extreme compression on that area of inflammation (where the IT band attaches) could exacerbate your symptoms.

Improving Knee Stability

When it comes to strengthening and stabilizing the knee joint, there are two common approaches: local and global.

Local approaches focus treatment at the site of symptoms. For example, some clinicians believe that knee pain can be caused by weakness in the VMO (inner quad muscle) based on research showing inhibition of this area of the quad in some subjects with patellofemoral pain syndrome. Due to the way its fibers run, the VMO works in sync with the lateral quads (vastus lateralis) to stabilize the kneecap and keep it tracking in proper alignment. For this reason, improper firing of this muscle is associated with tracking problems of the kneecap. Based on this notion, some clinicians recommend rehabilitation exercises that aim to strengthen the VMO in isolation, such as seated knee extensions, straight-leg raises, or wall sits while squeezing a ball between the knees.

QUAD ANATOMY

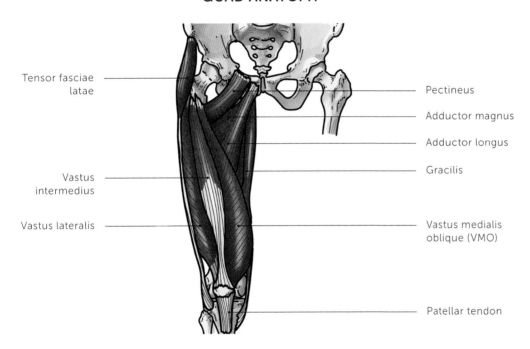

Tensor fasciae latae

Pectineus

Adductor magnus

Adductor longus

Gracilis

Vastus intermedius

Vastus lateralis

Vastus medialis oblique (VMO)

Patellar tendon

This theory is flawed. First, even if the VMO was shut down (relative to the other quad muscles), research shows that it *cannot* be strengthened in isolation! Contrary to what you may have read in the past, the VMO is *not* capable of firing independently.[41] When you contract your quad, the *entire quad* contracts.

The research is clear, however, that strength-based exercises are key for successful rehabilitation of a biomechanical dysfunction.[42] It comes down to choosing the *right* exercises. An "open chain" exercise is performed without bearing weight (such as a seated knee extension). A "closed chain" exercise is performed while bearing weight (such as a squat).

Closed chain exercises have two distinct advantages over open chain movements for fixing a biomechanical dysfunction. First, closed chain movements often create less compression and irritation on the patellofemoral joint. Let me explain why.

Many people assume that the entire kneecap remains in constant contact with the femur during movement. However, nothing could be further from the truth! As the knee flexes, the amount of contact between the back of the kneecap and the femur is constantly changing.[43] The more your knee bends, the more contact there is between these two bones, and any force placed on the knee can therefore be distributed over a greater surface area.

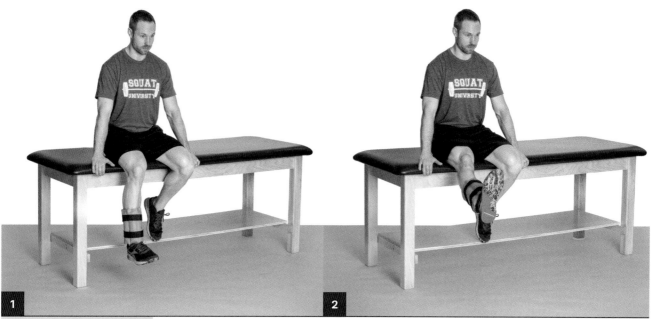

SEATED KNEE EXTENSION

If you're doing an exercise like a seated knee extension (open chain), your knee is moving from a flexed to an extended position. This means the amount of contact between the kneecap and femur in the groove is constantly getting smaller. The contraction of the quads to extend the lower leg pushes the kneecap into the femur, causing more compression. Therefore, the contraction of the quads places a high amount of compressive force on the joint that is distributed over a very small area under the kneecap. If the area under the kneecap is already inflamed and irritated, an exercise like this will only make things worse.

For this reason, you want to stick with exercises that can strengthen your quads but *also* spread the force of the joint compression across a greater surface area under the kneecap. Closed chain exercises have been shown to allow for more optimal loading and better tracking of the kneecap in the femoral groove than open chain exercises, potentially leading to less joint irritation for those dealing with certain kinds of knee pain.[44] For most people, a closed chain exercise such as a bodyweight squat to a pain-free depth is a better choice than an open chain knee extension.

If squatting to full depth is painful for you, modifying your depth early in the rehab process will be necessary. Never push into pain for the sake of achieving a full-depth squat. While your body dissipates compressive forces over a wider surface area during the squat compared to a seated knee extension, a deep squat still places a considerable amount of force on the knee joint. Research has shown that compression of the patella increases as the knee bends, maxing out at around 90 to 100 degrees of knee flexion.[45] For this reason, you want to start with bodyweight squats to a pain-free depth. As you work toward squatting to full depth without knee pain, you can slowly reintroduce the barbell (or any other load, such as a goblet squat) into your training.

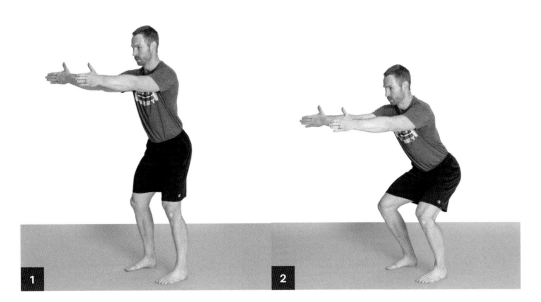

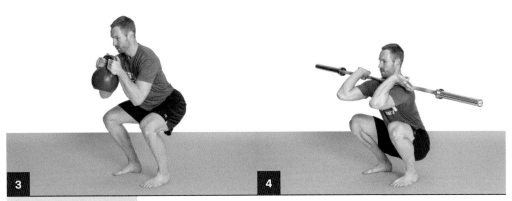

SQUAT PROGRESSION

The second reason closed chain exercises are more optimal than open chain exercises for rehabbing a biomechanical dysfunction is that they take a holistic approach to treating the full body but in a *functional* manner. Here's what I mean.

The lateral muscles of your hip "turn on" and control the position of your knee during movements like squatting, landing from a jump, and running. This is why research has linked lateral hip muscle weakness to poor knee mechanics, patellofemoral pain syndrome, and IT band syndrome.[46]

Some people will read that last line and think, "If the lateral hips are weak, we just have to strengthen them, and that will fix the knee control problem." This is why you often see side-lying exercises like clamshells and straight-leg raises prescribed. While these exercises can be helpful early in the rehab process when pain levels are very high, you eventually need to move past exercises like these to build the capacity of your lateral hip muscles. Let me explain.

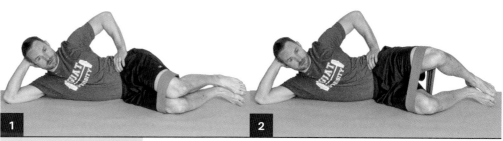

SIDE-LYING CLAMSHELL

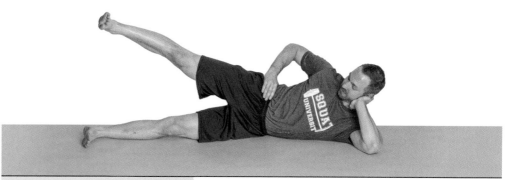

SIDE-LYING STRAIGHT-LEG RAISE

Research has shown that poor knee mechanics when landing from a jump can sometimes be altered with verbal instruction alone (e.g., "don't let your knees cave in").[47] These findings suggest that the quality of an athlete's lifting technique and ability to limit poor mechanics is often a "choice" and a learned movement pattern rather than *purely* a result of hip muscle weakness.

If hip muscle weakness was the *only* cause of poor knee control, then we would expect to see problematic movement patterns when simply overloading the muscles with a demanding task. However, this isn't always the case. For example, researchers have found poor mechanics to occur when running (a movement where the muscular demand at the hip is relatively low) in athletes dealing with IT band pain.[48] Studies have shown that people with patellofemoral pain often demonstrate poor landing strategies with single-leg hops.[49]

So what does this mean?

It means that improving knee control involves *more* than just strengthening weak muscles. Fixing a biomechanical dysfunction requires the use of exercises that improve both strength (the ability to produce force) *and* stability (the ability to limit excessive and unwanted motion).

Closed chain exercises such as a single-leg squat address both strength and stability. They incorporate lateral hip strength *and* lower body stability through movements that improve proprioception (the ability to sense and be aware of body position) and neuromuscular control (the unconscious response of the body to maintain stability). Therefore, a combination of strength exercises with movement reeducation is the optimal solution for improving knee stability.[50]

I want to introduce to you a five-step process for improving knee stability:

1. Correct squat technique from the ground up

2. Reawaken the glutes

3. Learn to single-leg squat

4. Improve your balance

5. Enhance lower body control

The Ground-Up Approach

The first move in addressing unstable knees is to correct squatting technique by establishing proper foot position. When you squat, lunge, receive a clean, or press a barbell overhead, your foot needs to be stable and maintain its natural arch. The arch of the foot moves in relation to the rest of the lower body. If the ankle, knee, and hip bow outward, the entire foot moves into a full arched position. If the ankle, knee, and hip fall inward, the foot collapses and the arch flattens out. This means you can manipulate the position of your feet by setting your hips and knees in a good position before initiating a squat.

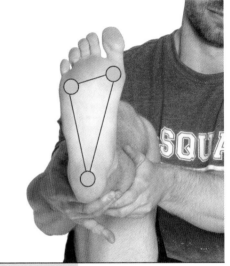

TRIPOD FOOT

Creating a good arch in your foot forms what is called a "tripod foot." The three points of the tripod are the heel, the base of the first toe, and the base of the fifth toe.

The foot is like a three-wheeled motorcycle. Your goal when squatting is to maintain the arch of your feet and distribute your weight evenly—like the three wheels of a motorcycle. If all three wheels are in contact with the ground, you get more power. If one wheel is lifted off the ground, or if the body of the motorcycle bottoms out, power is lost and the vehicle breaks down. Similarly, stability and power are lost when the foot is out of position (e.g., when the arch collapses).

Take off your shoes and assume a squat stance. Notice the position of your feet. Do you have equal weight on each of the three tripod points? Is your arch in a good position, or has it already collapsed? The goal is to become aware of how your feet are functioning.

From this position, squeeze your glutes and drive your knees out to the side while keeping your big toes in contact with the ground. Again, notice the position of your feet. Did anything change? Setting your knees in a stable position naturally brings your feet into a good position.

As you squat, do your best to maintain the tripod foot. Keep your foot strong and stable. Don't let the arch collapse. Notice how this feels. Your squat should feel more stable.

One of the most common cues coaches use is "drive your knees out." This cue teaches athletes to engage their hips properly and keep their knees from collapsing inward as they squat. However, it must be followed with "and keep your feet firmly planted." I find that some athletes overperform this cue and push their knees out too far without maintaining the tripod foot. Their weight shifts to the outside of the foot, allowing the base of the big toe to become unglued from the floor. Make sure your big toe remains firmly planted into the ground.

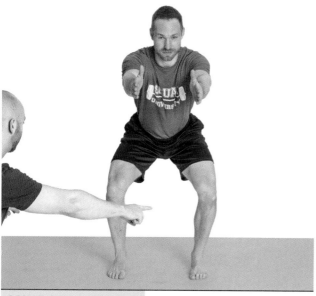

SQUAT WITH KNEES OUT

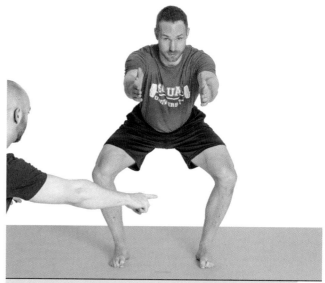

SQUAT WITH KNEES TOO FAR OUT & UNSTABLE FEET

After you adopt a better foot position, a lot of the other movement problems you have will take care of themselves. The body naturally starts to assume better positions because it is moving from a stable platform. Doing so not only improves movement quality but also decreases pain *and* improves performance. It all starts with solidifying the base.

For most athletes, I recommend performing 2 or 3 sets of 20 bodyweight squats to a pain-free depth every day. As your symptoms subside and your squat depth improves, you can slowly start adding weight.

If you can easily perform bodyweight squats and even light barbell squats without pain, you may continue to train, but be conscious of your technique and your symptoms. Remember, pushing through pain when lifting will only make things worse.

Reawaken the Glutes

The glutes (specifically the glute max) have two main jobs: hip extension and postural stability. Recall the single-leg bridge screen from page 194. Did you feel your glutes working the hardest on both sides, or did you feel a side-to-side difference—maybe your quads or hamstrings were working harder on the right side while the left side was all glutes? If this second option sounds like you, then you have a problem turning on the correct muscles at the right time.

If you felt your hamstrings cramping, your hamstrings are working double-time to produce hip extension because your glutes aren't pulling their weight. If you felt your quads working hard, you probably aren't sufficiently activating your posterior chain as you move.

When your body doesn't fire muscles in the proper sequence, it leads to inefficient movement that overloads certain parts of the body, creating microtrauma. Over time, this microtrauma can lead to a nagging injury. This is why some athletes develop pain. I recommend addressing inefficient glute activation with the double-leg bridge. Flip to page 74 in the Back Pain chapter and follow the instructions for performing this exercise. Once you master the double-leg bridge, you can progress to single-leg bridges.

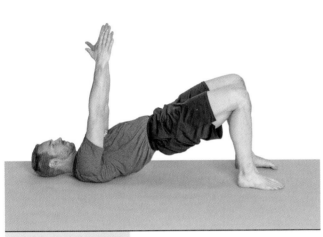

DOUBLE-LEG BRIDGE

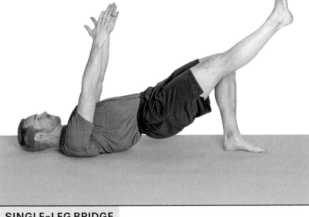

SINGLE-LEG BRIDGE

Just like a double-leg squat, many athletes can hide their glute activation problems with a double-leg bridge. If you have problems that are apparent on one side, try performing 15 to 20 single-leg bridges before training, focusing on holding the elevated position for 5 to 10 seconds and squeezing your glutes as hard as you can. Your goal is to get each side to activate equally.

I experienced a bout of knee pain years ago that I could not resolve until I applied this technique. The pain was located just above my patella. I tried *everything* I could think of: addressing technique, doing single-leg and Spanish squats, dry needling, soft tissue scraping, and more. It wasn't until I performed a single-leg bridge on each leg that my problem was exposed. On my pain-free leg, I could easily feel my glutes working hard. However, when bridging on my painful side, I noticed less glute activity and lateral quad activation! After I performed single-leg bridges for a week and focused hard on shifting the emphasis back into my glutes, my pain went away, and I was back to lifting.

LATERAL BAND WALK

As discussed earlier, the lateral hip muscles (primarily the gluteus medius) play an important role in stabilizing the knee. When you squat, land from a jump, or run, these muscles ensure that the knee stays in line with the foot and doesn't cave in. One of my favorite exercises for strengthening the lateral hip muscles is the lateral band walk.

The name of this exercise tells you pretty much everything you need to know about how to perform it. To start, place an elastic band around your knees or ankles. (Placing the band around your knees makes the exercise easier to perform.) Sit into a mini squat and screw your feet into the ground. Next, drive laterally through your trail leg. Keep constant tension on the band and make sure to take small steps. This exercise works the lateral hip muscles (specifically the glute medius) as they were designed to function, as a pelvis and hip stabilizer.

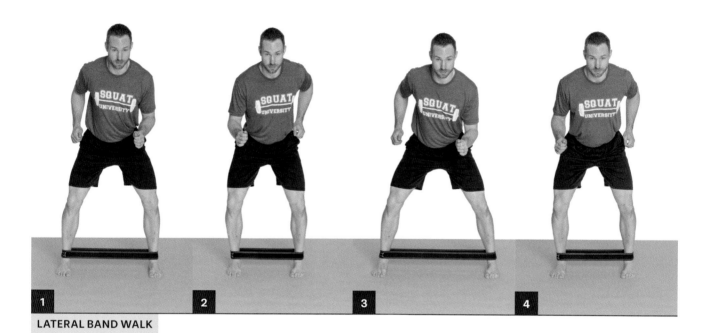

LATERAL BAND WALK

After walking 15 to 20 feet, stop and walk back the other direction. Eventually, you will start to feel fatigue in your lateral hip muscles.

UNILATERAL ABDUCTION

While the lateral band walk is a great exercise for addressing lateral hip strength/ stability while on two feet, you also need to address this "weak link" while in a single-leg stance. Unilateral hip abduction (a lateral kick out to the side) is a great exercise for working on single-leg balance while addressing glute medius strength.

To start, place an elastic band around your ankles. Stand on one leg before performing a mini squat on that leg. Push your hips backward and allow your chest to move forward. This small movement allows you to engage your posterior chain and remain balanced. The cue that I like to use to solidify this idea for every squat, even small ones like this, is "squat with the hips, not with the knees."

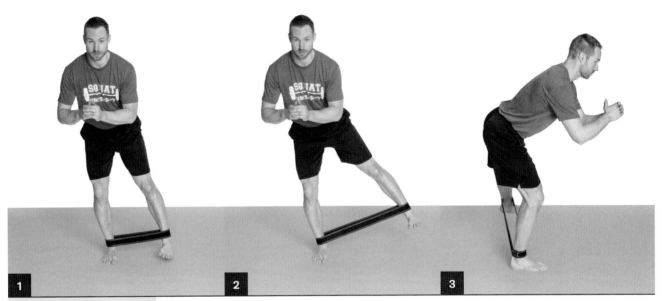

UNILATERAL ABDUCTION

Once you are in position, kick the non-stance leg out to the side and back in a slow, controlled manner. The distance your leg moves is *not* your main concern. Keep your focus on maintaining your stance leg in a stable and unwavering position throughout the entire exercise. Kick only as far as you can while keeping your pelvis level. Your ability to keep your pelvis from tipping and your stance leg from wobbling around as you kick is controlled by your lateral hip muscles (glute medius) working in tandem with a stable core. If you do this exercise correctly, you'll feel a good burn in the lateral hip muscles of your stance leg. You'll also feel your glutes on the kicking side.

Recommended sets/reps: 2 or 3 sets of 15 to 20 reps

Learn to Single-Leg Squat

In pursuit of squatting ridiculously heavy weight, you should strive to attain and maintain a quality single-leg squat. If you neglect unilateral training, you are likely to develop asymmetries in mobility/strength/stability and open yourself up to sustaining an injury. Implementing single-leg squats into your training is a good way to stay healthy. It can also be helpful for identifying any issues in knee control throughout your lifting career.

That being said, not every athlete needs to be able to perform a full-depth pistol squat. Doing so requires *amazing* mobility. However, *everyone* should have the ability to perform a quality single-leg squat to a height of 8 to 12 inches. This movement is called a *touchdown.*

If you're at the gym, you can stack one or two weighted plates. Assume a single-leg stance on top of the plates. From this position, drive your hips backward and bring your chest forward. This movement allows you to engage your posterior chain. If you do it correctly, you should feel a slight tension in your glute and hamstring muscles. Bringing your chest forward while driving your hips back will bring you into a balanced position with your body weight over the middle of your foot.

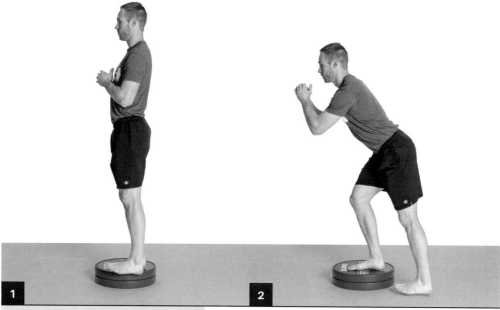

TOUCHDOWN SQUAT (TWO PLATES)

While keeping your knee in line with your foot, squat down until the heel of your free leg gently taps the floor before returning to the start position. I like to use the cue "pretend like you're tapping your heel softly onto an eggshell; don't break it!" If you are doing this exercise correctly, you will feel your glutes working hard after a few reps. You should *not* feel any pain or stiffness in your knee. If you do have pain, try using a smaller stack of plates or a box so that your touchdown is not as deep.

As you squat, focus not only on your knee but also on the position of your hips. Doing this movement in front of a full-length mirror can be helpful at first so you can see in real time what is happening at your pelvis. Most people who develop knee pain (regardless of whether it is around the front of the knee or even on the lateral aspect near the IT band attachment) are unable to keep their hips level and will allow the hip of their free leg to drop during the squat—often a compensation for poor coordination/strength of the glute medius in the stance leg.

It's also common to see the knee rotate inward toward the big toe. Work to keep your hips level and your knee in line with your third or fourth toe during the execution of this squat.

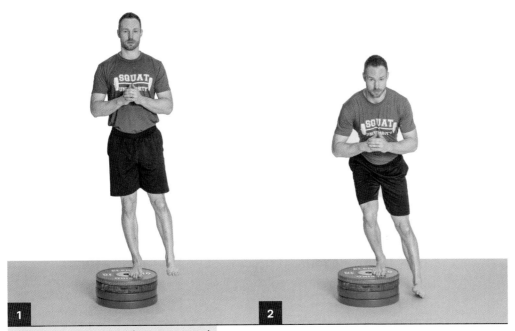

TOUCHDOWN SQUAT (FOUR PLATES)

As the smaller stack of plates or box becomes easier and easier for you, increase the difficulty by stacking more plates. A taller stack demands more control from the knee. The end goal is to perform a single-leg squat with great knee stability from a height of at least 8 inches (if not more!).

Recommended sets/reps: 2 or 3 sets of 15 to 20 reps

Improve Your Balance

While the touchdown is essential, it is only one part of a comprehensive plan to build knee stability. You must eventually increase the demand on knee stability by pushing your body into a number of positions and planes of motion. The balance and reach exercise is a great tool for this job.

Start by taping the pattern shown on the floor. Stand in the center of the "T" and perform a single-leg squat, just as you did with the touchdown. However, instead of squatting down and tapping the heel of your free leg next to a stack of plates, you simultaneously squat and reach out to the side down the length of the tape. Go as far to the side as you can without letting your knee cave. Hold the end position (with your free leg hovering just over the ground) for a few seconds before coming back to the start. Reaching your leg away from your body as you squat increases the demand on your core/hips in different planes of motion. The focus is to maintain good knee control and foot position in several planes. Perform a few reps in each direction.

TAPE PATTERN ON GROUND

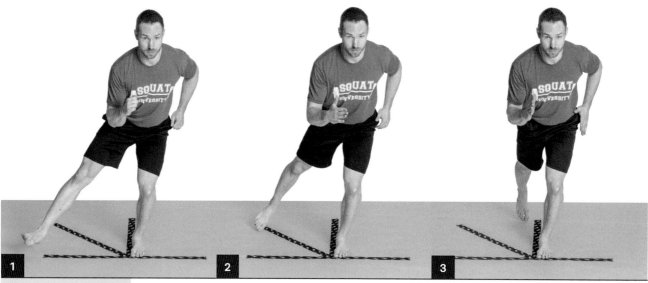

1   2   3

BALANCE AND REACH

Enhance Lower Body Control

The human body has an amazing ability to recognize and react to movements it identifies as familiar; this is known as *muscle memory*. With enough repetitions, the right corrective exercises used to enhance coordination and control will eventually teach the body to react correctly in real-life situations, thereby decreasing pain and future injury risk.

The next type of exercise I want to introduce to you, called *reactive neuromuscular training*, or RNT, is designed to improve coordination and control. First introduced by physical therapists Michael Voight and Gray Cook, RNT exercises are designed to help improve movement quality by teaching athletes to feel for how they are moving (known as *proprioception*).[51]

One of the easiest uses of RNT is a bodyweight squat with a hip circle band around your knees. Assume your natural squat stance and create the tripod foot. Jam your big toes into the ground and push your knees out to the side against the band resistance. As you squat, the band will attempt to pull your knees in (the motion of a valgus collapse). Don't let this happen.

To keep your knees from driving in the glutes (glute medius and glute max), you have to engage on both the descent *and* the ascent.[52] Therefore, this simple tool teaches your body how to squat with optimal technique!

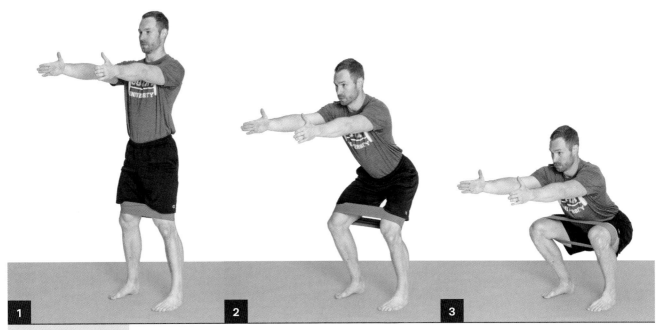

RNT BANDED SQUAT

I recommend using a very slow tempo with this banded squat and even performing 1½ movements. With constant tension against the band, perform a 5- to 10-second lower into the bottom of the squat. Pause for a second before ascending a few inches. Make sure your body weight remains directly over the middle of your feet. If your chest falls forward and your hips kick back, you'll feel your weight shift to your toes or heels. Ascend straight up and hold for a few seconds. Your lateral hips will be shaking in fatigue if you are performing this exercise with the right intensity.

After a few seconds, drop back down into the bottom of the squat. Perform three of these partial-ascent holds before standing all the way back up. This movement sequence teaches your body balance and control/coordination during the ascent, which is the most common time for knee collapse to occur.

Recommended sets/reps: 3 to 5 rounds of the 1½ squat sequence

Next up is the RNT split squat. For this exercise, you'll need to grab a friend and a light resistance band. (If you are unable to find a person to help, you can fasten a long resistance band around a rig.) Assume a lunge position, with one leg in front of the other and the heel of your back foot elevated off the ground. You should be barefoot; this will allow you to concentrate on how well your foot is maintaining stability over the three points of contact, aka the tripod foot.

Place the resistance band around your forward leg and have your friend pull the band inward as if they're trying to collapse your knee. To perform a good-quality split squat (with the knee in line with the foot), your body has to fight against the inward pull of the band. This process of the band pulling your body into a poor position stimulates the body's awareness of the knee during the squatting motion and teaches it to naturally turn on the appropriate glute muscles to prevent the knee from collapsing.

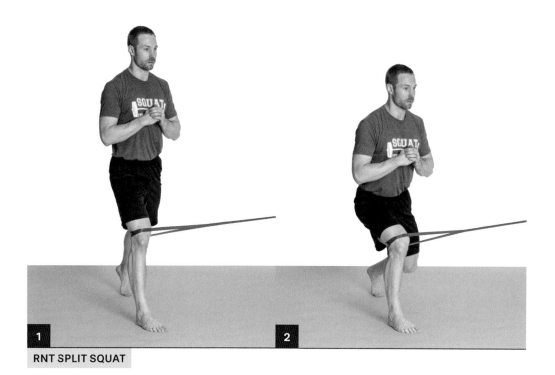

RNT SPLIT SQUAT

Recommended sets/reps: 3 sets of 10 reps

Improving Load Tolerance, Step 1: The Balancing Act

If your knee pain resembles a tendinopathy rather than a biomechanical dysfunction, your first step in treating this condition is to talk about load modification. As an athlete who competed in the sport of Olympic weightlifting for over a decade, I wholeheartedly understand the drive that most of us have to train despite aches and pains. Contrary to the advice of your doctor, not everyone has to stop training to fix a tendinopathy problem.

If you're dealing with tendon pain, you are in a reactive stage, regardless of whether it is the first "reactive" stage or later "reactive on disrepair/degeneration" stage. This pain is due to one simple mechanism: overload. The pain developed because you placed too much load on your patellar or quad tendon and surpassed its current load tolerance level.

Regardless of the exact cause or where you lie on the continuum of pathology, your first step in finding relief of your symptoms is to modify your training. Your body has experienced an abrupt overload of your tendon tissues and has responded negatively with pain. You need to look into *why* this occurred and make changes to decrease your pain.

Changing your training intensity and volume does not mean you're going to stay away from the gym and sit on the couch for the next week. You never want to rest a tendon completely!

The strength of your tendons follows the simple motto of "if you don't use it, you lose it."[53] If you take away all loading and *only* rest for a few weeks, you will set yourself up for the pain to eventually return. Tendinopathy occurs because your training surpassed your current load tolerance level. If you completely rest your body, it will adapt, and the tolerance level of your patellar and/or quad tendon will drop (because minimal load is being placed on it), making it even easier to overload when you return.

On the other hand, you don't want to ignore pain and continue pushing through painful exercises. If you do, the injury will only continue to get worse, and structural changes will eventually take place in the tendon. You must find the perfect amount of load that allows for healing to occur; too little or too much will only make things worse in the long run.

In my experience, a number of barbell athletes begin to experience this pain in the time leading up to an important weightlifting or powerlifting meet. Therefore, it isn't practical for everyone to stop training. You must, however, make a change to your training program (along with adding some of the exercises discussed later). The pain you're experiencing is your tendon telling you that it is not tolerating the loads you are placing on it. It is there for a reason. Listen to it.

Try changing one variable in your training program and see how your tendon responds. For example, if you currently train seven days a week, decrease the frequency by dropping one session. If you can't sacrifice one day of training, you must make a change to either the number of high-intensity loads or the total volume of your training. Regardless of which variable you choose, change only one at a time and wait to see how your body responds. Everyone will be slightly different, so there is no golden rule.

If your body does not respond well to this modification in training with the addition of corrective exercises, or if the pain has been ongoing for more than a few months (meaning your injury may be in the degenerative phase), it is highly recommended that you cease training and consult with a sports physical therapist or an orthopedic specialist (MD or DO).

Improving Load Tolerance, Step 2: The Rehab Plan

Exercise is the best treatment for any type of tendon pain. Period. If you have visited with a doctor or other medical practitioner who recommends injections or other passive treatments like electrotherapy or scraping techniques as the main mode of treatment, you have gone to the wrong person. While these kinds of treatments may decrease your pain in the short term, they will not be helpful in the long term because they do not address *why* your tendon became injured in the first place. You must strengthen the tendon and improve its ability to tolerate load.

Phase 1: Isometrics

The best tolerated of all strength exercises for tendinopathy is an isometric contraction. This is an exercise in which the muscle contracts but the joint doesn't move (e.g., squeezing your quad while standing or lying down). Isometrics have been shown to reduce pain for upwards of 45 minutes after being performed. They also spark the ability of the quad to kick back on, as it is usually inhibited in strength output due to pain (called *cortical inhibition*).[54] Think about it like this: If, every time you performed a jump, you experienced pain, your brain eventually would say, "Stop it!" This is why someone who has been dealing with tendon pain for a long time sees decreases in performance. Heavy isometric exercises have been shown to change this.

Isometrics should be relatively pain-free. While you may have a little pain at the start, it should decrease significantly by the third or fourth repetition.

For an isometric to be effective, it must be difficult to perform! This is where most people come up short. Research shows you must find a load that contracts your muscle(s) to 70 percent of its max capabilities. While there is no way to test exactly for this level by yourself, you can estimate it by finding the combination of intensity and load that makes an isometric difficult to hold for 45 seconds.

A low-level isometric for the patellar and quad tendons is a wall sit. With your back against a wall and your feet out in front of you, slide down the wall and sit with your knees bent to around 60 degrees. Perform 5 repetitions of a 45-second hold. If this exercise is too easy, try performing a single-leg wall sit.

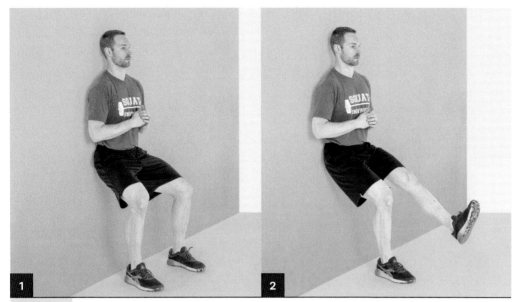

WALL SIT

If you finished these wall sits (either double or single leg) and thought to yourself, "I could have held that at least for 30 seconds more," you didn't have enough load on your tendon. This is a common response for athletes. It means the load from the wall sit is not enough to bring out the desired outcome, and you need to try the Spanish squat instead.[55]

Grab a thick rigid band and loop it around a squat rack or pillar. Place the band behind your knee at the top of your calf, with your toes facing the band attachment. Next, squat as deeply as possible while keeping your spine upright (think of this as a reverse wall sit). Don't hinge at your hips as if performing a normal squat, which would unload the desired force off your quads and transfer it to your hips. The Spanish squat places higher demand on the quads compared to the traditional wall sit exercise. It places more load on the patellar and quad tendons as well. Perform the hold for 5 repetitions of 45 seconds 2 or 3 times a day with 1 or 2 minutes of rest after each rep to help maximize your recovery.

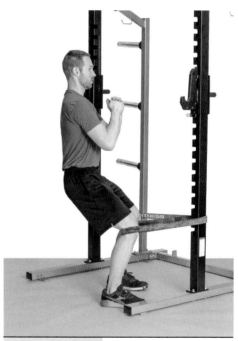

SPANISH SQUAT

Interestingly, isometrics like the Spanish squat hold can also be good diagnostic confirmation tests for patellar and quad tendinopathy. If performing these exercises does not decrease your knee pain afterward and instead increases your symptoms, you likely are dealing with a different type of injury, and you need to revisit the screening regimen from earlier in this chapter.

If you are continuing to train through this injury, use the Spanish squat hold isometric exercise before your workouts as a way to decrease pain and improve neuromuscular control and force generation during your lifting. Keep an eye on your body's responses to the amount of loading at this time!

Phase 2: Strength with Isotonics

Research has shown that tendons that are subjected to routine loading with an adequate strength program adapt by becoming stiffer.[56] For example, in 1986, a group of researchers performed a study on a 242-pound (110-kg) powerlifter squatting 550 pounds (250 kg). During this heavy lift, they estimated that the loads on the lifter's patellar and quad tendons reached 6,000 and 8,000 newtons, respectively.[57]

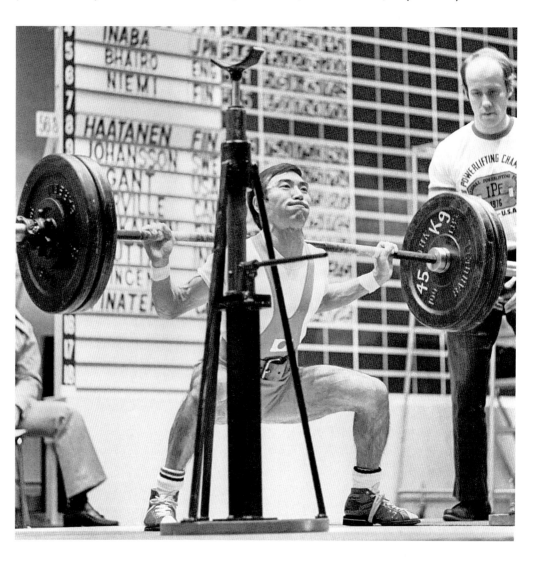

Powerlifter squatting tremendous weight.
Hideaki Inaba squat,
© Bruce Klemens

A newton (N) is an international unit for measuring force. Researchers have estimated that the patellar tendon can withstand forces of 10,000 to 15,000 newtons, which is around 13 to 19 times body weight for a smaller 176-pound (80-kg) athlete.[58] Estimating the ultimate strength of the quad tendon, however, is a little harder. Scientists have found the quad tendon to be 30 to 40 percent thicker than the patellar tendon; therefore, it can probably withstand much more force than the patellar tendon—a reason why overloading and creating a reactive quad tendon is rarer than patellar tendinopathy.[59]

Now, why is this so important? As I mentioned, routine loading can increase a tendon's stiffness, which gives it a higher capacity to bear load. While isometric exercises are great for decreasing pain and increasing strength temporarily through changes in cortical inhibition, they do little to improve the load-bearing capacity of the tendon. Eventually, your rehab must move past isometric exercises and start to incorporate traditional strength training exercises to accomplish this goal.

Most exercises performed in the gym have two phases: eccentric and concentric. The eccentric phase is the lowering portion of a movement where the muscle fibers are lengthened under tension. The concentric phase is where the muscle fibers are shortened under tension. In a traditional squat, for example, the vastus muscles of your quads lengthen as you descend (eccentric phase) and shorten as you stand back up (concentric phase).

Historically, physical therapists have treated tendinopathies at the knee with eccentric exercises.[60] One common exercise is a single-leg squat on a decline board for 3 sets of 15 reps twice a day. The athlete starts by standing on a decline board (usually on a 25-degree angle) and performs a slow single-leg squat while maintaining an upright chest. They then put their free leg down and stand back up with both legs. Placing the body on a decline targets the patellar tendon 25 to 30 percent more than performing this exercise on a flat surface.[61]

There are two problems with using this exercise. First, there is limited research to back it up.[62] Second, it may be too aggressive. Pain is a normal response to decline board single-leg squats, and using them with an athlete who is continuing to lift may cause excessive irritation and worsen the injury.

Also, if you think about it, the body moves using both eccentric and concentric muscle actions. Focusing strength efforts on only one phase of the movement does not strengthen it in a way that will carry over functionally to the activities you perform throughout the day and in training. Your muscles aren't performing *only* eccentric contractions when you sprint down a track. It's not that eccentrics don't work, but why ignore the other half of the movement?

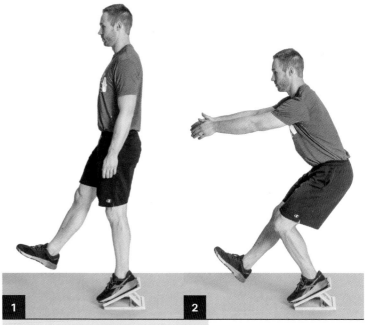

DECLINE BOARD SINGLE-LEG SQUAT

Recent research has shown that the type of contraction (eccentric-only versus normal eccentric and concentric loading) is irrelevant when it comes to driving the healing process with tendinopathies![63] Ultimately, it is the amount of load placed on the tendon that drives the injured tissue to return to a normal state.

In the early 2000s, research began to emerge on the use of heavy slow resistance (HSR) training in the rehabilitation of tendon injuries. HSR describes traditional exercises performed slowly with both concentric and eccentric muscle contractions (called an *isotonic movement*). The initial research showed that these heavy and slow exercises were just as effective as eccentric-only exercises in the rehab of tendinopathy.[64] They are excellent at building load tolerance during this phase of rehabilitation without using the tendon as a spring, which would otherwise overload the current capabilities of the tissues and exacerbate symptoms. As soon as your pain has decreased to a 3 out of 10 during normal day-to-day functions, I recommend starting HSR exercises.

BOX SQUAT

The squat is a great way to start loading the patellar and quad tendons. If you can squat to full depth without pain, by all means continue doing so. However, if extreme pain has limited your ability to squat to full depth, limiting your descent to a predetermined height is a necessary step.

For example, box squats allow you to load your body in a recognizable way while controlling for a few important factors. First, you can control the depth and limit pain by setting the box to a predetermined height. To maintain your balance as you descend into a full-depth squat, your knees must move forward toward (and sometimes over) your toes. While this forward knee position is not inherently dangerous for someone with healthy knees, the inclined shin angle can increase load on the patellar and quad tendons, creating pain. Performing a box squat to around parallel depth limits forward knee translation, enabling you to load the tendons without pain.

Box squats also decrease the total tension placed on the quad and patellar tendons because a powerful turnaround in the bottom of a free squat (which naturally stores and releases energy via the tendons) is not used. When doing a proper box squat, there is a pause between the descent and ascent. Normally, with a heavy squat, elastic energy is stored in the tendons. The pause eliminates the springlike loading and unloading of the tendons. Simply put, athletes with patellar tendinopathy will be able to tolerate box squats better than they can tolerate regular heavy squats.

The setup for the box squat is exactly the same as it is for your regular squat. Set your feet in a stable position. Take a breath and brace your core before initiating the squat with your hips.

While remaining balanced during the descent (barbell tracking over your midfoot when viewed from the side), sit straight down onto the top of the box. Do not rock back onto the box; instead, only pause in the bottom position.

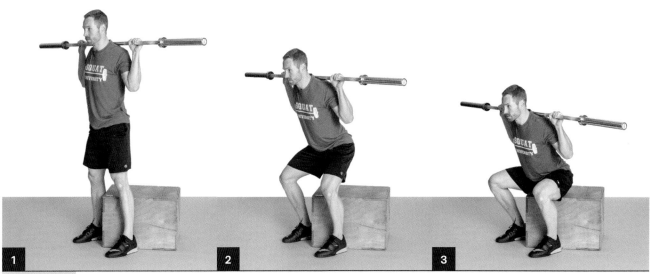

1   2   3

BOX SQUAT

Initiate your ascent by driving straight up. If you do it correctly, your knees will not travel forward as your hips rise from the box. Instead, your knees will remain in a stable position and remain aligned with your feet.

When you're starting the HSR phase of the rehab plan, start with 4 sets of 15 repetitions every other day. (On your off-days, continue to perform the isometrics from phase 1.) Perform your isometric exercises prior to any HSR, as the cortical inhibition benefits derived from the isometrics will enable you to access more motor units and therefore stimulate more strength.

How much weight should you use?

Unlike muscles, tendons require heavy loads to adapt and heal.[65] Research has shown positive changes in muscle size and strength with loads anywhere between 30 and 90 percent of one-rep max (1RM), whereas a much more significant load (greater than 70 percent) is needed to create the same adaptive changes in tendons.[66]

If this is your first time box squatting, I recommend starting with 50 to 70 percent of your back squat 1RM. The weight you choose for the box squat should be something you can control with good technique for each repetition but heavy enough that, after completing your fourth set, you are too fatigued to perform a fifth.[67] If you get done with your fourth set and feel like you have enough energy left to perform a fifth, add more weight! It is rare to have a lot of pain with HSR exercises if you're doing them slowly enough.

Researchers who have studied the use of HSR for tendinopathy recommend performing 4 sets of 15 repetitions of these strength exercises for a week before increasing the weight and dropping the volume to 4 sets of 12 reps for the next 2 weeks.[68] Eventually progress to 4 sets of 10 reps, followed by 4 sets of 8 and then 6 reps, each for 2 to 3 weeks.

How fast should you squat?

While the amount of weight on the bar is *the most* important factor in creating change in injured tendons, the speed at which you lift is a close second.[69] Researchers have recently found that manipulating the speed at which a squat is performed significantly changes the amount of stress and strain placed on the tendons of the knee.

Initially during the healing phase, moving quickly during a squat may elicit more pain. For this reason, performing strength exercises with a slow descent and ascent is ideal (a key component of HSR training). Ideally, you should take 3 seconds in the eccentric and 3 seconds in the concentric phase, meaning each rep takes a total of 6 seconds to complete.[70]

Most strength and conditioning programs write a tempo format like this as 3-1-3. The first number refers to the time it takes to perform the eccentric lowering. The second number refers to the length of the pause in the turnaround (a 0 means a fast or plyometric bounce at the bottom of the squat, whereas a 1 would be used for a 1-second pause). The third number refers to the time it takes to ascend (the concentric phase).

I recommend using this slow 3-1-3 tempo until you finish your 2 to 3 weeks of 4 sets of 6 repetitions. Eventually, you can start adding a faster-paced ascent. Using a slow descent (about 3 seconds) followed by a powerful drive upward places an increased demand on the tendons that can help increase load tolerance capacity to a greater degree compared to squatting slow on the way down *and* up.[71]

BULGARIAN SPLIT SQUAT

While the box squat is a great exercise, you can easily hide or cover up problems in side-to-side strength/coordination. Consciously or subconsciously, your body often changes the way it moves in the presence of pain. These compensatory movements may be very small and therefore hard for even the most well-trained coach to detect with the naked eye. For this reason, exercises performed mostly on one leg, like the Bulgarian split squat, will expose these asymmetries and ensure that you're loading the injured tendons adequately.

To set up for the Bulgarian split squat, kneel in front of a box or bench with your rear foot resting on the top of the platform behind you. Assume a stance where your torso angle mimics your shin angle of fairly vertical or leaning forward slightly. The knee that is in contact with the ground should be positioned slightly behind your hips (when viewed from the side). If you have access to a single-leg squat rack with a roller, as shown, it will allow your foot to move more easily during the next motion than a box or bench.

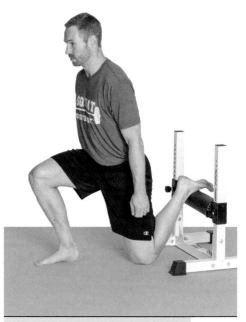

BULGARIAN SPLIT SQUAT SETUP

Grab a kettlebell or dumbbell and hold it by your chest in the goblet squat position. With your back foot resting lightly on the box, bench, or roller, perform a split squat by driving straight upward. Keep your shin as vertical as possible during this movement; just like the box squat, you want to limit forward knee translation. If you're doing it right, you'll feel the muscles of your forward leg working hard as you descend. I like to use the cue "put 90 percent of your body weight through your front leg while your back leg works only as a kickstand for balance."

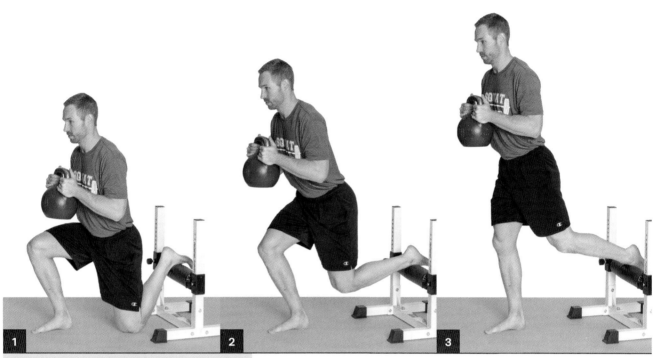

BULGARIAN SPLIT SQUAT WITH KETTLEBELL

Just like the squat, I recommend performing 4 sets of 15 repetitions for a week before increasing the weight and dropping the volume to 4 sets of 12 reps for the next 2 weeks.[72]

Eventually progress to 4 sets of 10 reps, followed by 4 sets of 8 and then 6 reps, each for 2 to 3 weeks. The weight you choose should be heavy enough that, after completing your fourth set, you are too fatigued to perform a fifth.[73] As the weight held at your chest in the goblet squat position becomes heavier and heavier and therefore harder to maintain for the full set, you may switch to holding a barbell on your back.

Testing Your Progress

When you start HSR training, a very small amount of pain—3 out of 10 maximum—is acceptable during and after the lift. If your pain was higher than a 3, then the weight was probably too much, or you moved too quickly.

I use the single-leg decline squat (the exercise previously used as a rehabilitation exercise in research) as a pain provocation test.[74] Using this test daily allows you to gauge how well your body is responding to the corrective exercises. Let me explain how.

It is normal to have a little pain during the process of rehabbing a tendon injury. To make sure you're healing as efficiently as possible, you need to place the right amount of load on your tendons. By using a pain provocation test, you can determine how well your tendons are tolerating the exercises; as discussed previously, this is called *load tolerance.*

Start by performing the single-leg decline squat before a training session and rating your pain on a scale from 0 to 10, 0 being no pain and 10 being the worst pain you can imagine. That number is your baseline score.

Perform the same test 24 hours after each training session to see if you were using the correct load for your body. If you were, your pain will stay the same or get better. If it gets better, increase the weight in the next session. If you are using too much weight, your pain will increase 24 hours later, and you will need to decrease the weight during your next session.

There isn't a set protocol for this progression, so getting with a strength coach and/or a physical therapist who has a background in weightlifting/powerlifting will be key to finding the optimal progression for your body.

Returning to Plyometrics

Along with the HSR component to strengthening the muscles/tendon complex, you also need to increase the ability of the tendon to absorb and store loads. The highest loads placed on the patellar and quad tendons occur when the tendons are used as a spring, utilizing what is called the *stretch-shortening cycle* (SSC).

Powerful movements like repetitive jumping use the tendons to store and then release energy to generate large amounts of power. Exercises that emphasize the storage of loads (such as stepping off a box and landing in a squat) are a bridge to eventually returning to the full energy storage *and* release capabilities of the tendons.

Stand on a small box, maybe 6 to 8 inches in height. (In the photos, opposite, I'm using a stack of plates.) Step off and land with both feet in a mini squat position. Don't land with stiff joints; make sure to absorb the force of impact. Perform 2 sets of 20 landings before progressing according to how your body responds to a taller box and eventually a single-leg landing.

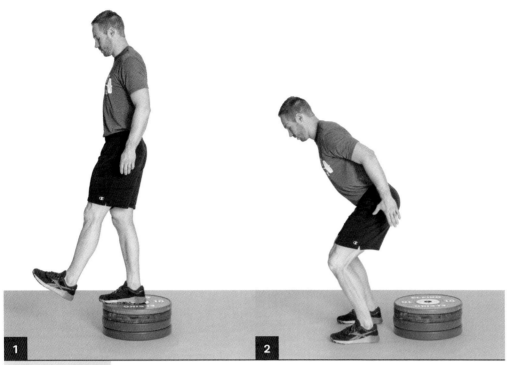

BOX DEPTH DROP

To start true plyometrics, where the tendon is used as a spring to store and release energy, you must first see profound improvements in muscle strength. The strength of the injured leg must be close to the capabilities of the uninjured one, and you should no longer have pain with the decline board single-leg squat.

If you pass the decline board single-leg squat and feel like your strength and control of your legs are fairly similar, perform a faster, more explosive movement like a single-leg hop on each leg. Originally, this movement was likely painful and difficult to perform on the injured leg. If you are ready to move on to the plyometric phase of rehab, you must have the ability to show good control of your body without pain during slow movements like the single-leg squat and a high-load functional movement like a hop.

The goal of this phase of rehab is to start using the tendon as a spring again to see how it responds. An example of an entry-level plyometric is double-leg pogo hops. Simply perform repetitive small jumps only a few inches off the ground, as shown in the photos on the next page. Start with 10 to 20 reps in a row before resting for a few minutes, and perform a total of 3 or 4 sets.

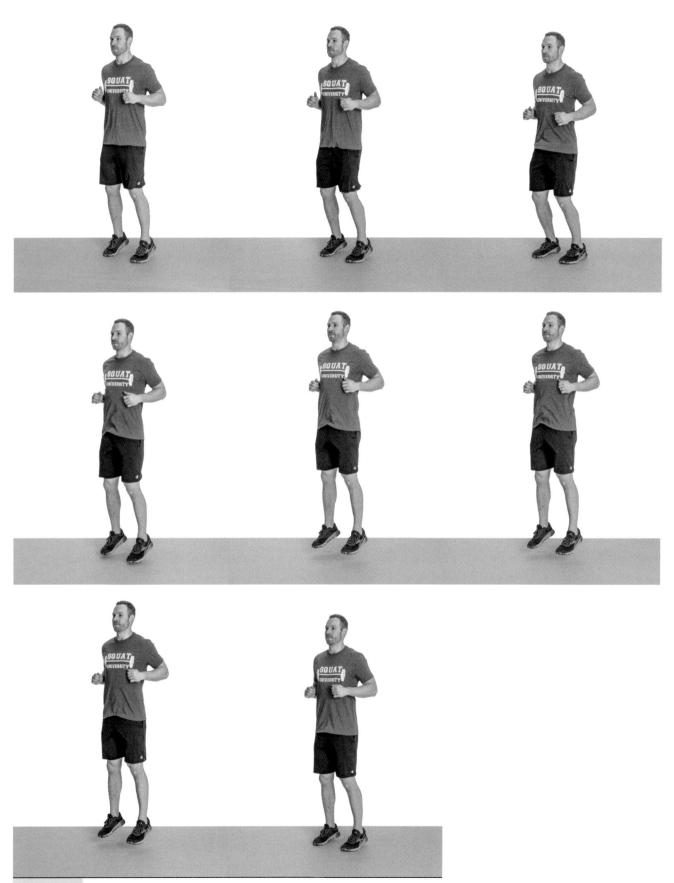

POGO HOP

Notice how your injured tendon responds to the loading during the session and over the next 24 hours. If you feel great during and do not have an increase in tendon pain or stiffness the following day, increase the training load in the next session. For the first few weeks, increase the volume of your loading by adding more jumps per set.

Recording every aspect of your plyometric program will allow you to progress and build this capacity as efficiently as possible. For example, suppose Athlete A and Athlete B both perform 3 sets of 15 jumps. Athlete A wakes up the next day and feels great, so they progress to 3 sets of 20 jumps in the next session. Athlete B, however, wakes up with a slight increase in patellar tendon pain. For this reason, Athlete B needs to modify the next plyometric session by decreasing the number of jumps.

Make sure to increase or decrease only one variable, whether it's volume or intensity, in each training session. If you change too many variables at the same time, you won't be able to go back through your notes to determine whether it was a change in volume or intensity that was too much for your tendon to handle.

Start with two or three sessions a week of these light plyometric exercises (one session every three days). At this stage of rehabilitation, the tendon cannot take plyometric loads every day without getting angry. For this reason, structure your weekly training by mixing in HSR days between plyometric sessions. If your tendon continues to respond well to the increases in plyometric loading every third day, you can continue to add more volume or start to increase the intensity.

Eventually, you'll be able to progress to medium-level plyometric exercises, including higher tuck jumps, depth drop jumps from a low to medium-height box (or stack of plates, as shown below), and multiple double-leg jumps for distance. If you are a runner (or your sport involves running), adding acceleration and deceleration drills along with cutting/change-of-direction movements may be a good option.

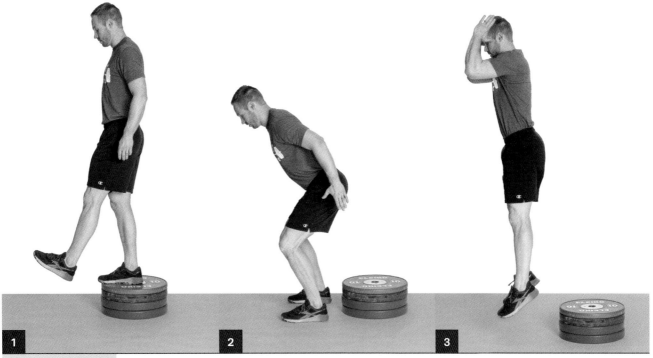

DEPTH DROP JUMP

After a few weeks of progressing these drills, you can move to even higher-level plyometric activities, including single-leg hops and depth drop jumps from a taller box. Eventually, you can start manipulating the frequency of loading by performing plyometrics every two days instead of three. As always, see how your tendon responds and adjust accordingly. There is no perfect recipe for how to progress through this plyometric stage. Everyone responds differently, and you need to find the loads that work best for your body. Be patient; this process can take several weeks or even months.

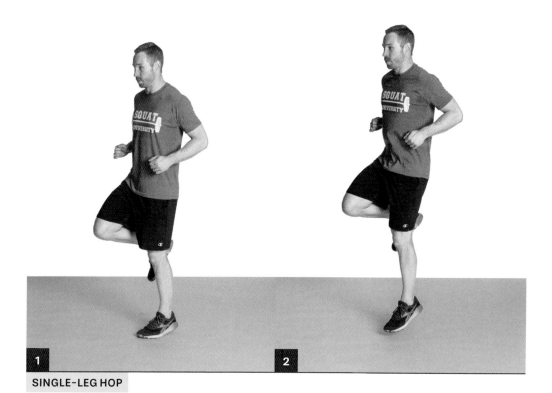

SINGLE-LEG HOP

Returning to Olympic Lifts

Ballistic lifts like the clean and snatch are the most aggravating movements to the tendons of the knee and, therefore, should be the last ones you reincorporate into your training during the rehab process. If you have returned to squatting heavy without pain, you can reintroduce these lifts. Start slowly on your progression, especially when it comes to the frequency of these lifts in your training. Giving yourself 48 to 72 hours between sessions is a good rule to start with to allow for proper healing.

Here is a simple training progression to use:

- **Day 1:** Olympic lifting
- **Day 2:** Isometric exercise (active rest)
- **Day 3:** Heavy slow resistance
- **Day 4:** Olympic lifting

Notice how there isn't a complete rest day. Some athletes feel worse after a day of full rest, so making sure to load the tendon with simple isometrics is a good idea.[75] At this time, continue to use isometric exercises as a warm-up before your Olympic lifts. Also use the decline board single-leg squat to test how well your body is responding to the newly added lifts.

Depending on where your injury lies on the tendinopathy continuum, the process of decreasing your pain could take a few days to several weeks or even months. Your progression for the exercises described will be guided by the amount of pain you experience in the pain provocation test (decline board single-leg squat) 24 hours after each session.

No two athletes will respond in the same way to these rehab exercises. Some will be able to add more weight in session after session. Others will require a more fluctuated load program to keep pain at bay. In the end, it is on you to regulate the weight based on how you feel. Don't be tough and push through pain if your knees hurt worse the next day. Listen to your body.

Once you have returned to pain-free training, you should continue to perform the isometric exercises, Bulgarian split squats, and coordination re-education exercises (if found to be a weak link) weekly to prevent the tendinopathy from returning. This is because the altered neuromuscular problems that arose in response to pain often persist even after the pain has resolved.[76] Once you have a tendinopathy, you are always susceptible to the pain returning if you don't stay on top of loading exercises or if you ramp up the intensity of your training too quickly.

"Passive" Treatments

I have had many patients come to me after failed treatment under the care of other rehabilitation professionals. It often revolved around some kind of passive treatment. "Passive" treatment refers to something that is done *to you,* whereas an "active" treatment is something you physically participate in. Passive treatments include ice, dry needling, and scraping techniques with tools made of metal, hard plastic, or bone.

While ice has been shown to be beneficial for controlling pain, it doesn't accelerate the healing process. (Turn to Chapter 7 for details on the limitations of icing.) If you really want to fix your injury, ditch the ice packs and address why your pain is present in the first place.

Passive treatment such as dry needling or IASTM (instrument-assisted soft tissue mobilization) can help address mobility deficits at the ankle or hip. For this reason, they can be beneficial additions to treatment for some forms of knee injury. However, there is no evidence that passive treatment effectively treats the patellar or quad tendon. You cannot "restart" the healing process by scraping or needling a tendon. Research has shown time and time again that proper loading of the tendon is the only way to permanently improve strength, decrease pain, and improve quality of life in people dealing with tendinopathies.

What About Straps or Braces?

The Cho-Pat and DonJoy Cross straps are two of the most commonly used braces for patellar tendon pain.[77] Each of these straps is simply a thick piece of material that wraps tightly around the patellar tendon and is used in an attempt to decrease strain on the painful tissue. While some people swear by these straps, research on their efficacy has been iffy.[78] My thought on patellar straps is that if using one decreases your pain with activity, you can continue using it. Just remember that using a strap should be a *supplement* to rehab exercises and not the sole method of treatment. The strap is not to be used as a Band-Aid to mask pain. You still have to address the issue with proper loading and smart rehab.

Should You Wear Knee Sleeves/Wraps?

Walk into any CrossFit box or Olympic weightlifting or powerlifting gym and you'll be sure to find a few athletes wearing knee sleeves or wraps while they work out. Wraps and sleeves are some of the most common accessories for barbell training. However, when it comes to how and when to use them, most people are clueless.

I want to set the record straight and tell you everything you need to know about these commonly misunderstood training tools. Let's start by addressing the most common question people have: what is the difference between knee sleeves and knee wraps?

Knee sleeves are compression garments (often made from a soft neoprene material) that surround the entire joint. They come in a variety of thicknesses, and their snug design allows your knees to stay warm during training. Some believe that the physical sensation of wearing knee sleeves can give athletes a better awareness of their knee positioning while lifting and potentially improve their technique.

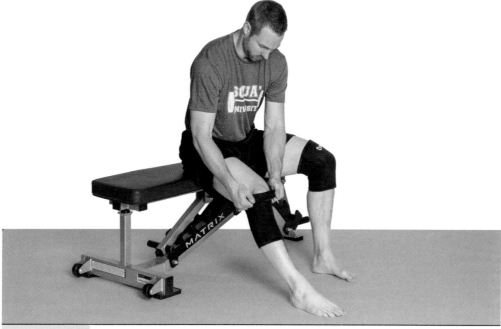

KNEE SLEEVES

Knee wraps are constructed from a thick polyester canvas that is interwoven with small rubber filaments.[79] These wraps, which are often 2 meters (78.7 inches) long and roughly 8 centimeters (3.1 inches) wide, are wrapped as tightly as possible around an athlete's knees, in either a spiral or a figure-eight configuration.

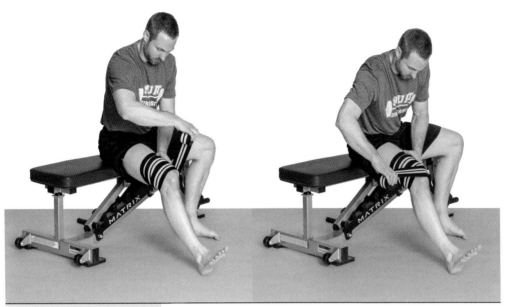

KNEE WRAPPING EXAMPLE

What generally makes a wrap different from a sleeve is the mechanical advantage that is created as the elastic material (rubber filament) is stretched during the lowering phase of a squat. Just like a spring being pulled into a stretched position, the elastic properties of the wrap allow it to store this energy and then transfer it to the lifter during the ascent. In fact, research has shown that wearing knee wraps can lead to 20 percent more speed out of the bottom of a squat.[80]

Now, there are sleeves on the market that are manufactured to fit extremely tightly around the knee, and these products can give a fair amount of elastic rebound compared to wraps. However, the majority of the knee sleeves that you see athletes wear do not.

Wraps are commonly used in the sport of powerlifting but not in the sport of Olympic weightlifting, as they can be very restricting for receiving the barbell in the bottom of the snatch and clean movements. While you may see some Olympic weightlifters wearing knee wraps that resemble the traditional thick powerlifting style, they are often constructed from a much softer cotton blend that keeps the knees warm but does not add any mechanical advantage to the lift.

Two traditional methods are used when wrapping the knees: a spiral and an "X technique," or "crossover figure-eight." In 2015, a study examined whether there was any significant difference in the amount of mechanical assistance (called *carryover*) between the two wrapping methods. Interestingly, the researchers did not find any difference between the two![81]

Because knee sleeves do not directly improve performance like tightly worn knee wraps do, you may wear them as often as you like. However, they should *not* be worn to cover up pain. Athletes often resort to buying a pair of sleeves in an attempt to fix aches and pains in the knee joint. This is *not* what they are meant for.

Knee wraps, on the other hand, need to be worn *sparingly*. Research shows that wearing wraps may change your squatting technique by forcing you into a more upright position.[82] This means your powerful hip extensors (glutes) may contribute less to the lift. For this reason, it is recommended that athletes who want to use knee wraps use them only for their heaviest training sessions and/or during powerlifting meets.

In the end, using knee wraps or sleeves is a personal decision. Many great barbell athletes do not use either, and some use either wraps or sleeves, depending on the goal of their training session. Knee wraps can be a great accessory to help you lift heavy weight. Remember, though, that knee wraps or sleeves should *not* be used as a crutch to cover up knee pain!

Notes

1. K. D. DeHaven and D. M. Lintner, "Athletic injuries: comparison by age, sport, and gender," *American Journal of Sports Medicine* 14, no. 2 (1986): 218–24.

2. B. P. Hamill, "Relative safety of weightlifting and weight training," *Journal of Strength & Conditioning Research* 8, no. 1 (1994): 53–7; M. H. Stone, A. C. Fry, M. Ritchie, L. Stossel-Ross, and J. L. Marsit, "Injury potential and safety aspects of weightlifting movements," *Strength and Conditioning Journal* 16, no. 3 (1994): 15–21; D. N. Kulund, J. B. Dewy, and C. E. Brubaker, "Olympic weight-lifting injuries," *Physician and Sportsmedicine* 6, no. 11 (1978): 111–9; G. Calhoon and A. C. Fry, "Injury rates and profiles of elite competitive weightlifters," *Journal of Athletic Training* 34, no. 3 (1993): 232–8.

3. Calhoon and Fry, "Injury rates and profiles of elite competitive weightlifters" (see note 2 above).

4. Calhoon and Fry, "Injury rates and profiles of elite competitive weightlifters" (see note 2 above).

5. T. Q. Lee, G. Morris, and R. P. Csintalan, "The influence of tibial and femoral rotation on patellofemoral contact area and pressure," *Journal of Orthopaedic & Sports Physical Therapy* 33, no. 11 (2003): 686–93.

6. F. A. Barber and A. N. Sutker, "Iliotibial band syndrome," *Sports Medicine* 14, no. 2 (1992): 144–8; D. B. Clement, J. E. Taunton, G. W. Smart, and K. L. McNicol, "A survey of overuse running injuries," *Physician and Sportsmedicine* 9, no. 5 (1981): 47–58; G. Linderburg, R. Pinshaw, and T. D. Noakes, "Iliotibial band syndrome in runners," *Physician and Sportsmedicine* 12, no. 5 (1984): 118–30.

7. M. Fredericson, M. Guillet, and L. DeBenedictis, "Quick solutions for iliotibial band syndrome," *Physician and Sportsmedicine* 28, no. 2 (2000): 52–68; J. W. Orchard, P. A. Fricker, A. T. Abud, and B. R. Mason, "Biomechanics of the iliotibial band friction syndrome in runners," *American Journal of Sports Medicine* 24, no. 3 (1996): 375–9.

8. J. Fairclough, K. Hayashi, H. Toumi, K. Lyons, G. Bydder, N. Phillips, T. M. Best, and M. Benjamin, "The functional anatomy of the iliotibial band during flexion and extension of the knee: implications for understanding iliotibial band syndrome," *Journal of Anatomy* 208, no. 3 (2006): 309–16.

9. B. Noehren, I. Davis, and J. Hamil, "ASB Clinical Biomechanics award winner 2006: prospective study of the biomechanical factors associated with iliotibial band syndrome," *Clinical Biomechanics* 22, no. 9 (2007): 951–6.

10. S. D. Rosengarten, J. L. Cook, A. L. Bryant, J. T. Cordy, J. Daffy, and S. I. Docking, "Australian football players' Achilles tendons respond to game loads within 2 days: an ultrasound tissue characterization (UTC) study," *British Journal of Sports Medicine* 49, no. 3 (2015): 183–7.

11. J. Cook, E. Rio, and S. Docking, "Patellar tendinopathy and its diagnosis," *Sports Health* 32, no. 1 (2014): 17–20.

12. K. M. Khan, N. Maffulli, B. D. Coleman, J. L. Cook, and J. E. Taunton, "Patellar tendinopathy: some aspects of basic science and clinical management," *British Journal of Sports Medicine* 32, no. 4 (1998): 346–55.

13. J. L. Cook, E. Rio, C. R. Purdam, and S. I. Docking, "Revisiting the continuum model of tendon pathology: what is its merit in clinical practice and research?" *British Journal of Sports Medicine* 50, no. 19 (2016): 1187–91.

14. Cook, Rio, Purdam, and Docking, "Revisiting the continuum model of tendon pathology" (see note 13 above).

15. H. Alfredson and J. Cook, "A treatment algorithm for managing Achilles tendinopathy: new treatment options," *British Journal of Sports Medicine* 41, no. 4 (2007): 211–6.

16. S. P. Magnusson, M. V. Narici, C. N. Maganaris, and M. Kjaer, "Human tendon behaviour and adaptation, in vivo," *Journal of Physiology* 586, no. 1 (2008): 71–81.

17. J. L. Cook and C. R. Purdam, "Is tendon pathology a continuum? A pathology model to explain the clinical presentation of load-induced tendinopathy," *British Journal of Sports Medicine* 43, no. 6 (2009): 409–16.

18. Cook and Purdam, "Is tendon pathology a continuum?" (see note 17 above).

19. J. L. Cook, K. M. Khan, P. R. Harcourt, M. Grant, D. A. Young, and S. F. Bonar, "A cross sectional study of 100 athletes with jumper's knee managed conservatively and surgically: the Victorian Institute of Sport Tendon Study Group," *British Journal of Sports Medicine* 31, no. 4 (1997): 332–6; M. Kongsgaard, V. Kovanen, P. Aagaard, S. Doessing, P. Hansen, A. H. Laursen, N. C. Kaldau, M. Kjaer, and S. P. Magnusson, "Corticosteroid injections, eccentric decline squat training and heavy slow resistance training in patellar tendinopathy," *Scandinavian Journal of Medicine & Science in Sports* 19, no. 6 (2009): 790–802.

20. A. Scott, Ø. Lian, R. Bahr, D. A. Hart, and V. Duronio, "VEGF expression in patellar tendinopathy: a preliminary study," *Clinical Orthopaedics and Related Research* 466, no. 7 (2008): 1598–604; H. Alfredson, L. Ohberg, and S. Forsgren, "Is vasculo-neural ingrowth the cause of pain in chronic Achilles tendinosis? An investigation using ultrasonography and colour Doppler, immunohistochemistry, and diagnostic injections," *Knee Surgery, Sports Traumatology, Arthroscopy* 11, no. 5 (2003): 334–8.

21. Cook, Rio, Purdam, and Docking, "Revisiting the continuum model of tendon pathology" (see note 13 above).

22. J. Cook, podcast interview, November 5, 2018.

23. S. I. Docking, M. A. Girdwood, J. Cook, L. V. Fortington, and E. Rio, "Reduced levels of aligned fibrillar structure are not associated with Achilles and patellar tendon symptoms," *Clinical Journal of Sport Medicine,* July 31, 2018, Volume Publish Ahead of Print - Issue.

24. Cook, Rio, Purdam, and Docking, "Revisiting the continuum model of tendon pathology" (see note 13 above).

25. E. K. Rio, R. F. Ellis, J. M. Henry, V. R. Falconer, Z. S. Kiss, M. A. Gridwood, J. L. Cook, and J. E. Gaida, "Don't assume the control group is normal—people with asymptomatic tendon pathology have higher pressure pain thresholds," *Pain Medicine* 19, no. 11 (2008): 2267–73.

26. J. Cook, podcast interview, November 5, 2018.

27. A. Rudavsky and J. Cook, "Physiotherapy management of patellar tendinopathy (jumper's knee)," *Journal of Physiotherapy* 60, no. 3 (2014): 122–9.

28. V. Graci and G. B. Salsich, "Trunk and lower extremity segment kinematics and their relationship to pain following movement instruction during a single-leg squat in females with dynamic knee valgus and patellofemoral pain," *Journal of Science and Medicine in Sport* 18, no. 3 (2015): 343–7; C. M. Powers, "The influence of altered lower-extremity kinematics on

patellofemoral joint dysfunction: a theoretical perspective," *Journal of Orthopaedic & Sports Physical Therapy* 33, no. 11 (2003): 639–46; T. A. Dierks, K. T. Manal, J. Hamil, and I. S. Davis, "Proximal and distal influences on hip and knee kinematics in runners with patellofemoral pain during a prolonged run," *Journal of Orthopaedic & Sports Physical Therapy* 38, no. 8 (2008): 448–56; Noehren, Davis, and Hamil, "ASB Clinical Biomechanics award winner 2006: prospective study of the biomechanical factors associated with iliotibial band syndrome" (see note 9 above) ; R. H. Miller, J. L. Lowry, S. A. Meardon, and J. C. Gillette, "Lower extremity mechanics of iliotibial band syndrome during an exhaustive run," *Gait Posture* 26, no. 3 (2007): 407–13; A. Chang, K. Hayes, D. Dunlop, D. Hurwitz, J. Song, S. Cahue, R. Genge, and L. Sharma, "Trust during ambulation and the progression of knee osteoarthritis," *Arthritis & Rheumatology* 50, no. 12 (2004): 3897–903; R. Cerejo, D. D. Dunlop, S. Cahue, D. Channin, J. Song, and L. Sharma, "The influence of alignment on risk of knee osteoarthritis progression according to baseline stage of disease," *Arthritis & Rheumatology* 46, no. 10 (2000): 2632–6; M. C. Boling, D. A. Padua, S. W. Marshall, K. Guskiewicz, S. Pyne, and A. Beutler, "A prospective investigation of biomechanical risk factors for patellofemoral pain syndrome: the joint undertaking to monitor and prevent ACL injury (JUMP-ACL) cohort," *American Journal of Sports Medicine* 37, no. 11 (2009): 2108–16; T. H. Nakagawa, E. T. Moriya, C. D. Maciel, and F. V. Serrão, "Trunk, pelvis, and knee kinematics, hip strength, and gluteal muscle activation during a single-leg squat in males and females with and without patellofemoral pain syndrome," *Journal of Orthopaedic & Sports Physical Therapy* 42, no. 6 (2012): 491–501; R. B. Souza and C. M. Powers, "Differences in hip kinematics, muscle strength, and muscle activation between subjects with and without patellofemoral pain," *Journal of Orthopaedic & Sports Physical Therapy* 39, no. 1 (2009): 12–9.

29. S. Sahrmann, D. C. Azevedo, and L. Van Dillen, "Diagnosis and treatment of movement system impairment syndromes," *Brazilian Journal of Physical Therapy* 21, no. 6 (2017): 391–9.

30. G. J. Sammarco, A. H. Burnstein, and V. H. Frankel, "Biomechanics of the ankle: a kinematic study," *Orthopedic Clinics of North America* 4, no. 1 (1973): 75–96.

31. C. M. Powers, "The influence of altered lower-extremity kinematics on patellofemoral joint dysfunction: a theoretical perspective," *Journal of Orthopaedic & Sports Physical Therapy* 33, no. 11 (2003): 639–46; M. T. Cibulka and J. Threlkeld-Watkins, "Patellofemoral pain and asymmetrical hip rotation," *Physical Therapy* 85, no. 11 (2005): 1201–7.

32. P. Devita and W. A. Skelly, "Effect of landing stiffness on joint kinetics and energetics in the lower extremity," *Medicine & Science in Sports & Exercise* 24, no. 1 (1992): 108–15.

33. L. J. Backman and P. Danielson, "Low range of ankle dorsiflexion predisposes for patellar tendinopathy in junior elite basketball players: a 1-year prospective study," *American Journal of Sports Medicine* 39, no. 12 (2011): 2626–33.

34. D. R. Bell, B. J. Vesci, L. J. DiStefano, K. M. Guskiewicz, C. J. Hirth, and D. Padua, "Muscle activity and flexibility in individuals with medial knee displacement during the overhead squat," *Athletic Training & Sports Health Care* 4, no. 3 (2014): 117–25; E. Macrum, D. R. Bell, and D. A. Padua, "Effect of limiting ankle-dorsiflexion range of motion on lower extremity kinematics and muscle-activation patterns during a squat," *Journal of Sport Rehabilitation* 21, no. 2 (2012): 144–50; A. Rabin and Z. Kozol, "Measures of range of motion and strength among healthy women with differing quality of lower extremity movement during the lateral step down test," *Journal of Orthopaedic & Sports Physical Therapy* 40, no. 12 (2010): 792–800; D. R. Bell, D. A. Padua, and M. A. Clark, "Muscle strength and flexibility characteristics of people displaying excessive medial knee displacement," *Archives of Physical Medicine and Rehabilitation* 89, no. 7 (2008): 1323–8.

35. J. Dicharry, *Anatomy for Runners* (New York: Skyhorse Publishing, 2012).

36. K. Bennell, R. Talbot, H. Wajswelner, W. Techovanich, and D. Kelly, "Intra-rater and inter-rater reliability of a weight-bearing lunge measure of ankle dorsiflexion," *Australian Journal of Physiotherapy* 44, no. 3 (1998): 175–80; "Ankle mobility exercises to improve dorsiflexion," MikeReinold.com, accessed April 30, 2020, https://mikereinold.com/ankle-mobility-exercises-to-improve-dorsiflexion/.

37. E. Rio, L. Mosley, C. Purdam, T. Samiric, D. Kidgell, A. J. Pearce, S. Jaberzadeh, and J. Cook, "The pain of tendinopathy: physiological or pathophysiological?" *Sports Medicine* 44, no. 1 (2014): 9–23.

38. Cook, Rio, and Docking, "Patellar tendinopathy and its diagnosis" (see note 11 above).

39. R. L. Baker and M. Fredericson, "Iliotibial band syndrome in runners. Biomechanical implications and exercise interventions," *Physical Medicine and Rehabilitation Clinics of North America* 27, no. 1 (2016): 53–77.

40. M. Fredericson, M. Guillet, and L. DeBenedictis, "Quick solutions for iliotibial band syndrome," *Physician and Sportsmedicine* 28, no. 2 (2000): 52–68.

41. K. Cerny, "Vastus medialis oblique/vastus lateralis muscle activity ratios for selected exercises in persons with and without patellofemoral pain syndrome," *Physical Therapy* 75, no. 8 (1995): 672–83; R. T. Jackson and H. H. Merrifield, "Electromyographic assessment of quadriceps muscle group during knee extension with weighted boot," *Medicine & Science in Sports & Exercise* 4, no. 2 (1972): 116–9; F. J. Lieb and J. Perry, "Quadriceps function: An electromyographic study under isometric conditions," *Journal of Bone & Joint Surgery* 53, no. 4 (1971): 749–58; G. S. Pocock, "Electromyographic study of the quadriceps during resistive exercise," *Physical Therapy* 43 (1963): 427–34; T. O. Smith, D. Bowyer, J. Dixon, R. Stephenson, R. Chester, and S. T. Donell, "Can vasus medialis oblique be preferentially activated? A systematic review of electromyographic studies," *Physiotherapy Theory and Practice* 25, no. 2 (2009): 69–98; J. Laprade, F. Culham, and B. Brouwer, "Comparison of five isometric exercises in the recruitment of the vastus medialis oblique in persons with and without patellofemoral pain," *Journal of Orthopaedic & Sports Physical Therapy* 27, no. 3 (1998): 197–204; C. M. Powers, "Rehabilitation of patellofemoral joint disorders: a critical review," *Journal of Orthopaedic & Sports Physical Therapy* 28, no. 5 (1998): 343–54.

42. K. E. DeHaven, W. A. Dolan, and P. J. Mayer, "Chondromalacia patellae in athletes: clinical presentation and conservative management," *American Journal of Sports Medicine* 7, no. 1 (1995): 5–11; J. McConnell, "The management of chondromalacia patellae: a long term solution," *Australian Journal of Physiotherapy* 32, no. 4 (1986): 215–23; S. A. Doucette and D. D. Child, "The effect of open and closed chain exercise and knee joint position on patellar tracking in lateral patellar compression syndrome," *Journal of Orthopaedic & Sports Physical Therapy* 23, no. 2 (1996): 104–10.

43. Powers, "Rehabilitation of patellofemoral joint disorders: a critical review" (see note 41 above).

44. Doucette and Child, "The effect of open and closed chain exercise and knee joint position on patellar tracking in lateral patellar compression syndrome" (see note 42 above) ; D. Kaya, M. N. Doral, and M. Callaghan, "How can we strengthen the quadriceps femoris in patients with patellofemoral pain syndrome?" *Muscles, Ligaments and Tendons Journal* 2, no. 1 (2012): 25–32.

45. R. F. Escamilla, G. S. Fleisig, N. Zheng, S. W. Barrentine, K. E. Wilk, and J. R. Andrews, "Biomechanics of the knee during closed kinetic chain and open kinetic chain exercises," *Medicine & Science Sports & Exercise* 30, no. 4 (1998): 556–69.

46. M. Fredericson, C. L. Cookingham, A. M. Chaudhari, B. C. Dowdell, N. Oestreicher, and S. A. Sahrmann, "Hip abductor weakness in distance runners with iliotibial band syndrome," *Clinical Journal of Sport Medicine* 10, no. 3 (2000): 169–75; S. F. Nadler, G. A. Malanga, M. DePrince, T. P. Stitik, and J. H. Feinberg, "The relationship between lower extremity injury, low back pain, and hip muscle strength in male and female collegiate athletes," *Clinical Journal of Sport Medicine* 10, no. 2 (2000): 89–97; P. E. Niemuth, R. J. Johnson, M. J. Myers, and T. J. Thieman, "Hip muscle weakness and overuse injuries in recreational runners," *Clinical Journal of Sport Medicine* 15, no. 1 (2005): 14–21; S. M. Souza and C. M. Powers, "Predictors of hip internal rotation during running: an evaluation of hip strength and femoral structure in women with and without patellofemoral pain," *American Journal of Sports Medicine* 37, no. 3 (2009): 579–87.

47. R. L. Minzer, J. K. Kawaguchi, and T. L. Chmielewski, "Muscle strength in the lower extremity does not predict postinstruction improvements in the landing patterns of female athletes," *Journal of Orthopaedic & Sports Physical Therapy* 38, no. 6 (2008): 353–61.

48. R. Rerber, B. Noehren, J. Hamill, and I. Davis, "Competitive female runners with a history of ilio-tibial band syndrome demonstrate atypical hip and knee kinematics," *Journal of Orthopaedic & Sports Physical Therapy* 40, no. 2 (2010): 52–8.

49. J. D. Willson, S. Binder-Macleod, and I. S. Davis, "Lower extremity jumping mechanics of female athletes with and without patellofemoral pain before and after exertion," *American Journal of Sports Medicine* 36, no. 8 (2008): 1587–96.

50. D. C. Herman, J. A. Onate, P. S. Weinhold, K. M. Guskiewicz, W. E. Garrett, B. Yu, and D. A. Padua, "The effects of feedback with and without strength training on lower extremity biomechan-ics," *American Journal of Sports Medicine* 37, no. 7 (2009): 1301–8.

51. G. Cook, L. Burton, and K. Fields, "Reactive neuromuscular training for the anterior cruciate ligament–deficient knee: a case report," *Journal of Athletic Training* 34, no. 2 (1999): 194–201.

52. K. F. Spracklin, D. C. Button, and I. Halperin, "Looped band placed around thighs increases EMG of gluteal muscles without hindering performance during squatting," *Journal of Performance Health Research* 1, no. 1 (2017): 60–71; R. C. A. Foley, B. D. Bulbrook, D. C. Button, and M. W. R. Holmes, "Effects of a band loop on lower extremity muscle activity and kinematics during the barbell squat," *International Journal of Sports Physical Therapy* 12, no. 4 (2017): 550–9.

53. K. Kubo, H. Akima, J. Ushiyama, I. Tabata, H. Fukuoka, H. Kanehisa, and T. Fukunaga, "Effects of 20 days of bed rest on the viscoelastic properties of tendon structures in lower limb muscles," *British Journal of Sports Medicine* 38, no. 3 (2004): 324–30.

54. E. Rio, D. Kidgell, C. Purdam, J. Gaida, G. Lorimer Moseley, A. J. Pearce, and J. Cook, "Isometric exercise induces analgesia and reduces inhibition in patellar tendinopathy," *British Journal of Sports Medicine* 49, no. 19 (2015): 1277–83.

55. E. Rio, C. Purdam, M. Girdwood, and J. Cook, "Isometric exercise to reduce pain in patellar tendinopathy in-season: is it effective 'on the road'?" *Clinical Journal of Sport Medicine* 29, no. 3 (2017): 188–92.

56. S. P. Magnusson, M. V. Narici, C. N. Maganaris, and M. Kjaer, "Human tendon behaviour and adaptation, in vivo," *Journal of Physiology* 586, no. 1 (2008): 71–81; M. Couppé, P. Kongsgaard, P. Aagaard, J. Hansen, J. Bojsen-Moller, M. Kjaer, and S. P. Magnusson, "Habitual loading results in tendon hypertrophy and increased stiffness of the human patellar tendon," *Journal of Applied Physiology* 105, no. 3 (2008): 805–10.

57. R. Nisell and J. Ekholm, "Joint load during the parallel squat in powerlifting and force analysis of in vivo bilateral quadriceps tendon rupture," *Scandinavian Journal of Sports Sciences* 8, no. 2 (1986): 63–70.

58. R. Zernicke, J. Garhammer, and F. W. Jobe, "Human patellartendon rupture: a kinetic analysis," *Journal of Bone & Joint Surgery* 59, no. 2 (1977): 179–83; R. F. Escamilla, "Knee biomechanics of the dynamic squat exercise," *Medicine and Science in Sports and Exercise* 33, no. 1 (2001): 127–41.

59. R. Nisell and J. Ekholm, "Patellar forces during knee extension," *Scandinavian Journal of Rehabilitation Medicine* 17, no. 2 (1985): 63–74.

60. M. Rutland, D. O'Connell, J. M. Brismee, P. Sizer, G. Apte, and J. O'Connell, "Evidence-supported rehabilitation of patellar rehabilitation," *North American Journal of Sports Physical Therapy* 5, no. 3 (2010): 166–78.

61. P. Jonsson and H. Alfredson, "Superior results with eccentric compared to concentric quadri-ceps training in patients with jumper's knee: a prospective randomized study," *British Journal of Sports Medicine* 39, no. 11 (2005): 847–50.

62. P. Malliaras, J. Cook, C. Purdam, and E. Rio, "Patellar tendinopathy: clinical diagnosis, load management, and advice for challenging case presentations," *Journal of Orthopaedic & Sports Physical Therapy* 45, no. 11 (2015): 887–98.

63. S. Bohm, F. Mersmann, and A. Arampatzis, "Human tendon adaptation in response to mechan-ical loading: a systematic review and meta-analysis of exercise intervention studies on healthy adults," *Sports Medicine-Open* 1, no. 1 (2015): 7.

64. Malliaras, Cook, Purdam, and Rio, "Patellar tendinopathy" (see note 62 above); M. Kongsgaard, K. Qvortrup, J. Larsen, P. Aagaard, S. Doessing, P. Hansen, M. Kjaer, and S. P. Magnusson, "Fibril morphology and tendon mechanical properties in patellar tendinopathy: effects of heavy slow resistance training," *American Journal of Sports Medicine* 38, no. 4 (2010): 749–56; K. Kubo, T. Ilebukuro, H. Yata, N. Tsunoda, and H. Kanehisa, "Time course of changes in muscle and tendon properties during strength training and detraining," *Journal of Strength and Conditioning Research* 24, no. 2 (2010): 322–31.

65. Bohm, Mersmann, and Arampatzis, "Human tendon adaptation in response to mechanical loading" (see note 63 above).

66. Bohm, Mersmann, and Arampatzis, "Human tendon adaptation in response to mechanical loading" (see note 63 above); R. W. Morton, S. Y. Oikawa, C. G. Wavell, N. Mazara, C. McGlory, J. Quadrilatero, B. L. Baechler, S. K. Baker, and S. M. Phillips, "Neither load nor systemic hormones determine resistance training-mediated hypertrophy or strength gains in resistance-trained young men," *Journal of Applied Physiology* 121, no. 1 (2016): 129–38.

67. J. Cook, podcast interview, November 5, 2018.

68. Kongsgaard et al., "Corticosteroid injections, eccentric decline squat training and heavy slow resistance training in patellar tendinopathy" (see note 19 above).

69. A. Arampatzis, K. Karamanidis, and K. Albracht, "Adaptational responses of the human Achilles tendon by modulation of the applied cyclic strain magnitude," *Journal of Experimental Biology* 210, Pt 15 (2007): 2743–53.

70. Kongsgaard et al., "Corticosteroid injections, eccentric decline squat training and heavy slow resistance training in patellar tendinopathy" (see note 19 above).

71. J. E. Earp, R. U. Newton, P. Cormie, and A. J. Blazevich, "Faster movement speed results in greater tendon strain during the loaded squat exercise," *Frontiers in Physiology* 7 (2016): 366.

72. Kongsgaard et al., "Corticosteroid injections, eccentric decline squat training and heavy slow resistance training in patellar tendinopathy" (see note 19 above).

73. J. Cook, podcast interview, November 5, 2018.

74. A. Rudavsky and J. Cook, "Physiotherapy management of patellar tendinopathy (jumper's knee)," *Journal of Physiotherapy* 60, no. 3 (2014): 122–9.

75. Malliaras, Cook, Purdam, and Rio, "Patellar tendinopathy" (see note 62 above).

76. J. Fairclough, K. Hayashi, H. Toumi, K. Lyons, G. Bydder, N. Phillips, T. M. Best, and M. Benjamin, "The functional anatomy of the iliotibial band during flexion and extension of the knee: implications for understanding iliotibial band syndrome," *Journal of Anatomy* 208, no. 3 (2006): 309–16.

77. M. Lavagnino, S. P. Arnoczky, J. Dodds, and N. Elvin, "Infrapatellar straps decrease patellar tendon strain at the site of the jumper's knee lesion," *Sports Health* 3, no. 3 (2011): 296–302.

78. M. D. Miller, D. T. Hinkin, and J. W. Wisnowski, "The efficacy of orthotics for anterior knee pain in military trainees. A preliminary report," *American Journal of Knee Surgery* 10, no. 1 (1997): 10–3.

79. E. Harman and P. Frykman, "Bridging the gap–research: The effects of knee wraps on weight-lifting performance and injury," *Journal of Strength Conditioning Research* 12 (1990): 30–5.

80. J. P. Lake, P. J. C. Carden, and K. A. Shorter, "Wearing knee wraps affects mechanical output and performance characteristics of back squat exercise," *Journal of Strength Conditioning Research* 26, no. 10 (2012): 2844–9.

81. P. H. Marchetti, V. de Jesus Pereira Matos, E. G. Soares, J. J. da Silva, E. Serpa, D. A. Corrêa, G. C. Martins, G. V. Junior, and W. A. Gomes, "Can the technique of knee wrap placement affect the maximal isometric force during back squat exercise?" *International Journal of Sports Science & Coaching* 5, no. 1 (2015): 16–8.

82. Lake, Carden, and Shorter, "Wearing knee wraps affects mechanical output and performance characteristics of back squat exercise" (see note 80 above).

CHAPTER 4

SHOULDER PAIN

The shoulder is the most dynamic and intricate joint in the entire body. Every time you pick up a barbell from the ground or drive one overhead, a complex network of muscles, ligaments, and bones must work perfectly in sync to keep the joint safe. For the shoulder to remain healthy, it must have sufficient mobility to move into a wide range of positions while being stable enough to maintain those positions.

In all my years of working with athletes, I have found the shoulder to be one of the most frequently injured joints. In fact, research shows that it is *the most* injured joint in those who lift weights either competitively or recreationally.[1] I want to begin this chapter by briefly going over the anatomy of the shoulder and covering some of the common shoulder injuries that I see in the weight room.

Shoulder Anatomy

Before jumping into the potential injuries that can occur at the shoulder, we must discuss its architecture (how the joint is designed) and its function (how the different parts work together to create movement).

The shoulder joint, or glenohumeral joint, is considered a ball-and-socket joint and is made up of three bones: the humerus, scapula, and clavicle. The end of the humerus (upper arm bone) is shaped like a small ball that fits into the socket of the scapula (shoulder blade). Unlike the relatively deep ball-and-socket joint of the hip, the socket of the shoulder is very shallow, which is why the joint connection is often compared to a golf ball sitting on a tee.

SHOULDER MUSCLE ANATOMY

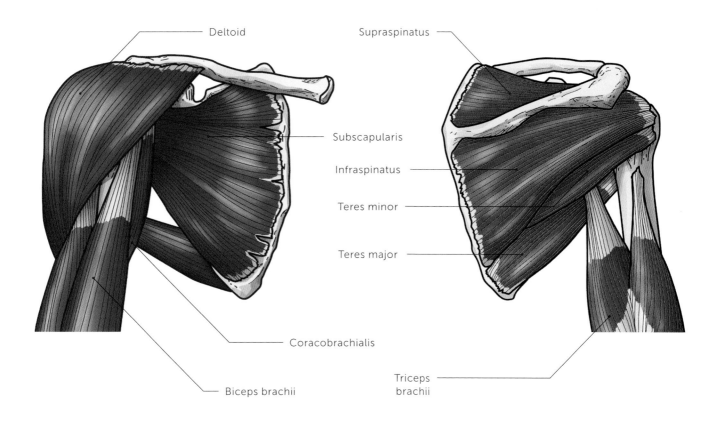

Deltoid

Supraspinatus

Subscapularis

Infraspinatus

Teres minor

Teres major

Coracobrachialis

Triceps brachii

Biceps brachii

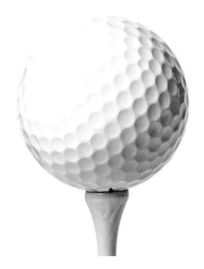

The shallow shoulder joint connection is often compared to a golf ball sitting on a tee. © TK

The "ball" of the humerus is held in place on the "tee" or socket of the shoulder blade, called the *glenoid*, by a number of small but very important tissues (ligaments and capsule). These tissues wrap around the joint like a tight-fitting glove and form an airtight hold.

LIGAMENTS AND CAPSULE SURROUNDING THE SHOULDER JOINT

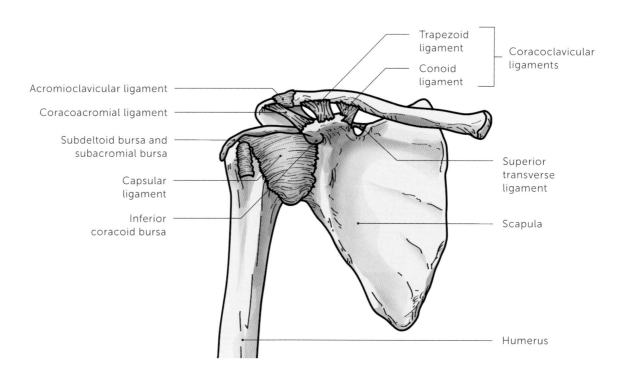

Right over the top of these ligaments and capsule runs the rotator cuff, a group of four small muscles that begin at the shoulder blade and attach to the humerus. Because these muscles lie close to the joint and act to compress the humerus in the socket as the arm moves, they are considered "primary stabilizers."

ROTATOR CUFF MUSCLES: PRIMARY STABILIZERS

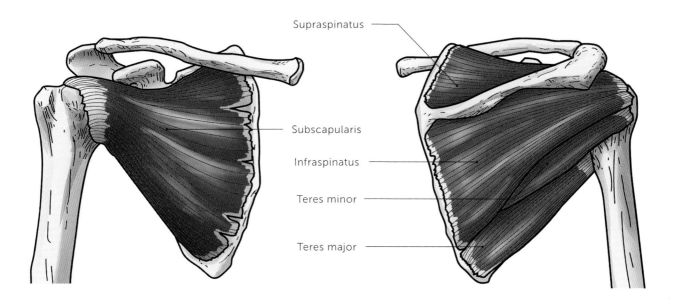

Supraspinatus

Subscapularis

Infraspinatus

Teres minor

Teres major

Then a number of large muscles attach to the shoulder blade and/or humerus to help move the arm. The lats, pecs, and deltoids are big muscles that are often referred to as "prime movers." You can walk into any gym and see people (especially young men) working religiously on getting these muscles bigger and stronger.

LATS, PECS, AND DELTOIDS: PRIME MOVERS

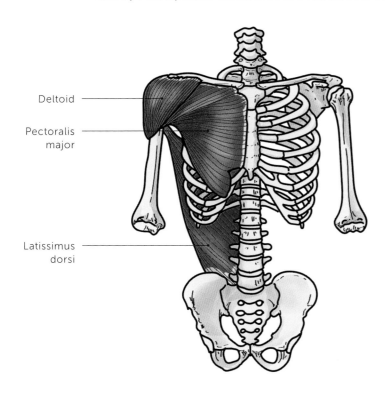

Deltoid

Pectoralis major

Latissimus dorsi

The shoulder joint is most efficient when the "golf ball" of the humerus remains in the center of the "tee." This is much easier said than done, however. As simple as this concept seems, only 25 to 30 percent of your "golf ball" is in contact with the "tee" at any given time.[2] However, a strong and healthy shoulder will maintain the ball of the humerus to within a few millimeters of the center of the socket throughout almost all arm movements.[3]

How is this movement precision possible? It is the result of a perfect interplay of two factors: static and dynamic (or active) forces.

Static and Dynamic Forces

Static forces are the pull or tension created by structures we have no control over, like the ligaments and capsule that surround the joint and the labrum that expands the joint socket. The combination of the tension that these tissues create and the shape of the joint socket is what dictates the degree of "passive stability" for the shoulder.[4]

If you've ever seen someone who is "double-jointed," that extreme flexibility is often due in part to very lax or loose static structures in the shoulders. It should come as no surprise that each of us has slight differences in our anatomy. Some people naturally have more or less ligament/capsular stiffness. Also, the shape/size of the scapular glenoid fossa (the tee in the golf ball analogy) varies from person to person. Some individuals have a deep glenoid fossa, while in others it may be flatter, resembling a plate. Both of these factors can have a great impact on the amount of stability a person has.

For example, as you pull a barbell over your head during a snatch or jerk, the shoulder joint capsule tightens or "winds up" to stabilize the joint and keep the humerus from sliding out of the socket. Those with a lax or loose capsule (or a shallow plate–shaped joint socket) have less natural passive stability and require even more "active stability" (from the muscles that surround the joint), or they risk injury.

While we obviously can't change how these static stabilizers work short of surgery, we can make sure the muscles that surround the shoulder joint (the active stabilizers) are doing their job. Therefore, *dynamic forces* are the pull or tension created by muscles—something we do have control over.

As mentioned earlier, the four small muscles that make up the rotator cuff—the subscapularis, supraspinatus, infraspinatus, and teres minor—surround the shoulder joint and create compression to maintain the center of the "ball" on the "tee" as you move your arm. These muscles work together with the larger muscles that attach to the arm and shoulder blade to produce safe and powerful movement whether you are picking up a bag of groceries or throwing a loaded barbell over your head.

To understand how the rotator cuff and prime movers work together to move your scapula and humerus, imagine a young boy helping his father set up a tall ladder. The boy kneels at the base of the ladder, securing it to the ground. The father then pushes the ladder upward, leaning it against the side of their house. (In the photo, opposite, that's me in the red shirt representing the boy in this analogy.)

This is precisely what happens at your shoulder every time you move your arm![5] Here's how each part plays out:

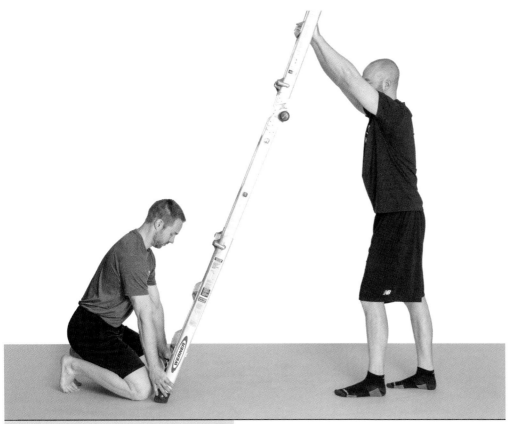

"BOY" AND FATHER SETTING UP LADDER

- **Father:** Prime movers (lats, pecs, and deltoids)
- **Boy:** Primary stabilizers (rotator cuff muscles)
- **Ladder:** Humerus bone
- **The ground:** Scapula socket

The boy (rotator cuff muscles) works to keep the ladder (humerus) in a stable position on the ground (scapula socket), while the father (powerful lat, pec, and deltoid muscles) focuses on moving the ladder into the correct position.

One person holding the base of the ladder in place while another person moves the ladder into place is a great analogy for how dynamic stability is created and maintained. Without sufficient passive and active stability, we risk injuries like rotator cuff tendonitis and tears, labrum tears, and shoulder instability injuries, to name a few.

Simple enough, right?

Unfortunately, the shoulder complex is a little more complicated. Not only do we need to understand the mechanics of the shoulder joint itself, but we also need to take into account how the shoulder blade is moving. As you move your arm over your head, your shoulder blade moves as well to maintain contact with the humerus.

Returning to the ladder analogy, think of what would happen if the father decided to grab the ladder and move it to a different part of the house. The ladder could topple over if the boy didn't get up from his kneeling position and move with the ladder to secure it in place again. Just as the boy moves to keep the base of the ladder connected to the ground, the shoulder blade must move to accommodate the changing position of the upper arm bone. This action comes from a number of muscles that connect to the shoulder blade, such as the rhomboids, trapezius, teres major, and serratus anterior.

There is one more important piece of the puzzle: the thoracic spine, or mid-back. Because the shoulder blade basically floats on top of the spine, the shape of the mid-back can dictate the efficiency of its movement (or lack thereof). To move correctly and be in the right place at the right time to provide stability for the arm, the shoulder blade has to glide easily over the upper back. This requires a certain amount of thoracic spine extension.

SCAPULA MOVING ON TOP OF THE THORACIC SPINE

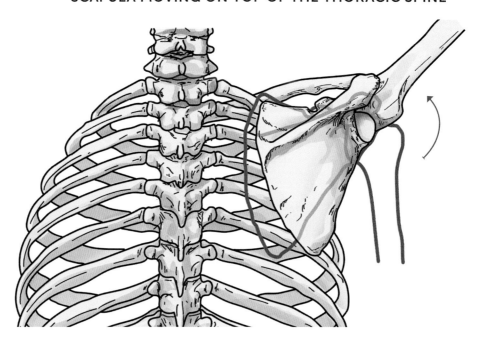

The architecture of the mid-back is naturally stiff and stable. It has to be stiff because many of the ribs that connect to it provide protection for the vital organs that lie underneath. Unfortunately, many of us assume poor postures throughout the day, which leads to the adaptation of a stiff or "kyphotic" and rounded upper back. When the upper back is rounded and unable to extend fully, the movement of the shoulder blades is limited.[6] An immobile shoulder blade affects the mechanics and stability of the shoulder joint. As you can see, there are many factors behind safe and efficient movement of the shoulder!

To wrap up this section, here are the basics of the shoulder complex that you need to remember: *If the shoulder blade moves as it should on top of a mobile thoracic spine, the rotator cuff muscles can do their job and maintain sufficient stability of the joint. The arm is then controlled by the large prime movers of the upper body. Basically, if every part performs its function correctly, the "ball" stays in the middle of the "tee," and injury is averted.*

Shoulder Injury Anatomy 101

What causes shoulder pain? The simplest answer is that pain is often the result of excessive stress or strain on the small structures that surround the shoulder joint. The normally harmonious shoulder complex can be derailed by a malfunction in one part (e.g., a weak rotator cuff or poor passive shoulder stability). For a strength athlete, pain usually comes from cumulative microtrauma due to three things:

- Imbalances between the prime movers and primary stabilizers
- Instability
- Poor movement and lifting technique

The specific injury that is sustained—rotator cuff tendinopathy, labrum tear, subluxation, and so on—depends on how balance and control are lost. Let me explain.

Imbalances and Instability

Let's begin by discussing commonly occurring problems from an anatomical perspective. For the shoulder to work correctly, the small primary stabilizers (rotator cuff muscles) must work in balance with the larger prime movers, like the deltoid. If these forces are not properly balanced, the joint loses stability and the mechanics of the shoulder are thrown off.[7]

A common injury that occurs due to an imbalance like this is impingement. Research shows that there are two kinds of impingement: external (or subacromial) and internal.[8] Because these classifications are based on where the impingement occurs, the two types often bring out pain in different parts of the shoulder.

When you look at the anatomy of the shoulder joint, you'll notice that there isn't a ton of space between the "ball" of the humerus and the structures that lie directly above it, like the acromion of the shoulder blade.

SHOULDER JOINT ANATOMY SHOWING EXTERNAL IMPINGEMENT

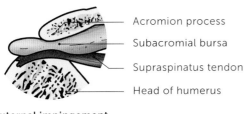

Acromion process
Subacromial bursa
Supraspinatus tendon
Head of humerus

External impingement

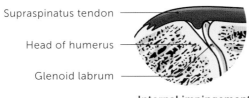

Supraspinatus tendon
Head of humerus
Glenoid labrum

Internal impingement

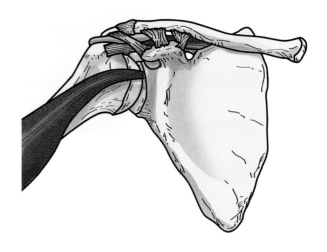

- **External impingement** describes the pinching of the bursa (a small, fluid-filled "bag") or rotator cuff tendons against the "ceiling" created by the acromion bone. (The space between the acromion and the rotator cuff/soft tissue structures is known as the *subacromial space*.) It often creates pain on the front of the shoulder as the arm is raised overhead.

- **Internal impingement** occurs when the tendons of the rotator cuff are pinched between the "ball" of the humerus and the edge (usually the back side) of the socket "tee." It creates pain on the back of the shoulder as the arm is elevated and externally rotated.

Impingement injuries can also be classified based on the cause of the pain (or *pathomechanics*). The pinching of the overlying structures in the joint can happen for two main reasons:

- Anatomy (primary impingement)

- Dynamic imbalances (secondary impingement)

The first factor is the anatomy of the shoulder blade. The acromion in most people is fairly flat or slightly curved. However, in some individuals, this bone has a hooked shape, which can leave less "free space" for the rotator cuff tendons and bursa as the shoulder moves. If someone who has this type of anatomy pushes through uncomfortable and painful positions, the rotator cuff tendons can become swollen and the subacromial space can become even narrower. Less space means more pinching of these tissues against the bony ceiling of the shoulder. With enough time, this microtrauma can turn into a big problem like a rotator cuff tear.

Unfortunately, we cannot change this anatomy short of surgery. Early recognition of symptoms is the key to getting ahead of this injury before it's too late. Working with a physical therapist or coach to modify your lifting technique to suit your anatomy, such as by taking a wider grip on the barbell for the snatch or jerk, might allow you to continue lifting overhead with less impingement.

Secondary impingement is more common in athletes in my experience. At the start of this chapter, I mentioned that the shoulder is a ball-and-socket joint. That statement isn't 100 percent accurate. You see, when the shoulder moves into extreme ranges of motion (such as when you lift your arm overhead), the arm not only rotates in the joint but also glides slightly forward, backward, and up or down. A secondary impingement doesn't occur because of a structural abnormality but because of a functional problem. Usually, an athlete will have a hard time maintaining adequate shoulder stability with overhead movements. In some cases, excessive movement of the humeral head ("ball") can lead to internal pinching.

Secondary impingements can be created by

- Muscle strength imbalances

- Mobility restrictions

- Coordination problems (shoulder blade and humerus)

- Instability

A muscle strength imbalance is one of the most common reasons for secondary impingement. If the rotator cuff is not firing correctly or is just plain weak, the stronger muscles that surround the shoulder (prime movers) will overpower the primary stabilizers (rotator cuff muscles). If we go back to the ladder analogy, the boy (rotator cuff) must stabilize the base of the ladder for the father (prime movers) to push the ladder up to secure it in place. If the base of the ladder is not secured, the ladder will wobble excessively, and the father will have a difficult time placing the ladder at the right location/height. Although the rotator cuff muscles are small, they have a *very big* job!

Mobility restrictions such as stiff lats, stiff pecs, and an excessively stiff thoracic spine can also create impingements. Any one of these restrictions can negatively impact scapula or humerus movement. Mobility restrictions can negatively affect an athlete's overhead barbell or dumbbell lifts. Here's one such example.

To maintain proper upper-body tension and stability for pulls and deadlifts, the body must activate the powerful lat muscles (the huge "V"-shaped muscles that run along the sides of the back). These strong muscles not only help create sufficient core stability and torso stiffness but also help maintain shoulder internal rotation to keep the bar close to the body as the barbell is pulled from the floor.

To move the barbell overhead also requires flexibility in the lats. To keep the head of the humerus in the center of the joint as the arm moves overhead, the humerus must externally rotate. If the lats are too stiff, the humerus will be unable to achieve adequate external rotation, which could lead to an impingement. Those who have limited overhead mobility due to flexibility restrictions yet continue to force their shoulders into poor positions when lifting end up with microtrauma, which can lead to shoulder injury and/or pain.

LAT FLEXIBILITY ALLOWS THE HUMERUS TO MOVE OVERHEAD

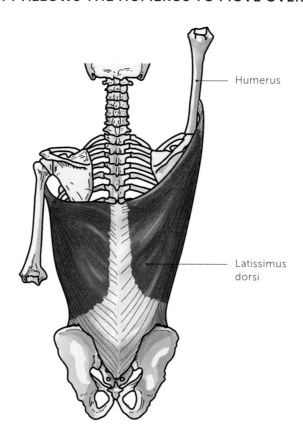

Humerus

Latissimus dorsi

Proper coordination between the shoulder blade and humerus is crucial for maintaining stability. As discussed earlier, the shoulder blade must move in sync with the arm. If the shoulder blade is unable to rotate upward enough when the arm is moving into an overhead position, the humeral head can shift excessively in the joint, and impingement can occur. A weak or poorly functioning serratus anterior muscle could be a cause for poor scapula upward rotation.

SERRATUS ANTERIOR MUSCLE

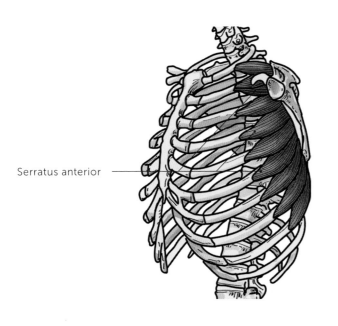

Serratus anterior

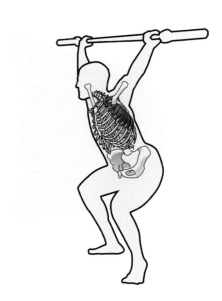

Normal serratus anterior

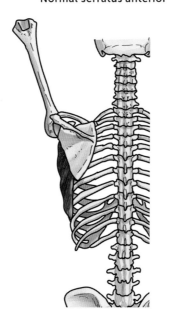

Weak serratus anterior

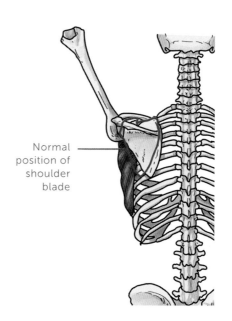

Normal position of shoulder blade

Lastly, secondary impingement, along with other serious shoulder injuries, could be caused by shoulder instability—a mechanical problem.[9] The term "shoulder instability" itself is fairly vague in part because it is difficult to determine whether the amount of mobility an athlete presents with is normal or problematic. Some athletes are extremely mobile, or "hypermobile." This hypermobility can be congenital or acquired:

- **Congenital** means you were born with it. Some people are born with "loose" joints due to lax connective tissue. Typically, they do well in activities such as gymnastics, cheerleading, and dance.

- **Acquired** hypermobility usually develops over a long period. The small structures of the shoulder are stretched or even torn due to repetitive micro-trauma. This kind of mobility is commonly seen in those who participate in sports that involve performing the same movements over and over, resulting in excessive stretching of the static structures that stabilize the joint. For example, it can develop in baseball players and swimmers due to the repetitive overhead motions used during training and competition.

Either congenital or acquired hypermobility can lead to injury if there is a significant deficiency in strength and/or stability.[10]

Research has shown that anywhere from 5 to 15 percent of people (more often women) are born with hypermobility.[11] An easy way to assess whether you fall into this category is to determine your Beighton score.[12]

Try these five screens. For each of the first four, test both sides of your body. Give yourself a score of 1 if you can perform the task or 0 if you cannot. Your total score then ranges from 0 to 9.

- Grab your opposite-hand pinky and pull it as far backward as possible. (Don't hurt yourself!) Can you move it past 90 degrees without pain?

- Grab your opposite-hand thumb and pull it toward your forearm. Can you touch your thumb to your forearm without pain?

- Straighten your elbow as far as you can. Does it hyperextend (move past 10 degrees)?

- Straighten your knee as far as you can. Does it hyperextend (move past 10 degrees)?

- Bend over at your hips and try to touch the ground without bending your knees. Can you rest your palms on the floor?

What did you find? Research has shown that those with a score of 2 or higher are likely to be hypermobile and are nearly two and a half times as likely to sustain an instability injury to the shoulder![13]

Now, here's what you need to understand. Joint hypermobility is not inherently dangerous. Plenty of athletes have hypermobility (either congenital or acquired) and go through their entire athletic careers without getting injured. If the rotator cuff fails to control a hypermobile shoulder joint during dynamic movements, however, the shoulder can become unstable, and injury is likely to occur. The ability to dynamically stabilize the shoulder is the difference between functional hypermobility and pathological instability.

So how does instability lead to injury when lifting weights?

CrossFitters and weightlifters are similar to baseball players and gymnasts in the sense that having the requisite shoulder mobility is paramount. The repetitive nature of lifting weights overhead can put the shoulder at increased risk for injury, especially in the presence of instability. Although you likely won't see a traumatic dislocation during overhead lifting (snatch, jerk, press, and so on), tiny amounts of trauma are sustained at the shoulder if stability is lacking.

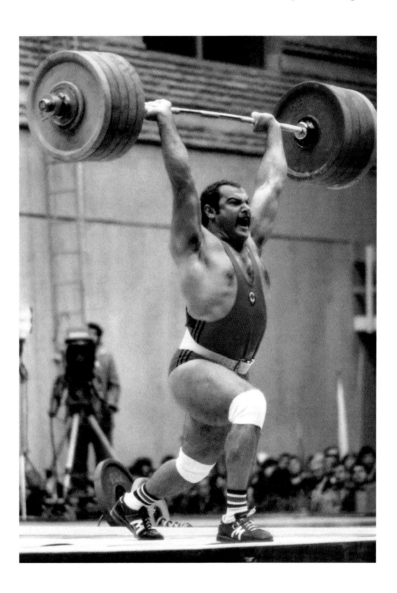

Elite weightlifter split jerk. *Anatoly Pisarenko, © Bruce Klemens*

Because the shoulder is a naturally mobile joint, the location and type of injury can differ from person to person. It all depends on the direction in which the "ball," or humeral head, moves off the "tee," or glenoid fossa. For example, let's go back to internal impingement. If someone has natural hypermobility of the shoulder joint and not enough muscular control, the tendons of the rotator cuff can be pinched against the back of the joint socket as they raise their arm overhead.

Instability can also result in a more serious injury to the labrum, which is a thick piece of tissue that expands or deepens the "tee" of the shoulder joint, allowing for more connection to the arm bone. Similar to placing a heavy block under a car's tire when parking on a hill to keep the car from rolling, the labrum acts as a passive restraint to help stabilize the shoulder joint.[14]

LABRUM

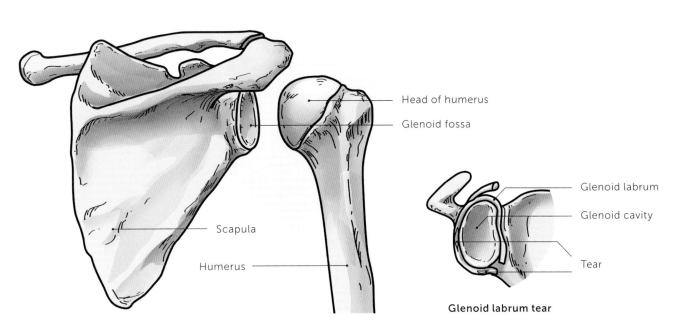

Head of humerus

Glenoid fossa

Scapula

Humerus

Glenoid labrum

Glenoid cavity

Tear

Glenoid labrum tear

The labrum works with the joint capsule to create an airtight seal over the joint. However, if sufficient dynamic stability is not maintained in the joint, excessive motion can occur, causing trauma to the labrum and eventual tearing. A tear in the labrum—even a slight one—results in a dramatic drop in pressure inside the joint and a huge loss of passive joint stability. The most common complaint among those who have this type of injury is a painful "catching" or "popping" of the shoulder when moving the arm overhead.[15]

Poor Movement and Technique

The final cause of shoulder injury should come as no surprise. Moving poorly, especially under load, increases your risk for injury. The most common technique flaw that leads to shoulder pain when lifting occurs when the barbell is pushed or held overhead (e.g., in the snatch, jerk/press, or overhead squat). Let's break down how it happens.

For the shoulder joint to remain safe during the snatch, jerk/press, or overhead squat, the wrists, elbows, shoulders/shoulder blades, and extended mid-back (thoracic spine) should be kept in a vertically stacked alignment. With the barbell positioned directly over the back of the neck, the shoulder muscles can work efficiently to stabilize the tremendous weight overhead. If everything is aligned properly, you should be able to sit in the bottom of a deep squat and press the bar vertically to the overhead position and back down to the tops of your traps, moving only your arms and keeping the rest of your body still.

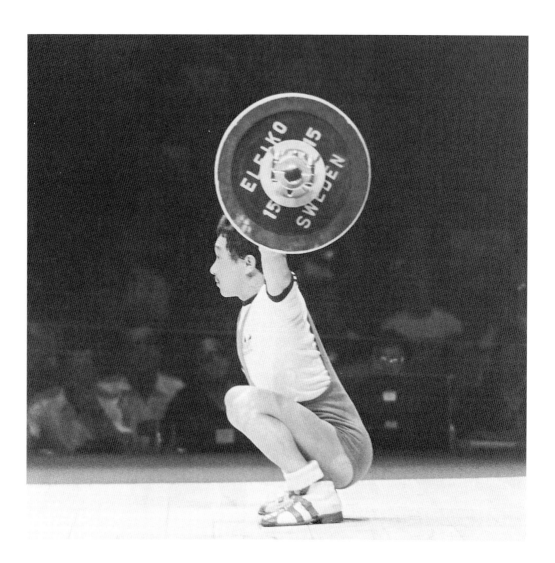

Overhead squat with proper vertically stacked alignment.
Kanybek Osmanaliev,
© *Bruce Klemens*

To maintain stability with overhead lifts, your shoulder blades must be in the proper position. For most athletes, the scapulae should be slightly retracted (pulled together) and rotated upward slightly, but not shrugged upward.

It is a common misconception that lifters should shrug their shoulder blades when the barbell is overhead. Some appear to have done so as they secure the barbell in the overhead position for two reasons. First, the shoulder blades naturally have to rotate upward to provide stability for the humeri. Second, the upper traps are engaged to help provide tension for the arms as they support the barbell overhead. The appearance of upwardly rotated shoulder blades and engaged upper traps gives the impression that the lifter is actively shrugging their shoulders upward. However, this is often not the case. Excessive shrugging of the shoulders can lead to early fatigue of the supporting musculature that stabilizes the joints. Simply put, over-emphasizing a shoulder shrug is an inefficient approach to stabilizing the barbell overhead.

Olympian Chad Vaughn explains this concept by telling athletes to envision doing a 100-meter overhead walking lunge with a barbell. If the shoulders are shrugged upward to support the barbell, the trap muscles will surely fatigue before the 100-meter distance is covered.

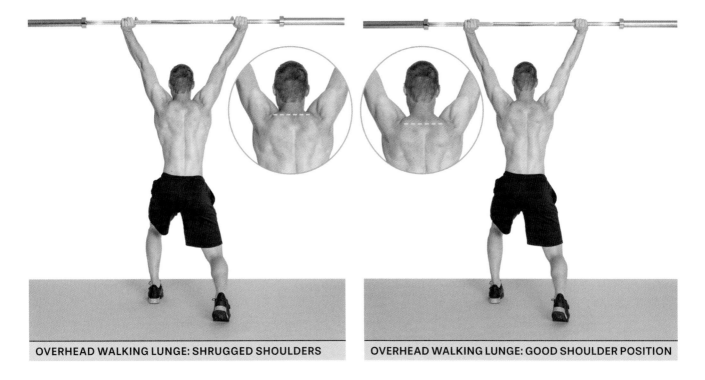

OVERHEAD WALKING LUNGE: SHRUGGED SHOULDERS

OVERHEAD WALKING LUNGE: GOOD SHOULDER POSITION

One of the most common technique flaws behind shoulder injuries when lifting overhead is excessive internal or external rotation of the joint. As you raise your arm (or toss a barbell over your head), your shoulder moves into slight external rotation to keep the "ball" centered on the "tee." Poor technique can shift the shoulder into excessive rotation to keep the body (and the weight overhead) in balance. If you drop your chest forward during an overhead squat, your arms will reflexively move farther behind your head to keep the barbell balanced over the mid-foot. This exaggerated position places your shoulders in significant external rotation and shifts the humerus too far forward in the joint. Lifting weights overhead in this unbalanced position (out of the ideal stacked alignment) subjects the small structures of the shoulder to microtrauma and can lead to pain.

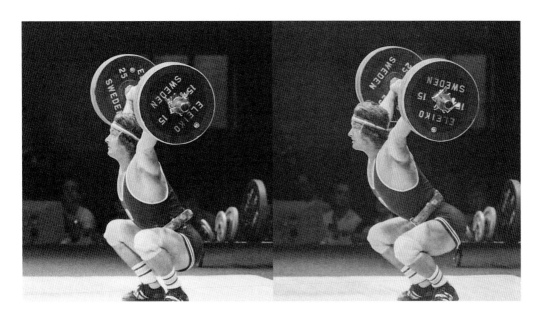

Overhead lifting technique with proper and poor positioning.
Kevin Winter, © Bruce Klemens

As a side note, a lot of people ask about coaches giving athletes the cue to internally rotate their shoulders in the overhead position. I think this is a misunderstanding of shoulder mechanics. I believe the problem lies in the appearance that some experienced athletes give as they squeeze their shoulder blades together and push their armpits forward with the barbell overhead, known as scapular retraction. While the shoulder may appear to be moving into internal rotation, the humerus itself is remaining externally rotated to stay in the middle of the shoulder socket.

Regardless of the cues your coach may give, your upper body must remain in a balanced stacked alignment for your shoulders to stay safe when lifting overhead. There will always be a little variation in how the overhead position looks from athlete to athlete due to individual anatomy, but we all must adhere to the foundation for safety and stability when lifting if we want to keep our shoulders injury-free.

How to Screen Your Shoulder Pain

By now, you should have noticed a common thread in how shoulder injuries occur. Safe and efficient movement is the combined action of mobility and stability. If you lack the proper stability or mobility, your joints can sustain microtrauma that can lead to a big injury over time.

The approach to screening shoulder pain is quite simple. Instead of trying to diagnose the specific part of the shoulder that may be injured (such as the labrum or rotator cuff), you need to uncover the root cause of the pain. By addressing the *why* behind the pain, you can (I hope) avoid tunnel vision in your rehab plan.

For example, an athlete who is dealing with rotator cuff irritation from performing high-volume push presses might start a rehab program that involves rotator cuff strengthening, with exercises found online or picked up from a gym-mate. If the inflammation was caused by an impingement because of poor thoracic spine extension (and therefore an inability of the shoulder blade to sufficiently glide upward), however, no amount of strengthening work for the rotator cuff muscles would truly fix the issue. The pain might subside in the short term but would likely return as soon as the athlete resumed lifting overhead.

Most clinicians are taught to screen the shoulder by performing a battery of tests to rule in or out specific injuries. However, many of these tests only serve to confirm the presence of an injury (such as a labrum or rotator cuff tear) rather than help identify the underlying injury mechanism. Knowing that someone has a rotator cuff tear doesn't necessarily tell you why they have pain or what needs to be corrected. Therefore, classifying an injury by the problem that is causing the pain (in this example, an inability to raise the arm overhead due to poor thoracic spine extension mobility) is more useful for driving the treatment process.

This doesn't mean we just ignore any findings from an MRI or other expensive scan! In fact, the movement-based model for screening (called the *kinesiopathologic model,* or KPM) does not dismiss or assume a specific anatomical problem as the cause of pain but, instead, treats any findings from an MRI as a piece of the pie in the overall decision-making process. By taking a big step back and looking at how athletes move in real time or in a videorecording, you can avoid tunnel vision. The radiology report provides useful information, but it shouldn't be the primary focus of rehab/treatment. Treat the person, not the injury, in other words.

I want you to think about which of the following categories best fits your shoulder pain:

- Poor movement/technique
- Limited mobility/flexibility
- Instability
- Strength imbalance/weakness

Your injury may fall into more than one category, so be sure to go through every section. Each area can give you clues on how to piece together a plan of action to fix your injury.

Movement and Technique Assessment

Assessing the quality of your lifting technique should be your first step toward uncovering the cause of your injury. Think about all of the repetitive lifts or movements you do in the gym that generate shoulder pain. Once you've placed your finger on the one or two things that lead to pain, can you find a common movement pattern or posture that you assume during those lifts or movements?

For example, a powerlifter might have shoulder pain when performing a back squat because their elbows are positioned too far behind their torso, causing the humerus "ball" to slide forward (to the anterior) in the socket "tee." If this sounds like you, see if your symptoms change when you lower your elbows so that your arms are in alignment with your trunk.

When you assess your lifting technique, make sure you observe everything from your wrists down to your low back. Each of these components (which you will read more about soon) can have an impact on the forces sustained at the shoulder joint. Also look for subtle side-to-side differences if you are experiencing pain in only one shoulder. Having a skilled coach serve as another set of eyes can be helpful for identifying these small technique problems that could be causing your symptoms.

A key area to focus on during this assessment is the action of your shoulder blades. If you can, remove your shirt or wear a tight-fitting shirt that leaves your back visible. Lift your arms straight forward and out to the sides. Perform a press with a barbell and do a pull-up. During each movement, assess whether the shoulder blade on your painful side is moving excessively or not as much as the one on the pain-free side. Limited upward rotation can be a sign of a poorly functioning serratus anterior muscle, whereas excessive scapular motion can be due to instability and posterior rotator cuff weakness.

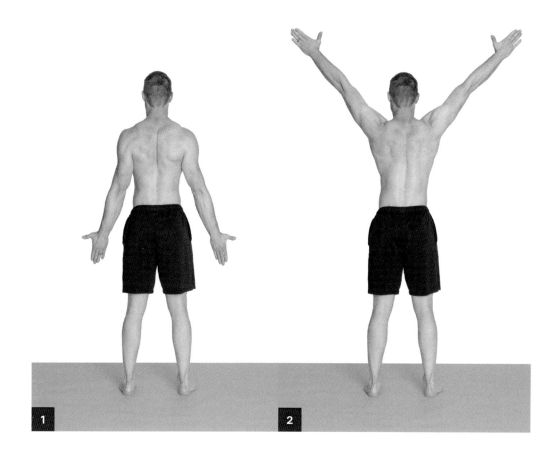

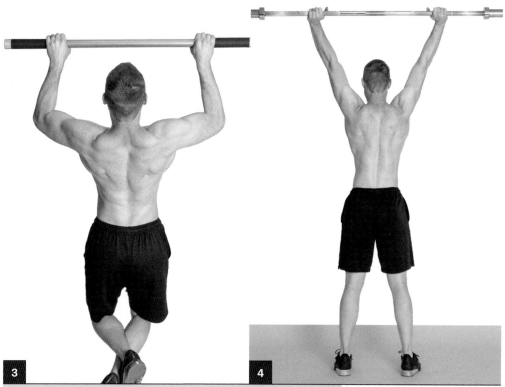

SHOULDER BLADE MOVEMENT: ABDUCTION, PULL-UP, PRESS

Mobility and Flexibility Assessment

Seated Mobility Assessments

In the sports of weightlifting and CrossFit, athletes perform a ton of overhead lifting in a variety of positions: for example, a wide grip with the snatch and a close grip with the jerk or press. If an athlete does not have adequate mobility to perform these lifts correctly, a number of injuries can eventually occur.

I first saw this screen demonstrated by physical therapist Dave Tilley of Shiftmovementscience.com. Start by sitting with your back against a wall. Your head, upper back, and hips should all be in contact with the wall. Your lower spine should be neutral (meaning you don't need to jam your low back into the wall).

With your arms extended in front of you and your palms facing the ground, raise your arms as high overhead as you can. If you'd like, you can do this with a PVC pipe (or broomstick) and the same grip you would use for a clean and jerk or an overhead press. Keep your core braced and your ribs from flaring out as you perform this movement.

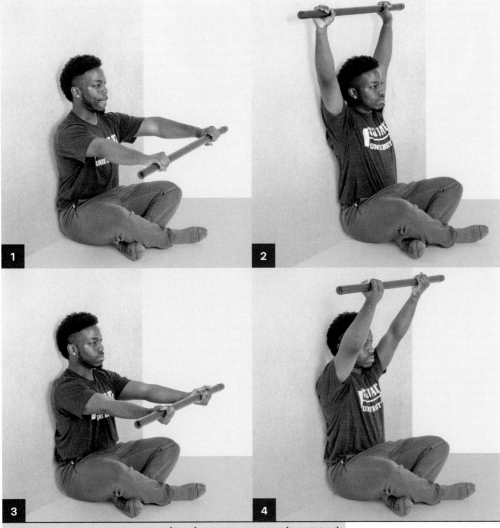

WALL SCREEN: PALMS DOWN (TOP) AND PALMS UP (BOTTOM)

Could you get your hands all the way to the wall without your arms bending? If you were able to touch the wall behind you, did it require a ton of effort?

If you answered yes to both questions, try the same movement but with your palms facing toward the ceiling, a more externally rotated shoulder position. Were you able to still reach the wall? Did your elbows end up bending? Did your head pop forward off the wall, or did your arms move out to a "Y" position to touch your hands to the wall? If you didn't have a PVC pipe to hold, did your thumbs want to turn toward your head (shoulder internal rotation) as you raised your arms?

Ideally, your arms should end up close to your ears, similar to a narrow grip on an overhead press. This should be an effortless motion that doesn't require much grunt force to complete. If this was you, congratulations. You have adequate overhead mobility!

Next, place your arms against the wall in an "L" position, with your elbows bent at a 90-degree angle. Slide your arms as far down the wall as you can without losing contact.

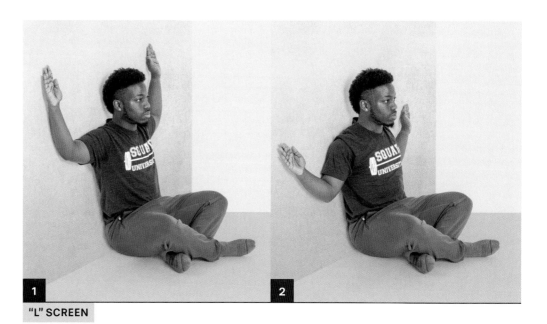

"L" SCREEN

What did you experience?

This motion mimics the arm positions necessary to efficiently hold a barbell on your back during a back squat. If you were unable to slide your arms to at least a 45-degree angle without compensation (flaring your ribs or arching your low back), you're likely missing mobility somewhere. This could be due to limited shoulder external rotation, thoracic spine extension, or pec major/minor flexibility (something I'll go over soon).

Standing Mobility Assessment

While the past few screens focused on the importance of shoulder external rotation, weightlifters and CrossFitters must also have sufficient shoulder *internal* rotation to keep the bar close to the body during Olympic lifts, especially the snatch. An athlete who is lacking adequate internal rotation will have to compensate by rolling the entire shoulder complex forward (moving the shoulder blade excessively) to keep the bar from looping away from the body.

To screen for internal rotation, stand up, assume the same "L" position with your arms, and rotate your hands as far toward the ground as you can without your shoulder blades rolling forward. Ideally, you should be able to internally rotate your shoulders so that your forearms at least reach parallel to the ground.

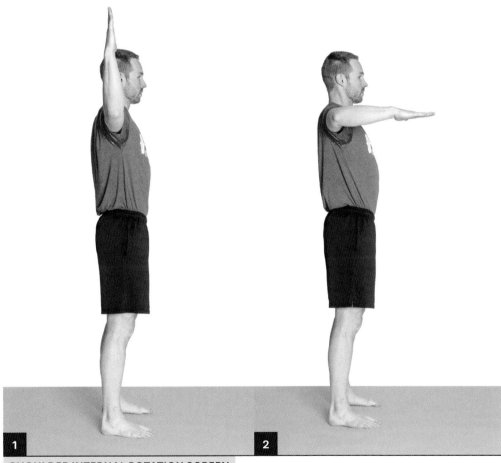

SHOULDER INTERNAL ROTATION SCREEN

If you were unable to pass any of these screens, proceed to the following assessments to determine what is limiting your mobility.

Lat/Teres Major Flexibility Screening

While lying on your back, have a friend raise your arm overhead while holding your shoulder blade in place with their other hand. Perform this movement with your thumb facing the sky and with your thumb facing away from your head so that you're assessing shoulder elevation in both an internally and an externally rotated position.

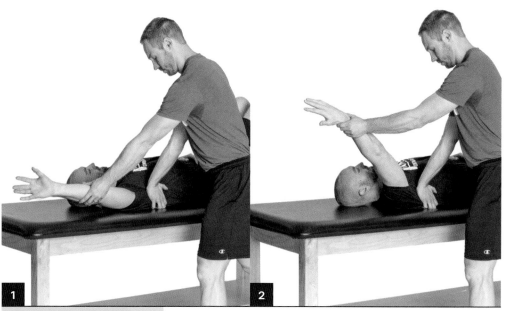

LAT FLEXIBILITY SCREENING

Were you able to move your arm higher overhead when your thumb was facing skyward? This internally rotated position takes slack off of the lats and teres major muscles and therefore allows someone with flexibility limitations in these muscles to move the arm farther overhead.

If your arm elevation is limited, with no significant difference between the two hand positions, the mobility restriction may be coming from deeper in the joint, such as a stiff/restricted joint capsule. That kind of restriction would require a rehabilitation professional to address appropriately.

Pec Minor and Major Flexibility Screening

Sufficient flexibility of the pectoralis minor muscles is imperative for proper shoulder blade mechanics when lifting. An inflexible pec minor will render the shoulder blade unable to move adequately, leaving it protracted and anteriorly tilted, and could result in impingement of the small structures in the shoulder joint.

To assess the flexibility of your pec minor, lie on your back with your hands on your stomach and your elbows bent. Placing your hands in this position takes slack off of the coracobrachialis and the "short head" portion of the biceps brachii, two small muscles that attach to the top of the shoulder and could contribute to a false positive in this test.

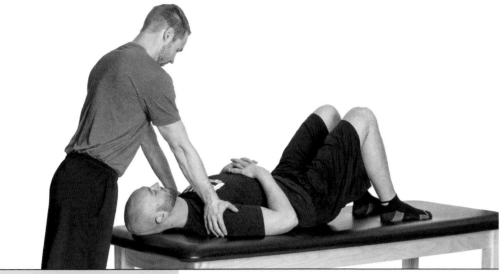

PARTNER PEC FLEXIBILITY TEST

Have a friend place their palms across the tops of your shoulders (over the bony part that sticks out, called the *coracoid process*) and push down. If there is sufficient flexibility of these small muscles, the shoulders should be easily pushed without any sensation of excessive muscle stretch in the upper chest.[16]

PECTORALIS MAJOR AND MINOR MUSCLES

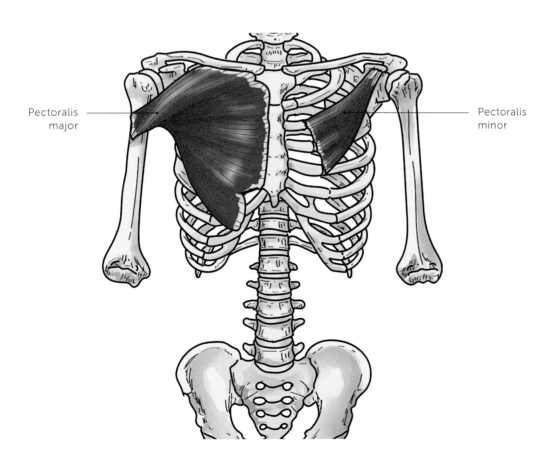

Pectoralis major

Pectoralis minor

While the pec minor attaches to and affects the position and movement of your shoulder blade, the pec major attaches directly to your arm bone (humerus). Stiffness in this muscle will roll the arm and shoulder joint forward into a poor position.

To assess the flexibility of your pec major muscles, lie on your back with your hands clasped behind your head. Allow your elbows to relax as far toward the ground as possible. If you cannot easily touch your elbows to the ground, you have short/stiff pec major muscles.[17]

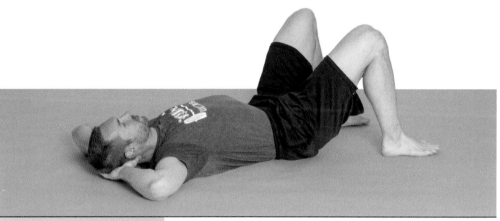

PEC MAJOR FLEXIBILITY TEST

Thoracic Spine Mobility Screening

Mobility of the thoracic spine can be difficult to assess, as the T-spine is composed of multiple spinal joints. The architecture of this portion of the spine is naturally stiff to keep our vital organs safe. However, too much stiffness in this area will affect the movement of the shoulder blade and compromise mobility and stability of the shoulder joint.

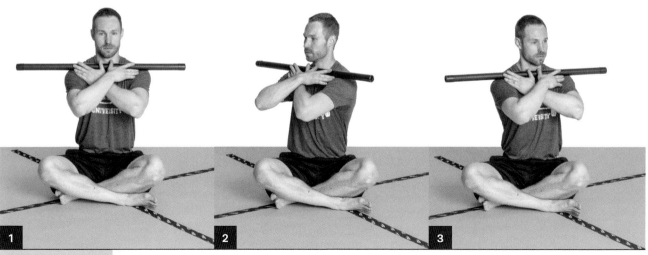

T-SPINE ROTATION

Perform the thoracic spine mobility assessment on pages 55 and 56. Ideally, you should be able to rotate your T-spine 45 degrees in each direction. This will align the PVC pipe with the tape on the ground.[18]

Instability Testing

Stability in the shoulder joint is created and maintained by both active and passive forces. Active stability is something we can work on and modify by increasing or decreasing muscle force. We have zero control over passive stability (e.g., ligaments, shoulder capsule, labrum, and the bony anatomy of the shoulder joint).

A simple test to determine whether you have shoulder laxity is the sulcus test. While seated or standing with your arm relaxed by your side, have a friend grab your arm at the elbow and gently pull down. The goal is to see if this downward pull creates a noticeable gap between the humerus and the top of your shoulder. This test is considered positive if the gap created between these two areas is wider than a finger width (8 to 10 millimeters).[19]

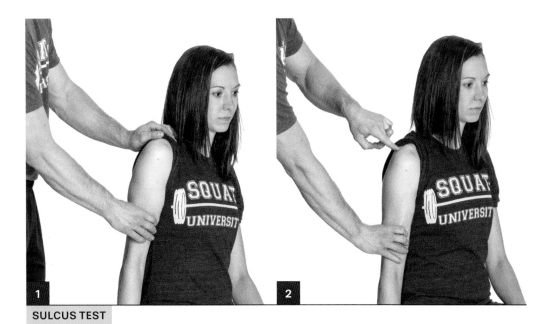

SULCUS TEST

Even though the sulcus test assesses the laxity of the lower or inferior capsule of the shoulder joint, several researchers have noted that those with instability in this direction almost always have excessive movement in other directions, called multidirectional instability, or MDI.[20] For this reason, those with a positive sulcus sign should do stability and strength exercises to improve their control of the joint. These athletes almost always have normal range of motion in their shoulders and therefore should not be stretched, even if they "feel tight"; stretching would likely lead to even more instability.

Strength Imbalance Testing

One of the most common strength imbalances that leads to shoulder pain is anterior dominance. Poor posture and training habits (focusing too much on developing the chest and deltoids) lead to the anterior muscles overpowering the weaker back muscles. The back muscles include the posterior rotator cuff, rhomboids, mid/lower trapezius, teres major, and lats.

MUSCLES OF THE BACK

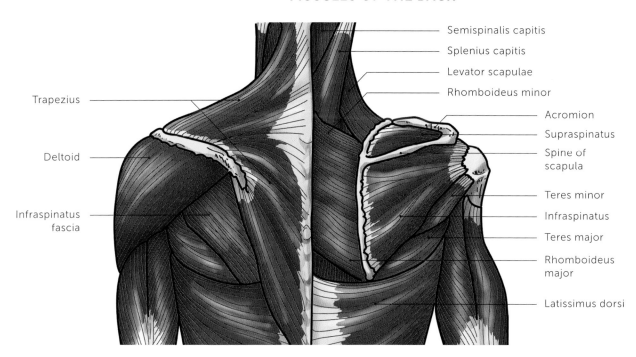

Trapezius

Deltoid

Infraspinatus fascia

Semispinalis capitis

Splenius capitis

Levator scapulae

Rhomboideus minor

Acromion

Supraspinatus

Spine of scapula

Teres minor

Infraspinatus

Teres major

Rhomboideus major

Latissimus dorsi

MUSCLES OF THE CHEST/DELTOIDS

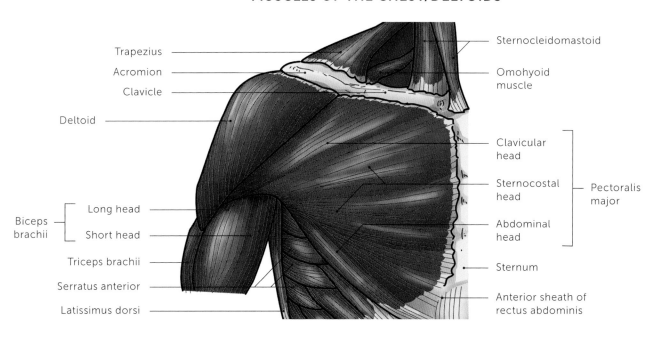

Trapezius

Acromion

Clavicle

Deltoid

Biceps brachii
  Long head
  Short head

Triceps brachii

Serratus anterior

Latissimus dorsi

Sternocleidomastoid

Omohyoid muscle

Clavicular head

Sternocostal head

Abdominal head

Pectoralis major

Sternum

Anterior sheath of rectus abdominis

Too often, regular gym-goers and athletes overtrain their pecs and deltoids without devoting enough time to training their scapular and back muscles. Strength in these back muscles ensures proper stability of the scapulae and prevents poor posture (such as forward shoulders). The posterior rotator cuff also ensures that the shoulder joint is properly stabilized. Two simple tests you can do at home to assess the strength of these posterior shoulder muscles are the "T" and "Y" tests.

Lie on your stomach on an elevated flat surface, or get in a quadruped position (on your hands and knees). Hold one arm directly out to your side as if making one side of the letter "T," with your palm facing the ground. Then have a friend push down on your outstretched arm for three seconds. Resist that force! Did your arm drop easily, or were you able to stabilize it against the force your friend was exerting?

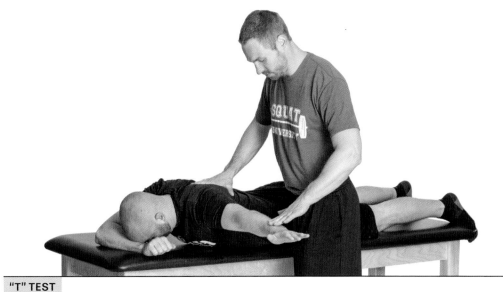

"T" TEST

Next, take your outstretched arm and move it into an elevated position, as if making one side of the letter "Y." Again, have your friend push down on your outstretched arm for three seconds. Resist this force as much as you can!

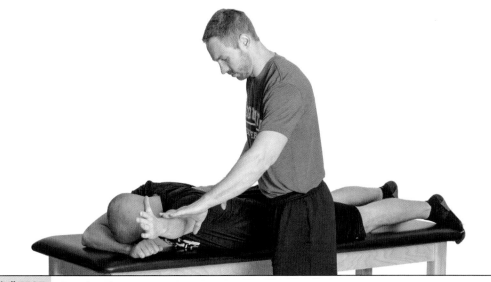

"Y" TEST

What did you feel? If you had a hard time keeping your arm from moving in either position, you may have poor scapular stability due to weakness in your posterior shoulder and mid-back muscles. The "T" position is designed to test for weakness in the middle portion of your trapezius muscle, whereas the "Y" position is used to expose weakness in the lower portion. If you had more trouble with the "Y" test, you're not alone. A weakened lower trap is a common imbalance found in those who develop shoulder pain.

If any of the smaller muscles that attach to the shoulder blade are weak, the stronger muscles that surround the shoulder (such as the deltoids) can overpower the smaller cuff muscles, leading to poor movement of the joint; eventually, injury can occur. If you found weakness with either of these tests, I recommend adding the prone lateral raise exercise found later in this chapter to your plan.

Poor shoulder external rotation strength is a big culprit in the vast majority of shoulder pain cases. Most clinicians screen for this problem with the athlete's arms at their sides. With your elbows bent in a 90-degree "L" position, try to resist any movement of your arms as a friend tries to force your hands together.

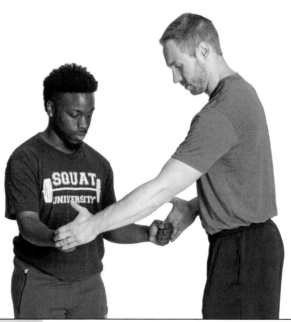

EXTERNAL ROTATION TEST

Were you able to hold your arms straight forward, or did your hands readily collapse inward? Was one side weaker than the other?

Try this test with your arm in that same "L" position but with your elbow at shoulder height as if you were giving a high-five. Have your friend stand behind you and push your hand forward into shoulder internal rotation. Do your best to resist this force.

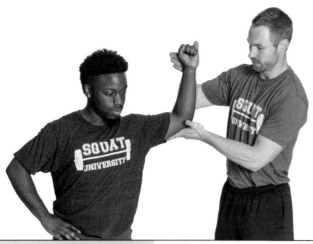

EXTERNAL ROTATION TEST AT 90 DEGREES

Was it harder to control your arm with it elevated? If so, your shoulder is more likely to get injured in an elevated or overhead position. The elevated position increases the challenge for the rotator cuff muscles to provide stability for the shoulder joint. On an interesting side note, the vast majority of shoulder dislocations occur when the shoulder is in an elevated, externally rotated position. If you found weakness with either of these screens, I recommend including the external rotation strength and stability exercises found later in this chapter to your plan.

Another common screen to assess rotator cuff strength and stability (specifically of the supraspinatus muscle) is the full can test.[21] While standing, raise your arms to shoulder height in a "V" shape, with your thumbs pointed toward the ceiling. Hold this position as a friend attempts to push your hands down toward the ground. If you have a weak and/or injured rotator cuff, you will be unable to keep your arm from moving!

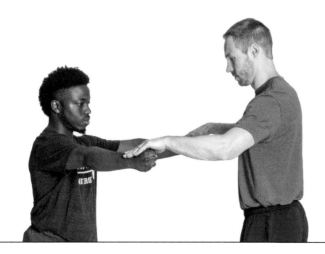

FULL CAN TEST

This last strength test is for the serratus anterior muscle. As the arm elevates above the head, the serratus anterior works with the trapezius muscles to move the shoulder blade into an efficient position to provide stability for the shoulder joint, aiding specifically with upward rotation and posterior tilt of the scapula. If the serratus isn't working optimally, the shoulder blade will fail to rotate upward and tilt appropriately, which could limit overhead range of motion and create impingement of the shoulder. Athletes with weakness in this muscle often overcompensate with their upper traps when pushing a barbell overhead.

To assess the strength of this muscle, stand with your shirt off (or wear a tank top). Raise your arm in front of you to just above shoulder height and hold it there. Have a friend grab your arm with one hand while feeling for the bottom angle of your shoulder blade (called the *inferior angle*) with their other hand. Have your friend apply a force down and back (toward your body) while you resist. Watch what happens to your shoulder blade.

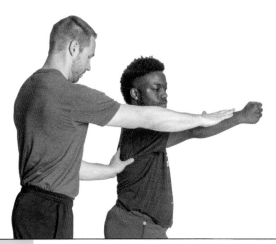

SERRATUS STRENGTH TEST

If your serratus muscle is weak, the inferior angle of your shoulder blade will rotate down and pop off the back (a motion called *winging*), or your upper trap will shrug upward as a compensation. Also perform this test with your arm elevated to ear level to ensure that you're evaluating the strength of this muscle in similar positions needed for overhead barbell training.

If you do not notice a side-to-side difference with this strength test, but you do notice that your painful-side shoulder blade does not rotate upward as much as your pain-free side, it's a good idea to add some of the serratus anterior strength exercises presented later in this chapter to your rehab plan.

When to Seek Professional Help

If you have any pain or numbness/tingling down your arm (which can reach your fingers), I recommend checking out the nerve tests in the Elbow Pain chapter. The information presented there will help you determine whether the symptoms you are experiencing are stemming from your neck, which would benefit from further testing with a medical practitioner. If you do not have symptoms that seem to be coming from the neck, the nerve gliding exercises presented in the Elbow Pain chapter (see pages 337 and 338) may be helpful additions to your plan.

If your pain is severe or your shoulder weakness is significant (for example, you are unable to raise your arm to shoulder height), I recommend seeking advice from your medical doctor.

The Rebuilding Process

Now that you have made your way through the screening tests, it's time to address any weak links you may have found, starting with mobility restrictions.

Improving Thoracic Spine Mobility

To have great technique when lifting and to decrease your risk of shoulder injury, you need sufficient thoracic spine mobility.

When addressing weak links in your upper body, you should always tackle mobility restrictions in the thoracic spine before moving on to other areas that need help, such as lat flexibility or rotator cuff strength/stability. Think about it like this: If you're going to spend time and energy fixing up a run-down house, you want to address the cracks in the foundation before painting the walls. Just like the concrete that supports the walls of a house, your mid-back sets the foundation for the entire shoulder joint.

I want to share with you six exercises that help promote mobility in the thoracic spine. I recommend performing each exercise and then retesting your mobility afterward. Doing so will help you figure out which of these exercises are the most efficient for your body.

Self-Mobilization with a "Peanut"

One of the best tools for improving thoracic spine mobility is a "peanut." Some manufacturers make fancy peanuts that cost a pretty penny. However, you can save a lot of money by simply taping two tennis or lacrosse balls together.

To perform a thoracic spine joint mobilization, lie on your back with your arms crossed in front of your chest. This pulls your shoulder blades (scapulae) "out" to the sides, creating space for the peanut. The balls should rest on either side of your spine.

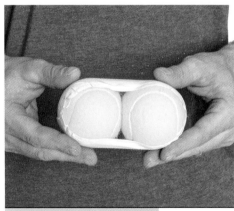

TWO TAPED TENNIS BALLS

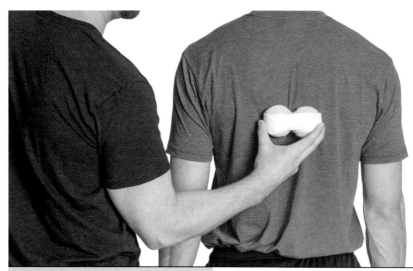

PEANUT PLACEMENT ON MID-BACK

Perform a small crunch by raising your shoulders a few inches off the ground.[22] Hold this position for a few seconds before returning to the start position. Make sure not to hyperextend your low back during this movement. You want to move only from the mid-back.

The peanut acts as a fulcrum on the spine during this movement, much like the anchor in the middle of a teeter-totter. Applying this force to a stiff joint can help improve mobility.

Recommended sets/reps: 2 or 3 sets of 15 reps for each segment of your mid-back that feels stiff

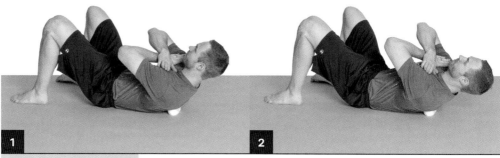

PEANUT MOBILIZATION

If you don't feel any stiffness in a particular part of your spine during the movement, move the peanut up or down to another segment. It is normal to have restrictions in some, but not all, areas of the thoracic spine.

You should not feel intense pain during this mobility drill. If you do, stop immediately and see a medical professional to find out why.

Prayer Stretch

This mobility exercise is similar to the classic yoga posture called child's pose. Start in a kneeling position. Sit your hips back on your heels and push your hands out in front of you, with one hand on top of the other. Next, let your chest drop to the floor. Continue to reach with your arms together overhead while you let your breath out slowly. Try to sink your chest toward the floor.

Recommended sets/reps: 3 or 4 reps of a 30-second hold (about 5 deep breaths in and out)

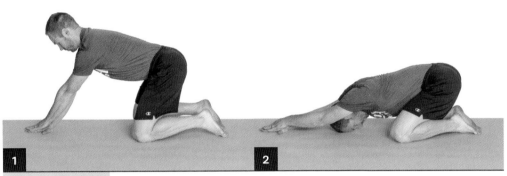

PRAYER STRETCH

If you have a stiff mid-back, this exercise should bring out a good stretch in your spine. Those who also have poor lat muscle flexibility may feel a good stretch on the sides of the back where these muscles run and attach to the underside of the arm, near the armpit.

To increase the intensity of the stretch, place your hands on top of a foam roller, which allows you to stretch further into thoracic spine extension.

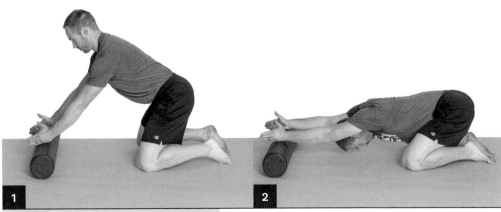

PRAYER STRETCH WITH FOAM ROLLER

Box T-Spine Stretch

Assume a kneeling position close to a box or bench. Grab a PVC pipe (or broomstick) and place your elbows on top of the box. Perform a similar motion to the prayer stretch on the previous page by sitting your hips back on your heels and simultaneously dropping your chest toward the ground. This motion should bring out a good stretch to your mid-back (and possibly your lat muscles).

Recommended sets/reps: 3 or 4 reps of a 30-second hold (about 5 deep breaths in and out)

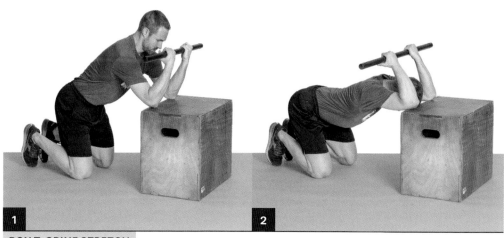

BOX T-SPINE STRETCH

Quadruped Downward Rotation Stretch

Because the spinal joints of the mid-back move on top of each other in a similar fashion during rotation and extension, you can also work to improve thoracic spine mobility with rotational exercises. The quadruped downward rotation stretch is an exercise that anyone can perform no matter what their current level of mobility.

Start in a quadruped position (on your hands and knees). Take your right hand and slide it as far under your left arm as possible. Dropping your right shoulder to the ground in an attempt to reach across your body should bring out a light stretch in your mid-back. Return to the start position and then repeat the same action with your left hand sliding under your right arm.

Recommended sets/reps: 10 reps of a 10-second hold on each side

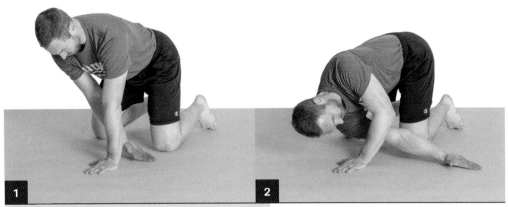

QUADRUPED DOWNWARD ROTATION STRETCH

To increase the intensity of this stretch, you can use a resistance band. Set up in the same quadruped position a few feet from a resistance band attached to a rack. Reach under your body with the hand farther from the rack and grab the band. There should be enough tension in the band that, when you attempt to rotate, the resistance assists in creating more mid-back rotation.

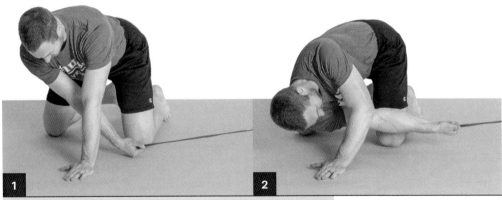

QUADRUPED DOWNWARD ROTATION STRETCH WITH BAND

Seated Rotation and Side Bend

Sit on top of a box or bench with a PVC pipe (or broomstick) on your back, as if you were performing a high-bar back squat. Squeeze a small foam roller between your knees to stabilize your lower body.

Start by rotating as far to the right as you can. When you hit your end range, perform a side bend to the right. This should be a small motion; too much side bend will cause your hips to rise from the seated position and your low back to move. It should bring out a good stretch in your mid-back and possibly to your lats on the sides of your torso as well.

After returning to an upright position, repeat the same action to the left. Did you notice a difference from one side to the other? After three to five rotations with bends to each side, you may notice that you're able to move farther than before.

Recommended sets/reps: 3 to 5 rotations with 3 consecutive side bends

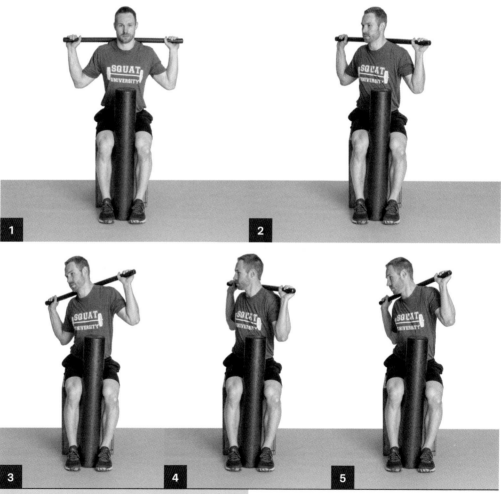

SEATED ROTATION AND SIDE BEND STRETCH

Deep Squat with Rotation

This last T-spine exercise is an advanced movement that requires you to have full mobility in the squat motion. In a deep bodyweight squat, take your left hand and grab your right foot. Next, drop your left shoulder as far to the ground as you can while rotating your right arm up toward the sky. Hold this position for 5 seconds before reversing the movement on the other side.

Recommended sets/reps: 3 to 5 rotations with a 5-second hold on each side

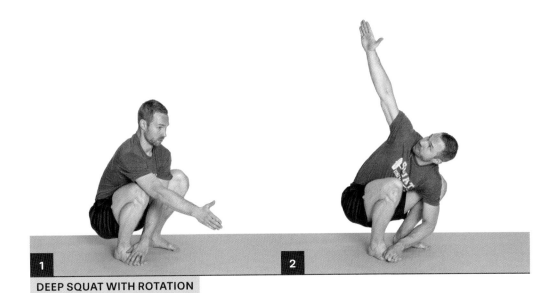

DEEP SQUAT WITH ROTATION

Making It Stick

Once you get that new thoracic spine mobility and range of motion, how do you maintain it? Try this exercise I first saw from Gray Cook, the founder of the FMS screen and author of the book *Movement*. Start by assuming a quadruped position and rock your hips back onto your heels. It's okay if you round your low back a little to get into this position; doing so will "lock in" your low back so you can concentrate on your upper back. Bend your left elbow and place it between your knees. Take your right hand and place it on your low back.

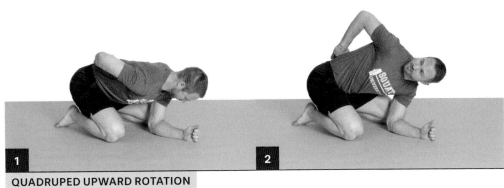

QUADRUPED UPWARD ROTATION

Next, rotate your torso to the right and do your best to keep the left side of your rib cage glued to your left thigh; this prevents excessive low back rotation. This action works many of the muscles that provide stability for the mid-back. After holding the position for a few seconds, rotate back to the start position and repeat on the other side.

Recommended sets/reps: 10 to 20 reps on each side

If your pecs and lats are especially tight, try placing your right hand on your left shoulder and then perform the maneuver.

Always use the test-retest method to see if the exercises you performed are putting you on the right track to improve your mid-back mobility. The exercises that I have shared here are not a magic pill for improving mobility. They will not fix stiffness in one session. If you do notice a small change in movement quality after retesting your motion, consider adding these corrective exercises to your daily schedule. Consistency is key for progressing mobility.

Improving Pec and Lat Flexibility

After you have addressed mobility restrictions in your thoracic spine, it's time to move on to the muscle groups that limit shoulder mobility from both the front and the back side of the body: the latissimus dorsi, teres major, and pectoralis major/minor. To show great technique during any overhead barbell lift (and even get a proper hold of the barbell when you place it on your back when squatting), you need a sufficient amount of flexibility in these muscles.

Lat and Teres Major Flexibility

Here are three simple and efficient methods to help you improve the flexibility of your lats and teres major muscles.

SOFT TISSUE MOBILIZATION

Soft tissue mobilization with a foam roller can be a great way to improve the flexibility of stiff lats/teres major muscles.[23] Start by lying on your side with your bottom arm raised over your head and a foam roller pinned under the outside of your armpit. Because these muscles are strong internal rotators of the shoulder, you want to mobilize these tissues in the position of desired change (external rotation). To accomplish this task, have the palm of your extended arm facing upward toward the sky as you lie on the foam roller.

Roll up and down this muscle until you find a tender area. Pause on this spot for a few seconds before moving on. You can take this mobilization one step further by pausing on the tender area and then moving your arm over your head and back for a few repetitions. Make sure to move slowly on the foam roller; moving too quickly will have little effect on improving flexibility.

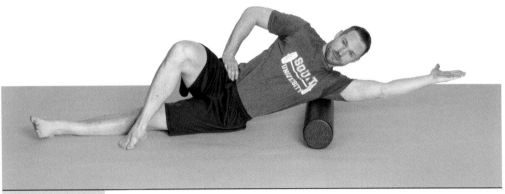

FOAM ROLL LATS

You can also perform soft tissue mobilization on these two muscles with a small ball (lacrosse or tennis ball). The smaller surface area of a ball allows you to focus your treatment on a more specific area and create more change in the underlying tissues compared to a foam roller. Stand next to a wall and trap a ball between the outside of your armpit and the wall. Slowly move around until you find a stiff, tender area. From this position, you can again pin the tender area and slowly move your arm up and down over your head.

Recommended sets/reps: 1 set of rolling for 1 to 2 minutes

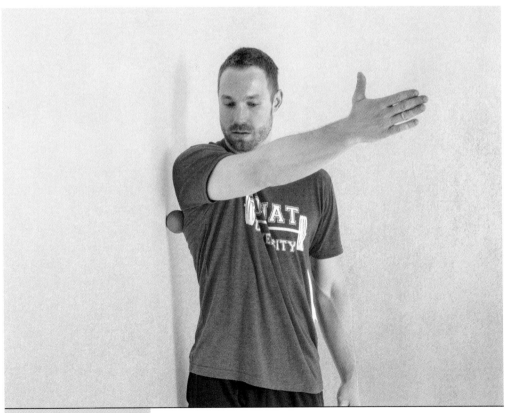

LACROSSE BALL TO LATS

BOX LAT STRETCH

Assume a kneeling position behind a box or bench. Grab a PVC pipe (or broomstick) and position your arms in a "V": hands grabbing wide with elbows held close together. Place your elbows on top of the box.

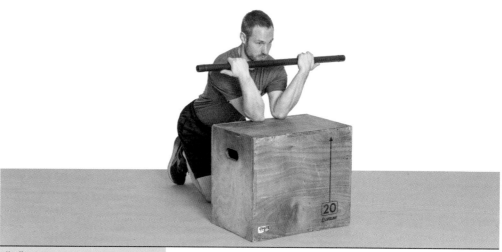

"V" POSITION SETUP ON BOX

Next, sit your hips back on your heels and simultaneously round your upper back and pull your hips under your body as you elevate your arms over your head. (Notice that this box stretch is performed slightly differently than if trying to increase thoracic spine mobility.)

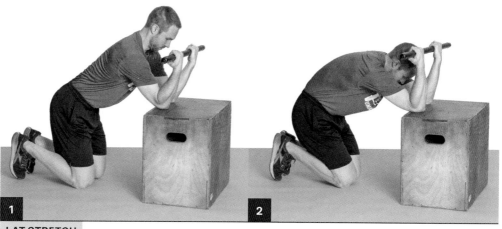

LAT STRETCH

Because the lats run the length of your spine, rounding your back as you sit your butt on your heels stretches these muscles. If you're doing it correctly, you should feel a stretch along the lateral part of your back and into the lateral armpit region (where these muscles attach to your arms); you should not feel a stretch in your shoulder joints. Hold this end-range stretch for five deep breaths in and out before returning to the start position.

Recommended sets/reps: 3 to 5 reps

ECCENTRIC CURL-UP

While a large majority of the research and practical understanding of how to improve the flexibility of a stiff/short muscle rests with stretching and soft tissue mobilization, a growing amount of scientific research supports the use of eccentric exercises to help lengthen muscles.[24] In fact, some studies have shown that eccentric training can lead to significant improvements in flexibility in as little as six weeks.[25]

An *eccentric contraction* describes the action of a muscle lengthening under tension. This is the opposite of what happens when a muscle shortens as it contracts (called a *concentric contraction*), such as when you perform a biceps curl.

One way to eccentrically lengthen stiff lat muscles is with eccentric curl-ups. With an underhand grip on a pull-up bar (an externally rotated position to place a stretch on the lats), jump up to the top position and slowly lower yourself back to the ground. Fully extending your arms should take you no less than five seconds.

Recommended sets/reps: 2 or 3 sets of 5 reps with a 5-second lower

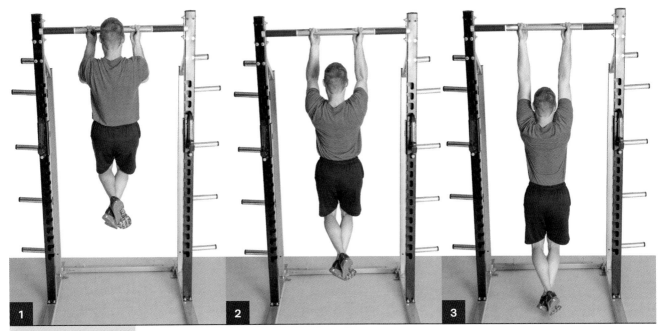

ECCENTRIC CURL-UP

If you do not have adequate strength to perform this exercise on a pull-up bar, I recommend using a lat pull-down machine. Stand next to the machine and grab the bar, holding it close to your body (as at the top of a pull-up). Keep your hold on the bar as you sit down before slowly letting your arms rise back to an extended position over your head against the resistance of the machine. Stand back up and perform the same sequence again.

Pec Flexibility

Next, let's look at three methods for improving the flexibility of the pectoralis muscles (major and minor).

SOFT TISSUE MOBILIZATION

To mobilize the pec muscles, grab a lacrosse or tennis ball and trap it between your chest and a wall. Slowly move the ball around your muscles until you find a tender area. Pause on the tender spot for a few seconds before moving on to another.

You can add some active movement to this mobilization. Once you find a tender area, start moving your arm out to the side (away from your body) and back. This movement can increase the effectiveness of the exercise.

Recommended sets/reps: 1 set of 1 to 2 minutes

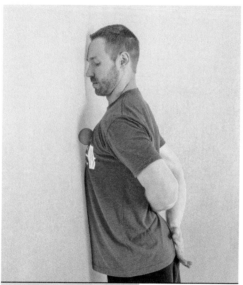

LACROSSE BALL TO PEC

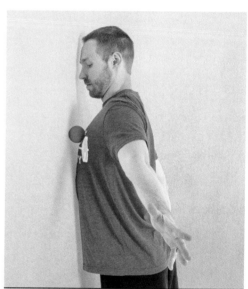

WITH ARM MOVEMENT

CORNER PEC STRETCH

Find a corner and place your arms out to the sides with your elbows bent in an "L" position. Place your hands on the walls and slowly lean into the corner, keeping your core slightly braced and your back completely flat. This movement should bring out a good stretch in your chest if you have stiff pecs (especially the pec minor muscles).[26]

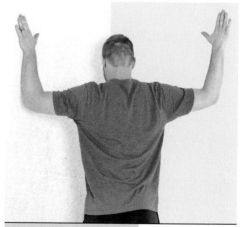

CORNER PEC STRETCH

Do not push too hard with this stretch; doing so can place harmful forces on your shoulder joints. You should feel a stretch only in your pec muscles, not on the fronts of your shoulders!

Recommended sets/reps: 3 reps of 10 to 30 seconds

FOAM ROLLER PEC STRETCH

For some people, the corner pec stretch may be too intense. You can modify it by using a PVC pipe.

Lie faceup on a foam roller or bench. Holding a PVC pipe (or broomstick) in your hands, extend your arms toward the ceiling. Then, keeping your elbows straight, move your arms as far over your head as you can. Keep your core braced to prevent your low back from arching and your ribs from flaring out as your arms move.

This should bring out a light stretch in your chest as your arms reach their end position over your head. Hold this low-load stretch for 30 seconds.

Recommended sets/reps: 3 reps of 10 to 30 seconds

I caution against performing this stretch with a barbell or other heavy object in hand because it can place excessive force on the shoulder joints. If you feel tingling or numbness down your arms/fingers, you are probably stretching too aggressively. (Be sure to check out the nerve testing section of the Elbow Pain chapter if these symptoms persist.)

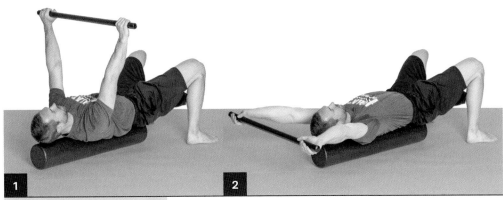

FOAM ROLLER PEC STRETCH

Making It Stick

After you perform the prior exercises—whether to improve the flexibility of your lats/ teres major muscles, your pec muscles, or both—it's time to learn how to control this new range of motion you have created. You can accomplish this in two ways.

HALF-PRONE ANGEL

Start by lying on your stomach with your hands positioned by your shoulders and your palms facing down. Brace your core to ensure sufficient trunk stability. Next, lift your arms from the ground and push your hands as far above your head as you can. (This mimics the motion of a standing barbell press.) Once your arms are fully extended, rotate them so that your palms are angled upward toward the sky.

From this position, raise both arms as far off the ground as you can, keeping your elbows straight. After holding for three seconds, lower your arms back down before rotating them to the original palms-down position and then return to the start position. After performing a few reps correctly, you should feel a good amount of fatigue in your posterior shoulder muscles.

Recommended sets/reps: 2 sets of 5 to 10 reps

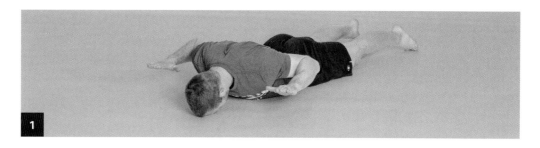

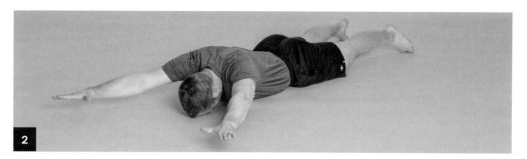

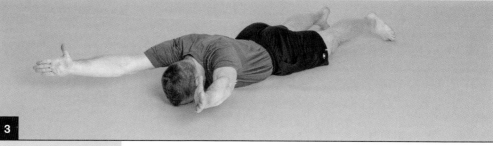

HALF-PRONE ANGEL

WALL HANDSTAND

Performing a handstand is a great way to work the same muscle groups that are used during lifts such as the barbell push-press and the jerk. Handstands improve your core stability, shoulder proprioception, and shoulder endurance and highlight any faults you have from your wrists down to your hips. The wrists are extended with your arms locked out and stacked directly in line with your shoulder blades and torso. Because most of us lack the balance needed to perform an unassisted handstand, we can use a wall to modify the movement and still get the same great benefits.

Walk your feet up a wall as you push yourself into an inverted position. The goal is to walk your hands as close to the wall as possible to bring your body into a vertical position, mimicking the unassisted handstand. In the end position, you want to be able to draw a straight line from your wrists through your upper body. You can perform this exercise with your body completely extended or with your hips and knees flexed against the wall (mirroring what a deep overhead squat would look like).

Recommended sets/reps: 3 reps of 20 to 30 seconds

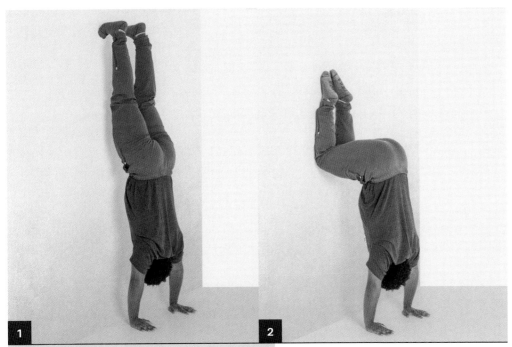

WALL HANDSTAND, EXTENDED OR HALF SQUAT

It's no wonder that gymnasts can make a smooth transition to Olympic lifting and CrossFit. Gymnasts usually have the prerequisite shoulder stability, core strength, and overhead mobility to achieve ideal technique with lifts like snatches, clean and jerks, and push-presses.

Training Program Considerations

If the flexibility restrictions you have developed are severe and have led to shoulder pain, consider modifying your training program. Overworking certain muscle groups by performing the same exercises over and over again can create imbalances that produce mobility issues. For example, countless pull-ups may lead to lat stiffness, and excessive push-ups/bench pressing could develop overly stiff/tight pecs. Removing or decreasing the volume and intensity of the following exercises while you work on overhead mobility/stability is a great way to hit the reset button. Once you have the newfound overhead mobility and your shoulder stability has improved, you can slowly reintroduce these exercises into your program:

- Deadlift
- Snatch and clean deadlift or pull
- Pull-up
- Rope climb
- Bench press or push-up
- Ring dip
- Push-press

Obviously, these exercises are crucial for weightlifters, powerlifters, and CrossFitters. You should not perform them at the expense of shoulder mobility, and you should not push through sharp, intense pain.

As you can see, improving flexibility of your upper body muscles isn't only about which exercises you perform, but also about which exercises you avoid or modify. Improvements in flexibility will not happen overnight. If you are consistent with these mobility drills and you modify your training program, though, you should start to notice progress in shoulder mobility and an improvement in pain (if you had any). Sometimes when we run into a wall, it's smart to take a step back and hit the reset button.

Do You Need More Internal Rotation?

One of the most common questions people ask me in reference to the shoulder is, "Do I need more internal rotation?" The answer is, "It depends."

If you hold your arm by your side with your elbow bent to 90 degrees, internal rotation is the movement of your hand toward your stomach. If you raise your arm to the side (as if giving a friend a high-five) internal rotation is the movement of lowering your hand toward the ground.

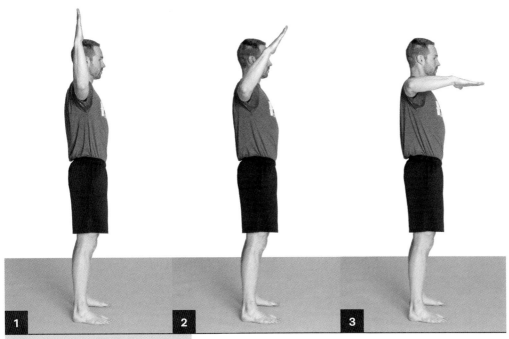

SHOULDER INTERNAL ROTATION

More mobility isn't always a good thing, especially when it comes to overhead athletes, who often have excess motion at the shoulder joint. In addition to weight-lifters who regularly perform overhead lifts such as the snatch and jerk, "overhead athletes" also describes those who participate in sports such as baseball, softball, tennis, volleyball, or any other repetitive activity performed above head level. We can't assume that someone who lacks internal rotation (especially an overhead ath-lete) needs to stretch to gain more motion. Instead, we need to assess and address why there is a lack of internal rotation in the first place. Let me explain.

In the screening section of this chapter, I described a simple test to assess your level of active shoulder internal rotation. While sitting against a wall with your arms in an "L" position, you rotate your shoulders and forearms as far toward the ground as possible without allowing your shoulder blades to pop off the wall. Most people should have the ability to rotate their forearms to a parallel position (relative to the ground), if not farther.

If you passed this screen easily, congratulations. You likely have sufficient shoul-der internal rotation. You do not need the flexibility and mobility exercises described in the rest of this section. In fact, for you, performing stretches to create more motion could lead to instability. However, if you were unable to pass this mobility screen, ask yourself, "Did I feel pain or stiffness when performing this motion?"

A loss of shoulder internal rotation can be due to many factors, such as limited muscular flexibility (stiff or tight soft tissues), excessive tightness in the joint capsule, or poor alignment of the shoulder complex (such as poor posture and muscular imbalances). Deficits in shoulder internal rotation can also be caused by natural adaptations from sports, such as the throwing motion in baseball or the hitting motion in volleyball.

For example, research has shown that many lifelong baseball players develop a backward "twist" of the humerus bone (called *humeral retroversion*) over time due to the forces sustained during the repetitive overhead throwing motion.[27] Much like twisting and wringing out a wet towel, the humerus twists backward at the growth plate, causing a permanent adaptation to the bone structure. This change creates a situation where the athlete shows excessive shoulder external rotation and very limited internal rotation. It is not pathological or harmful!

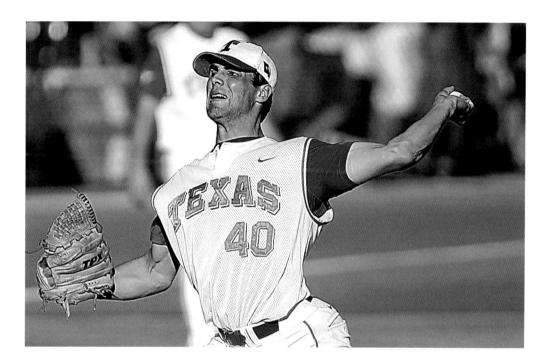

Lifelong baseball players can develop a backward "twist" of the humerus.

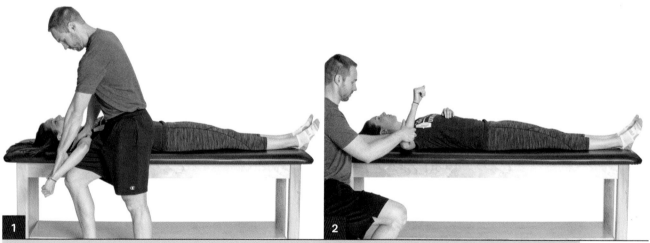

HUMERAL RETROVERSION SHOWING EXCESSIVE EXTERNAL ROTATION AND LIMITED INTERNAL ROTATION

Regardless of what is limiting your internal rotation, if actively moving into internal rotation is painful, the last thing you want to do is try to stretch into that range. Doing so will only perpetuate the pain cycle and further irritate the symptomatic tissues. Instead, I recommend focusing your attention on addressing other factors that contribute to your symptoms, such as muscular imbalances (flip to page 286).

If you had less-than-perfect shoulder internal rotation but no pain with the "L" screen, ask yourself if you *need* full range of motion in that direction. While limited internal rotation may not hinder your bench press, squat, or deadlift technique, it can have a dramatic effect on the quality of your Olympic lifts. For example, sufficient internal rotation of the shoulder is needed to keep the barbell close to the body during the later phases of the pull into the turnover, especially with the snatch lift. Athletes who are missing this motion often compensate in one of two ways.

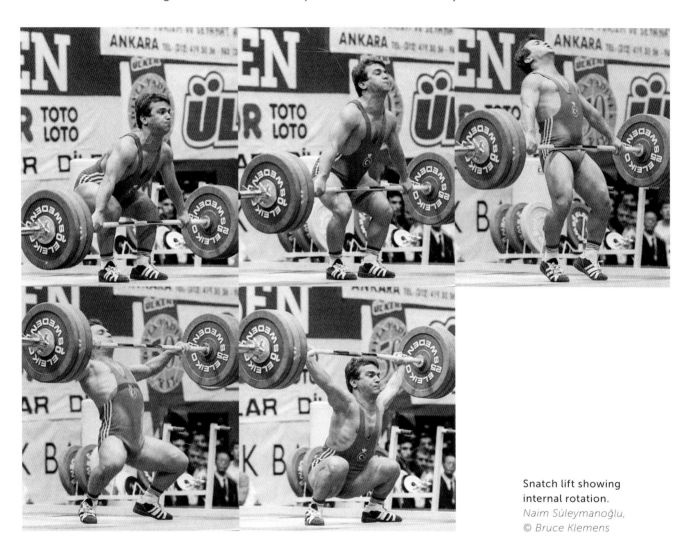

Snatch lift showing internal rotation.
Naim Süleymanoğlu,
© *Bruce Klemens*

The first is an exaggerated looping of the bar away from the body, killing the efficiency of the lift and causing most athletes to miss heavy attempts. In an effort to combat this obvious technique fault and keep the bar close to the body, athletes often compensate for a lack of internal rotation by rolling the entire shoulder complex forward (excessively moving their shoulder blades). If you find yourself committing either of these faults, you will probably benefit from working on improving your shoulder internal rotation range of motion.

Finding the Right Stretch

If Olympic lifting is a staple of your training and you found yourself with limited shoulder internal rotation, the next step is to find the right exercises/stretches to fix your range of motion deficits. One of the most popular stretches prescribed to fix internal rotation deficits is the classic sleeper stretch. You perform this stretch by lying on your side and pushing your shoulder into internal rotation. Ideally, it would bring out a gentle stretch to the back side of the shoulder. This exercise is so popular, in fact, that a number of medical doctors have asked me specifically for this stretch for some patients. However, I'm not a big fan of this exercise, and for a few reasons, I caution you against using it.

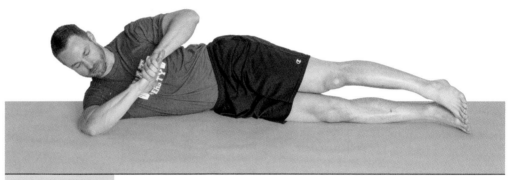

SLEEPER STRETCH

The first is that the stretch is easy to perform incorrectly. I often see athletes roll too far onto their shoulder and aggressively crank their hand toward the ground. Doing so places excessive stress on certain tissues of the joint (posterior capsule), which can lead to more problems down the road.

The sleeper stretch also looks very similar to a test used to confirm shoulder impingement injuries, the Hawkins-Kennedy test. Internally rotating the arm in this position closes off the available room for the rotator cuff muscles and biceps tendon in the joint, impinging the structures in some people and provoking pain. If you took a photo of this test being performed and flipped it on its side, it is a mirror image of the sleeper stretch. Physical therapist Mike Reinold argues that the sleeper stretch closely mimics the Hawkins-Kennedy test, which is designed

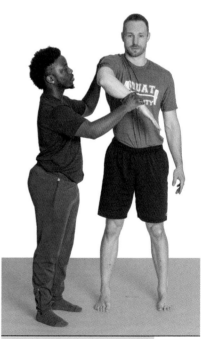

HAWKINS-KENNEDY TEST

to elicit pain in someone who has anterior shoulder pain,[28] so he generally recommends *against* using the sleeper stretch for athletes.

Even if you do the sleeper stretch correctly, I believe other alternatives may be more effective and generally less irritating to the shoulder. For example, a 2007 study published in the *Journal of Orthopaedic & Sports Physical Therapy* compared the sleeper stretch to a simple cross-body stretch and found that the cross-body stretch was actually more effective at eliciting improvements in shoulder internal rotation.[29]

To perform the cross-body stretch, grab your arm (around the elbow) with your opposite hand and pull it across your chest. Doing so should bring out a stretch on the back side of your shoulder. To make this stretch even more efficient, lean against a rig or doorway and wedge the side of your shoulder blade against the rig or door jamb to keep it from moving as you pull your arm across your body.

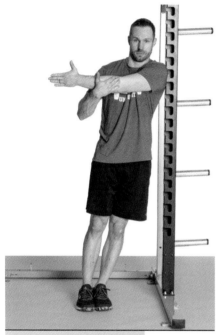

CROSS-BODY STRETCH

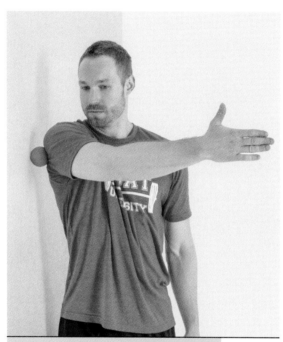

POSTERIOR SHOULDER SOFT TISSUE
MOBILIZATION WITH LACROSSE BALL

Another helpful way to improve shoulder internal rotation is to perform soft tissue mobilization with a small ball such as a lacrosse or tennis ball. Stand next to a wall and pin the ball between the wall and the back side of your shoulder. Slowly roll the ball around until you find tender areas. Pause on these areas while you slowly pull your arm across your body.

Final Thoughts on Internal Rotation

Your individual needs, problem areas, and goals in lifting must be taken into account when determining whether you require more shoulder internal rotation. You can put yourself in a bad position if you blindly perform internal rotation stretches without doing the appropriate screening first.

Athletes require just enough mobility to meet the demands of their sport and its required movements. Athletes with extreme mobility walk a thin line between normality and dysfunction. "Just enough" mobility provides endless movement options and can maximize performance, whereas pushing too much can create instability, leading to uncontrolled movement and putting the athlete on a fast track to injury.

Ask yourself these questions:

- Do I have sufficient shoulder internal rotation?

- If my internal rotation is limited, is it due to pain or stiffness?

- Do the activities and lifts that I participate in require more internal rotation?

If you can navigate your way through these simple questions, you'll be in a much better position to answer the larger question of "Do I need more internal rotation?"

Addressing Muscular Imbalances

Now that you have addressed any mobility and flexibility restrictions that may be contributing to your symptoms, it's time to tackle deficits in muscular strength, endurance, and coordination that lead to instability and poor mechanics. If you failed any of the stability tests from earlier in this chapter, pay close attention to this section. It covers a few of my favorite exercises that address these problems.

Many of the exercises discussed in this section are performed with a paused hold at certain ranges. Pausing allows you to emphasize shoulder stability. Remember, strength is not the same as stability. Strength is the ability to produce force, whereas stability is the ability to limit excessive or unwanted motion. If a muscle is strong but can't maintain adequate tension and can't work in coordination with the surrounding muscles, joint mechanics will break down, and injury can ensue.

Stability also requires muscular endurance. This is why many corrective exercises to enhance stability are initially performed with high-repetition sets. This helps build the capacity of these muscles to "turn on" and maintain adequate stability from your first to your last set in a training session, as well as during everyday movements outside the gym.

Side-Lying External Rotation

If you exposed a weakness in external rotation strength and stability in the screening section of this chapter, side-lying external rotation is a good exercise to start with. Research has shown that the posterior rotator cuff muscles (infraspinatus and teres minor) are most efficiently activated with this simple exercise.[30] These two muscles keep the humerus compressed and centered in the joint socket during arm movement (in other words, keeping the "golf ball" centered on the "tee").

Lie on your side with a rolled-up towel pinned between your top-side arm and your rib cage, which places that arm in the optimal position.[31] Start with your arm parallel to the floor and your shoulder blade pulled back and down (scapular retraction and depression). Without allowing your shoulder blade to move, push your hand up toward the sky (the motion of external rotation) before returning back down.

Recommended sets/reps: 2 or 3 sets of 15 to 20 reps

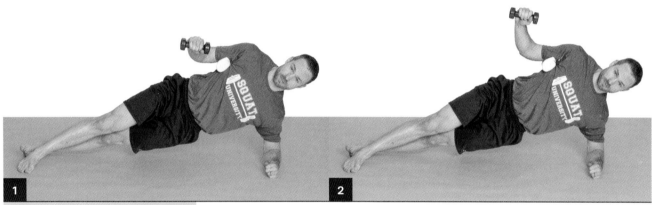

SIDE-LYING EXTERNAL ROTATION

Depending on your current level of strength, you may need to perform this exercise without weight at first. Once you can perform the recommended number of sets and reps without significant fatigue or pain, start adding weight.

If you are unable to externally rotate through a full range of motion due to shoulder pain, you can start with partial reps within a pain-free zone. These "short arc" motions will allow you to benefit without furthering the injury process or increasing your symptoms. As the pain subsides, continue to progress how far you can externally rotate without pain as you increase the resistance.

Banded "W"

One of my favorite exercises, and one that I perform during my own daily warm-up regardless of whether I'll be performing any of the Olympic lifts or squatting, is the banded "W." This progression from the previous side-lying external rotation exercise not only addresses rotator cuff strength and stability but also activates the often underutilized lower portion of the trapezius muscle.[32]

One of the most common imbalances seen in athletes is between the upper and lower trapezius muscle fibers. The upper traps are highly active during movements such as the pulling motion of the clean and snatch and therefore have a tendency to become overly dominant, which can lead to poor mechanics of the shoulder complex. Research has shown that the banded "W" is one of the best exercises for concentrating on the lower traps to address this imbalance.[33]

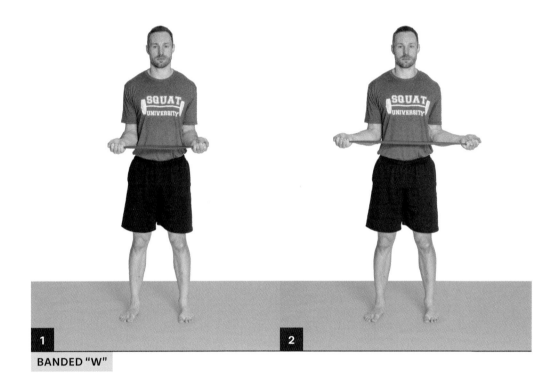

BANDED "W"

Start by grabbing an elastic band in both hands with your arms by your sides and your elbows bent to a 90-degree "L" position. Your thumbs can be facing upward or outward, as shown. As you pull your hands away from your body against the resistance of the band (the motion of external rotation), make sure your elbows remain in the same bent position by your ribs. Hold the end position for 5 to 10 seconds before returning to the start.

Recommended sets/reps: 2 or 3 sets of 15 to 20 reps

External Rotation Press

While the prior two exercises are great for strengthening the posterior rotator cuff, many of the movements that athletes perform in training sessions take place above shoulder height in positions where the joint is more vulnerable to instability and injury. This is why I advise you to test for external rotation strength and stability in the screening section with your arm by your side *and* at shoulder height! For this reason, corrective exercises to enhance shoulder stability must also be performed at different angles of shoulder elevation.

Start by tying a resistance band around a rig or rack. Grab the band and pull it toward you in a rowing motion. Your hand should finish directly in front of your elbow with your arm parallel to the ground. This locks your shoulder blade into a good position by activating muscles like the rhomboids and middle portions of the trapezius.[34] Hold this position for three seconds.

Next, rotate your shoulder backward—the motion of external rotation. Doing so activates the posterior rotator cuff (particularly the infraspinatus) similarly to the turnover catch phase of a snatch.[35] Your fist should be facing the ceiling with your elbow bent 90 degrees, and your shoulder blade should not move at all during this rotation. Again, hold this end position for three seconds.

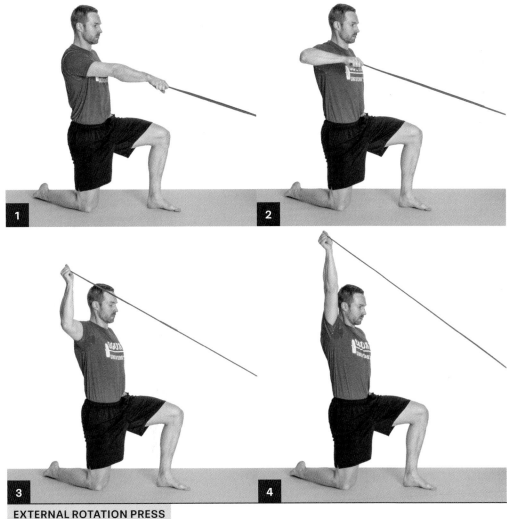

EXTERNAL ROTATION PRESS

Lastly, push your hand overhead and hold this end position for another three seconds. (If you perform the Olympic lifts, your hand should be stacked directly over the back of your head to mimic the barbell jerk.) With your arm extended, the muscles that stabilize your shoulder blade will be working hard against the band resistance to keep your arm from falling forward. Interestingly, this exercise not only recruits the rotator cuff but also produces a high degree of serratus anterior activation to help stabilize the shoulder blade against the rib cage.[36]

After the brief hold, reverse the pattern with the same pauses in each position as you return to the start.

Recommended sets/reps: 2 or 3 sets of 10 reps

Prone Lateral Raise

As I mentioned earlier, one of the most common muscular imbalances that athletes present with is upper trap dominance. A great exercise to strengthen the lower and middle portions of the trapezius muscle is the prone lateral raise. If you failed the "T" and "Y" strength imbalance tests (see page 261), this exercise should be a part of your rehabilitation plan!

Start by lying on your stomach on a bench or bed with one arm hanging over the side. With your elbow locked in a straight position, raise your arm to the side until it is parallel to the ground, as if making one side of the letter "T." As you raise your arm, think about simultaneously pulling your shoulder blade in toward your spine (the motion of scapular retraction). You can perform this exercise with your palm facing the ground or with your thumb pointed toward the ceiling (the motion of shoulder external rotation). Hold the end position for five seconds before lowering back down.

Recommended sets/reps: 2 or 3 sets of 10 to 15 reps

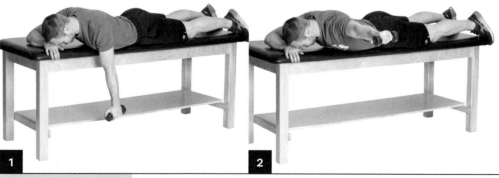

PRONE LATERAL RAISE

Prone Floor Angel

This exercise is a progression from the half-prone angel from earlier in the chapter (see page 278). Start by lying on your stomach with your hands positioned by your hips and your palms facing down. With your elbows locked in a straight position, pull your hands up off the ground as you simultaneously squeeze your shoulder blades together. This motion of shoulder extension is great for activating the rhomboid muscles of the mid-back that help control your shoulder blades.[37]

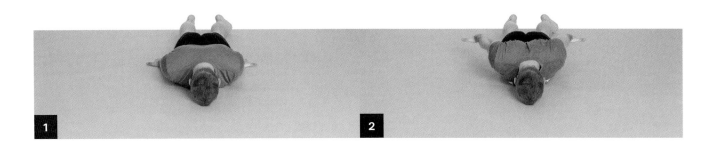

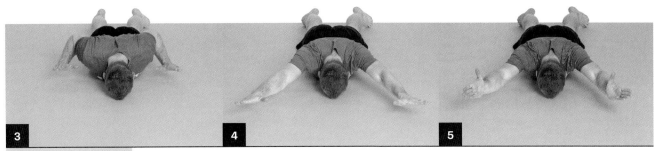

PRONE FLOOR ANGEL

Next, while keeping your shoulder blades pulled together and depressed, rotate your hands upward into what will end up looking like a back squat hold position. Then push your hands as far above your head as you can; this mimics the motion of a standing barbell press. Once your arms are fully extended, rotate your arms upward so that your palms are facing the sky. From this position, raise both arms off the ground as far as you can, making sure to keep your elbows straight. After holding for three seconds, lower your arms back down before rotating them to the original palms-down position and then returning your hands to your hips.

Recommended sets/reps: 2 or 3 sets of 10 reps

Suspension Trainer Row

The row is an excellent exercise for addressing weakness in the posterior shoulder complex. You can perform it with a suspension trainer or a set of gymnastics rings. If you've never done inverted rows before, a good teaching cue is to start the exercise from the end "row" position.

While grasping the grips of the suspension trainer or the rings, squeeze your shoulder blades together and start walking your feet forward as you lower your body toward the ground, creating a more difficult angle of pull. Stop when you find a position where it is challenging to hold yourself up but not too difficult to maintain your posture. You should be able to draw a straight line from your feet to your head.

From this position, lower yourself down until your arms are fully extended. Keep your core braced and your body in a straight line throughout this movement—no low back or hip sag!

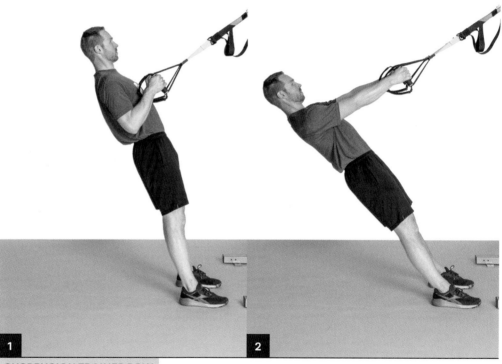

SUSPENSION TRAINER ROW

To increase the difficulty of this exercise, continue to lower your body toward the ground until you are close to parallel. If you don't have a suspension trainer or a set of gymnastics rings, you can perform the inverted row with a barbell positioned in a rack. You can also place your feet on a bench or box to increase the challenge.

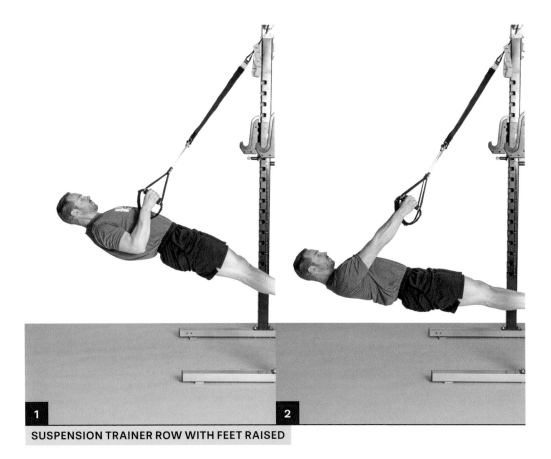

SUSPENSION TRAINER ROW WITH FEET RAISED

Recommended sets/reps: 2 or 3 sets of 10 reps with a 3-second hold at the top "row" position

Rhythmic Stabilizations

Muscle fatigue can hinder your ability to create stability at the shoulder joint. It can also negatively influence proprioception (joint/body awareness).[38] The more fatigued you become, the less control you have over your body, and the more likely it is that your form/technique will break down. This is why fatigue combined with poor muscular stability sets off a cascade of events that creates eventual joint instability and injury.

Rhythmic stabilization exercises are great for improving proprioception and joint stability. The goal with these exercises is to improve muscular co-contraction (turning on all of the surrounding muscles simultaneously).[39] You'll need a partner.

Lie on your back on a bench or bed with one arm extended straight toward the sky. Have a friend push your arm in different directions while you try to prevent it from moving. Have your friend push lightly at first before speeding up and applying more force as your control of the arm improves. If you're doing these exercises with the right amount of force, your shoulder should be fairly fatigued after 20 seconds.

Recommended sets/reps: 4 or 5 sets of 20 seconds

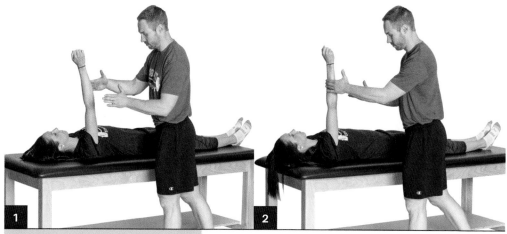

RHYTHMIC STABILIZATION SUPINE

Rhythmic stabilization exercises can be performed in a number of positions, such as with your hand placed against a Swiss ball and your arm fully extended.[40] Explore different positions and try to perform these rhythmic stabilizations in the positions you find most unstable.

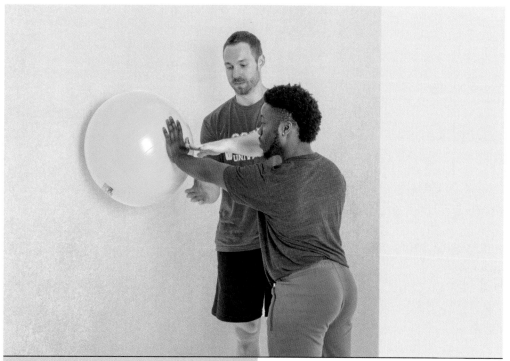

RHYTHMIC STABILIZATION WITH SWISS BALL

If you show signs of shoulder instability, you should include rhythmic stabilization exercises in your rehab program. I have found rhythmic stabilizations to be a great tool for my patients who couldn't get better with standard PT exercises alone (banded exercises, dumbbells, cable machines, etc.).

Bottoms-Up Kettlebell Press

The bottoms-up kettlebell press is one of my favorite stability-based exercises for the shoulder because it carries over to many of the movements we perform as strength athletes.

Start in a half-kneeling position. With your wrist straight (knuckles up) and your elbow bent 90 degrees, hold a kettlebell upside down. Press the weight above your head and hold it there for five seconds before slowly bringing it back down. The pressing motion should be performed in the scapular plane, which means that your elbow should be positioned around 30 degrees to the side, not straight forward or completely out to the side.

Holding the kettlebell upside down places the weight's center of gravity farther from your hand as compared to a dumbbell. If your shoulder is unable to meet the stability demands of holding the kettlebell in this unbalanced position, the kettlebell will fall over.

Recommended sets/reps: 2 or 3 sets of 10 reps

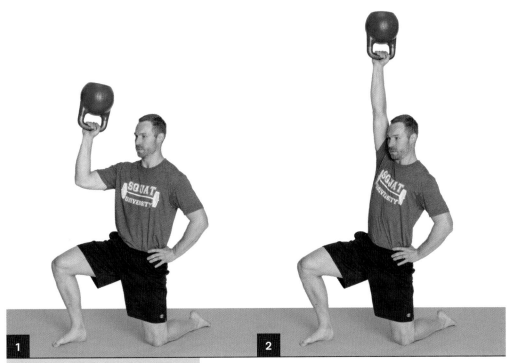

BOTTOMS-UP KETTLEBELL PRESS

You can increase the difficulty of this exercise by adding a resistance band around your wrist that pulls in toward the midline of your body, as shown on the next page. You can attach the band to a rig or have a partner hold the other end of the band. This variation requires your lateral and posterior shoulder muscles to work even harder to maintain balance and coordination of the kettlebell.

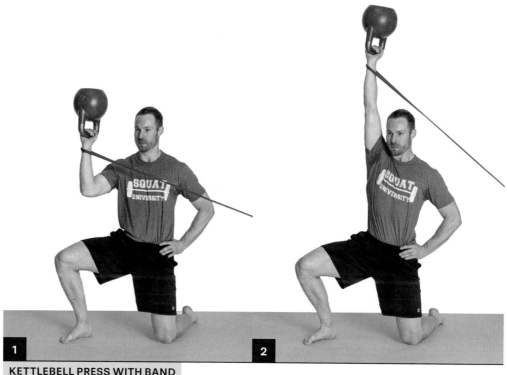

KETTLEBELL PRESS WITH BAND

Kettlebell Turkish Get-Up

The get-up takes the preceding kettlebell exercise one step further and requires you to move your body (and therefore your shoulder complex) through a variety of positions. During each transition, every muscle that stabilizes your arm must work to keep the weight from falling forward or backward.

Start by lying on your back with your left leg straight and your right knee bent. Hold a small kettlebell in your right hand with your arm extended toward the sky. Twist your upper body to the left, propping yourself up on your left elbow. Try to keep your left foot from coming off the ground during this transition.

Next, lift your hips off the ground by activating your glutes. Pause during this transition, feel for the position of your scapula, and work to keep the weight from falling forward. To help with this transition, imagine yourself balancing a glass of water in the hand that is holding the weight. If your arm falls forward, the water will spill from the glass.

Pull your left foot under your body and shift your weight onto your left knee. Pause in this position for a few seconds. Next, shift yourself into a stable half-kneeling position with the kettlebell still directly overhead. Feel the muscles in the back of your shoulder working hard. Lastly, stand straight up, keeping your arm locked out above your head. Reverse this same order of movements until you are lying on the floor again.

To progress this exercise, you can use a heavier kettlebell or barbell, perform a longer hold at the end of each transition, or hold the kettlebell upside-down.

During this movement, remember to look straight forward rather than up at the kettlebell (which is how some coaches teach this exercise). The goal of any corrective exercise is to have direct carryover to barbell lifts. Because no single exercise ends with you staring up at the barbell, the corrective exercise must reflect this and should train your ability to sense joint position without needing to see the weight above your head.

Recommended sets/reps: 2 or 3 sets of 10 reps

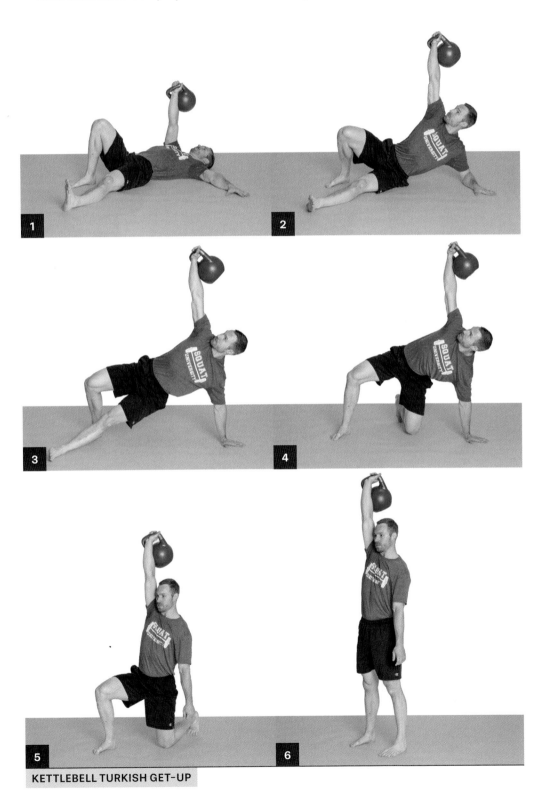

KETTLEBELL TURKISH GET-UP

If the full get-up is too difficult for you to perform, you can regress the movement to a windmill. Start in the half-kneeling position with your arm extended overhead and holding a weight; an upside-down kettlebell works great. Slowly lean over until your free hand is on the ground. The weight should remain pointed toward the sky and your arm should be locked out straight.

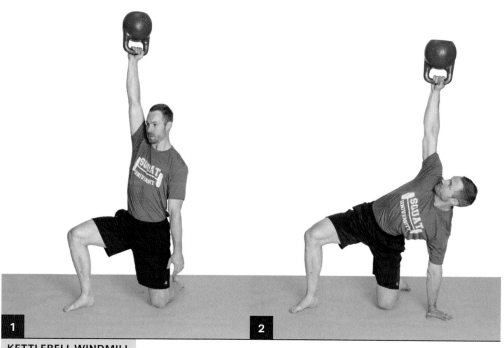

KETTLEBELL WINDMILL

Feel the back of your shoulder working hard to stabilize the weight overhead as you hold this position for a few seconds. Eventually, you can rotate back up to the start position. Make sure your shoulder blade transitions back into a stable position and does not shrug upward excessively.

"Full Can"

Traditionally, two exercises are performed to target the supraspinatus muscle of the rotator cuff. Both are done with the arms extended and elevated in a scapular plane (about 30 degrees from the front of the body). The difference between them is how the arms are positioned.

The "empty can" is performed with the thumbs pointed toward the ground, as if pouring liquid from a can. The "full can" is performed in the opposite manner, with the thumbs pointed toward the sky.

While medical professionals often use the empty can clinically to rule out a shoulder impingement injury, suggestions to use the empty can as an exercise can be traced back to the early 1980s.[41] While the empty can exercise may activate the supraspinatus just as much as the full can version, it might also bring out a high amount of deltoid muscle activation. This is problematic for two reasons:

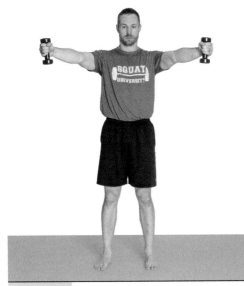

FULL CAN

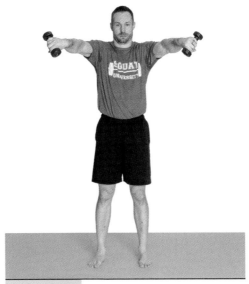

EMPTY CAN

- Trying to strengthen a weak rotator cuff with exercises that produce high levels of deltoid activation can lead to unfavorable joint mechanics. For example, the empty can exercise creates more upward pull on the humerus than the full can, leading to a greater risk of joint impingement.[42] This is why the empty can movement often elicits pain in athletes dealing with shoulder injuries.

- It is common to see scapular winging during the internally rotated empty can exercise as compared to the full can.[43] When the shoulder blade wings out to the side (the movement of protraction and anterior tilting), the available space deep inside the shoulder joint for the humerus to move is closed off, increasing the risk for impingement.

In contrast, pulling your shoulder blades together (retraction) as you perform the full can exercise in combination with the externally rotated thumbs-up position increases this joint space and allows you to strengthen your rotator cuff in a mechanically efficient position.

To perform the full can exercise, raise your arms to shoulder height in an extended position in the scapular plane. Hold this position for three to five seconds before lowering back down.

Recommended reps/sets: 2 sets of 15 to 20 reps

As your strength builds, you can increase the resistance and drop to 3 or 4 sets of 10 reps.

You can progress this exercise in two ways, both shown on the next page. The first is by either adding weight or looping a resistance band around your wrists. The second is to perform static holds. Hold one arm out in the scapular plane while raising and lowering the other arm. For example, you would hold your right arm elevated at shoulder height while performing the full can for 20 reps with your left arm before switching and holding your left arm at shoulder height while performing the movement with your right arm.

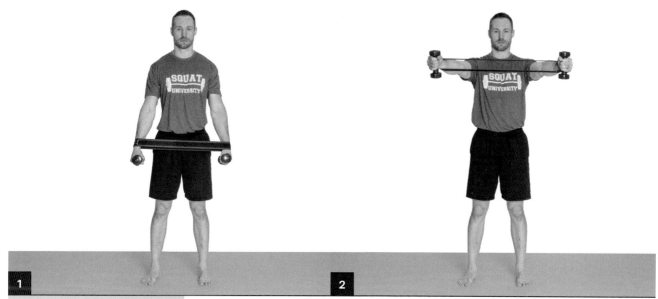

FULL CAN WITH BANDED LOOP

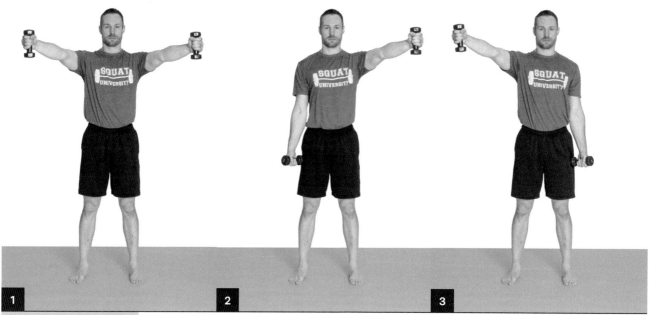

FULL CAN STATIC HOLD

Improving Overhead Coordination

Proper coordination between the shoulder blade and arm as a barbell is moved overhead is crucial for maintaining joint stability and limiting potential impingement. If the shoulder blade does not rotate upward properly as the arm moves overhead, the humerus can shift excessively in the socket, and impingement can occur. If you have tested and cleared up potential mobility restrictions and you still have a problem with scapular coordination, it may be related to a weak or poorly functioning serratus anterior muscle.

The serratus anterior upwardly rotates and protracts the shoulder blade (moves it away from the midline of the body). It also assists in keeping the shoulder blade close to your rib cage and prevents it from winging out to the side.[45] If this muscle becomes weak or fatigued, it can lead to unwanted movement within the shoulder joint (excessive humeral elevation and anterior translation), poor mechanics, and eventual injury, such as an impingement.

Traditionally, rehab specialists have prescribed exercises like the press-up (or punch) and the push-up plus to improve the strength of the serratus anterior.[46] While there is nothing wrong with performing these exercises to try to improve serratus strength and coordination, I have found two disadvantages to their use.

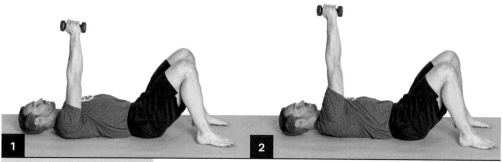

SUPINE SERRATUS PUNCH

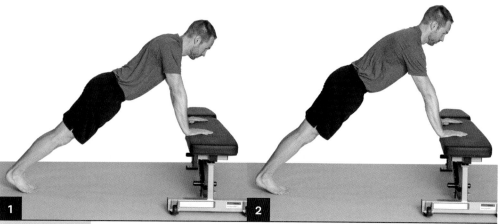

PUSH-UP PLUS

First, both exercises are performed with a pressing motion away from the body. While this may strengthen the serratus anterior, the pressing action also tends to reinforce overactive pec muscles.[47]

Second, these exercises activate the serratus anterior in a fixed position (90 degrees of arm elevation).[48] Most athletes do not show problematic shoulder mechanics until their arms are elevated past this range of motion. Therefore, strengthening this particular muscle at this height will have limited carryover for athletes who need help when their arms are overhead.

I want to share with you three exercises that are intended to enhance serratus anterior activation, strength, and endurance through a full range of motion and in a way that won't reinforce currently overactive muscles like the pecs. With these exercises, you can work to restore and improve ideal and pain-free coordination between the scapula and humerus during overhead lifts.

Scapular Raise

Raising your arms in a scapular plane of motion (about 30 degrees from the front of your body) is a great early-stage rehab exercise for the serratus anterior that also recruits the commonly underactive muscles of the lower trapezius.[49] Start by lying on the floor with your knees bent. Place your hands on your thighs with your thumbs pointed toward your head. Pull your shoulder blades toward the ground to depress and tip them slightly posteriorly. Some people respond well to the cue "tuck your shoulder blades into your back pockets" to create the ideal setup for this exercise.

    With your elbows straight, slowly raise your arms as far over your head as you can while maintaining that 30-degree angle from your body. As you lift your arms above your head, try to keep your shoulder blades pinned to the ground. Brace your core slightly, and don't allow your lower back to move at all during this exercise. Those who really need this exercise will notice a tendency to arch their back and cheat to get their arms overhead. Fight this tendency and go only as far as you can without low back compensation!

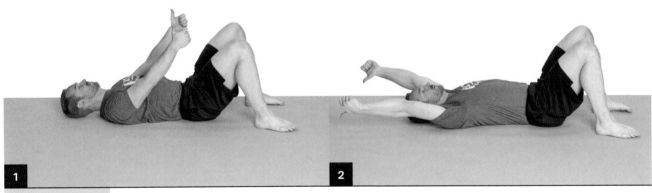

SCAPULAR RAISE

    As you raise your arms, feel for both shoulder blades pushing into the ground with the same amount of force. Using this cue will help you sense the position of your shoulder blades and better recognize if one is winging out to the side more than the other or is not moving symmetrically.

    Maintaining this posture (shoulder blades into the ground) requires your serratus anterior to kick on to move your arms overhead efficiently. If proper scapular motion does not take place, impingement of the shoulder joint can occur, meaning you'll feel a pinching pain in the front or back of your shoulder.

    To guarantee that you're creating sufficient movement of your shoulder blades, you must elevate your arms past shoulder height. Prior to this range, the scapula remains relatively stable on your back.[50] Research has shown that the most serratus anterior activity occurs as your arm moves from your chin to your ears (roughly between 120 and 150 degrees).[51]

Perform this exercise at first with the goal of reaching your thumbs all the way to the floor above your head. As it gets easier, tuck your thumbs into your palms and then try to reach your fists all the way to the floor. The end goal is to reach the floor behind you with open hands (palms to the sky) and lay your entire arm flat on the ground without your low back arching or your ribs flaring out as compensation.

Recommended sets/reps: 2 or 3 sets of 15 to 20 reps

Supine Floor Angel

Once you master the floor scapular raise and can reach your arms all the way to the floor with your palms up, you can move on to floor angels.

Start by lying on your back with your arms in a 90-degree "L" position to your sides. Your entire forearm and back of your hand should be in contact with the floor. (If you cannot achieve this position, I recommend working on improving your thoracic mobility/lat flexibility and focusing on serratus raises before attempting floor angels.)

Then slide your arms above your head (as if you're performing an overhead press) without allowing your arms to pop off the ground. Actively pressing your arms into the floor will deactivate the commonly overactive anterior shoulder muscles like the pecs. To raise your arms completely overhead, your shoulder blades will need to rotate upward and tip posteriorly.

Recommended sets/reps: 2 or 3 sets of 10 reps

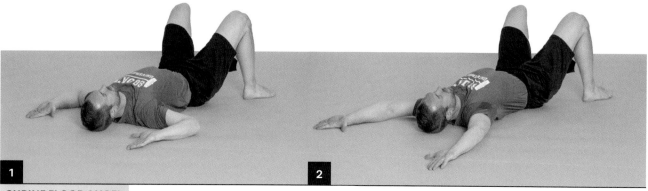

SUPINE FLOOR ANGEL

Make sure that the backs of your shoulders stay pinned to the ground throughout the entire movement. It is common to compensate for a lack of upward rotation of the shoulder blades by shrugging the shoulders (recruiting too much upper trap) in an attempt to elevate the arms farther overhead. To avoid this fault, think about moving your shoulder blades out and away from your body (rather than straight up) as you slide your arms over your head.

Performing this exercise in the supine position allows you to home in on your technique and exposes compensations that could go unnoticed if you performed it in other positions, such as standing by a wall. For example, as with the previous exercise, it is common to arch the low back in an effort to move the arms overhead. Resist this urge! As you master the floor angel, you can move on to other positions, such as sitting with your back against a wall.

In a seated position, place your head, upper back, and hips in contact with a wall. Your low back should be in a neutral, slightly arched position and not flattened completely against the wall. As you perform the angel movement in this position, focus on keeping your low back from arching and your ribs from flaring outward. Those who have stiff lats should perform flexibility exercises before doing this exercise, as restrictions in flexibility can lead to compensations (a low back arch, for example) as the arms move overhead.

Recommended sets/reps: 2 or 3 sets of 10 reps

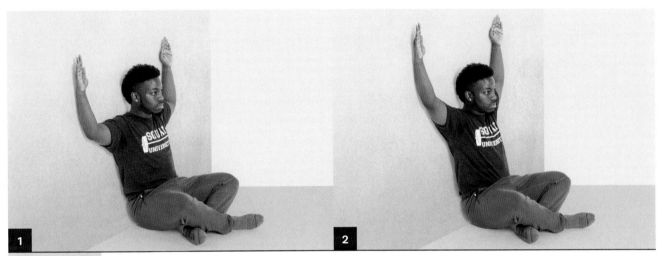

SEATED ANGEL

Wall Slide

The wall slide has been cited as one of the best exercises for activating the serratus anterior.[52] What makes it so much better than the punch or push-up plus is that it can help strengthen the serratus anterior and improve scapular coordination with the arm elevated position above shoulder height. Most athletes report shoulder pain when the arm is overhead and less pain (or no pain) when the arm is below shoulder level.

To perform this exercise, raise your arms to shoulder height with your elbows bent to 90 degrees and place your forearms against a wall. Your arms should be just outside of shoulder width and your forearms parallel. A cue that I learned from strength coach Eric Cressey to achieve the desired movement of the shoulder blades is "reach, round, and rotate."

Start by sliding your forearms slowly up the wall. Reach your shoulder blades out and around your torso as your arms slide upward. This action of shoulder blade protraction (moving the scapulae away from the midline of the body) should push your upper back slightly away from the wall. Because many athletes who need serratus anterior work often have a flat upper back, cueing to "round the upper back" can help you hug your shoulder blades to your torso.

Lastly, think "rotate shoulder blades around armpits" (the motion of upward rotation). If you have a friend to help, they can assist this motion by pushing on the medial border of your shoulder blade.

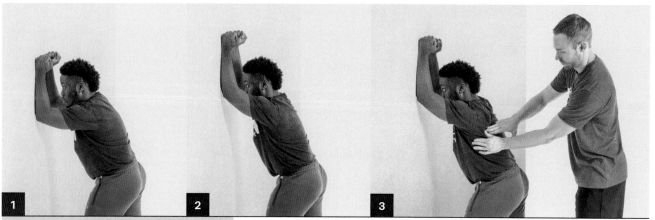

WALL SLIDE WITH PARTNER ASSISTANCE

The arms do not need to extend completely to make this drill effective. You've gone too far with the arm elevation if you notice pain in your upper traps or anterior shoulder. If you do it correctly, you'll notice muscle fatigue around your lateral armpit.

Keep your core slightly braced during this motion as it is common to let the low back arch excessively as the arms slide up the wall. Staggering your feet (one in front of the other) and shifting your body weight from the back foot to the front may allow you to complete the appropriate weight shift while keeping your back in a neutral flat position.

As you elevate your arms, it is normal to see a small amount of upper trap activation. This is expected and desirable as the upper trapezius muscle works hand in hand with the serratus anterior to rotate the scapula upward. But any exaggerated use of the upper traps (seen as a shrugging of the shoulders) is discouraged because it would excessively elevate the scapula and possibly re-create impingement symptoms if you are dealing with shoulder pain. This upper trap compensation is normal, especially in weightlifters and CrossFitters who perform the Olympic lifts.

The traditional wall slide exercise has two small limitations. The first is that you can raise your arms only so high above your head before your forearms pop off the wall. This limits your ability to work on serratus anterior strength at the end ranges of arm elevation, which is where many barbell athletes truly need it to perform a snatch, press, or jerk. Second, actively pulling your arms back down against the friction of the wall can reinforce overactive pecs, especially the pec minor.

For these reasons, try this exercise with a small twist. Assume the same start position but place your hands on top of a foam roller against the wall, holding the roller just above eye level so you don't run out of room during the next step. Again, brace your core slightly as you lean forward and slide your arms up the wall. The roller enables you to slide your arms back to the start position easily, and you don't have to worry about reinforcing an overactive pec minor.

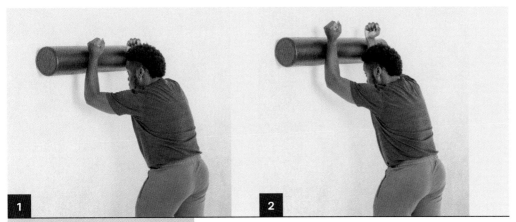

WALL SLIDE WITH FOAM ROLLER

Another muscle that commonly becomes overactive in the presence of a weak serratus anterior is the subscapularis, one of the rotator cuff muscles that lies on the anterior, or front, side of your shoulder blade. To reciprocally inhibit or "turn off" this muscle during the wall slide exercise, simply loop a small resistance band around your arms. Creating external rotation torque (an action performed by the posterior rotator cuff muscles) while you slide your arms up the wall allows you to home in on the serratus anterior in an optimal manner. This resistance band does not need to be super strong; a light band works great.

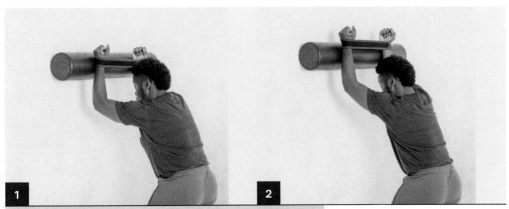

WALL SLIDE WITH FOAM ROLLER AND RESISTANCE BAND

To progress this exercise, you can start slowly backing your feet away from the wall. A greater lean will increase the challenge for your body to maintain all of the prior cues. Again, staggering your feet during this exercise can help ensure that you don't end up over-recruiting your pec minor muscles by dragging your arms down from the elevated position.

Recommended sets/reps: 2 or 3 sets of 10 to 20 reps

Final Thoughts on Overhead Coordination

At first glance, the few exercises described here may not appear that difficult to perform. In fact, if you go through them lackadaisically, they will seem extremely easy! With the right attention to detail, however, these exercises can be quite challenging and will work for you.

Notes

1. G. Calhoon and A. C. Fry, "Injury rates and profiles of elite competitive weightlifters," *Journal of Athletic Training* 34, no. 3 (1999): 232–8.

2. G. C. Terry and T. M. Chopp, "Functional anatomy of the shoulder," *Journal of Athletic Training* 35, no. 3 (2000): 248–55; K. E. Wilk, C. A. Arrigo, and J. R. Andrews, "Current concepts: the stabilizing structures of the glenohumeral joint," *Journal of Orthopaedic & Sports Physical Therapy* 25, no. 6 (1997): 364–78.

3. Wilk, Arrigo, and Andrews, "Current concepts: the stabilizing structures of the glenohumeral joint" (see note 2 above).

4. Wilk, Arrigo, and Andrews, "Current concepts: the stabilizing structures of the glenohumeral joint" (see note 2 above).

5. Terry and Chopp, "Functional anatomy of the shoulder" (see note 2 above).

6. M. Kebaetse, P. McClure, and N. A. Pratt, "Thoracic position effect on shoulder range of motion, strength, and three-dimensional scapular kinematics," *Archives of Physical Medicine and Rehabilitation* 80, no. 8 (1999): 945–50.

7. Wilk, Arrigo, and Andrews, "Current concepts: the stabilizing structures of the glenohumeral joint" (see note 2 above).

8. A. M. Cools, D. Cambier, and E. E. Witvrouw, "Screening the athlete's shoulder for impingement symptoms: a clinical reasoning algorithm for early detection of shoulder pathology," *British Journal of Sports Medicine* 42, no. 8 (2008): 628–35.

9. M. L. Gross, S. L. Brenner, I. Esformes, and J. J. Sonzogni, "Anterior shoulder instability in weight lifters," *American Journal of Sports Medicine* 21, no. 4 (1993): 599–603.

10. M. F. Saccomanno, M. Fodale, L. Capasso, and G. M. Cazzato, "Generalized joint laxity and multidirectional instability of the shoulder," *Joints* 1, no. 4 (2013): 171–9; F. A. Cordasco, "Understanding multidirectional instability of the shoulder," *Journal of Athletic Training* 35, no. 3 (2000): 278–85.

11. Saccomanno, Fodale, Capasso, and Cazzato, "Generalized joint laxity and multidirectional instability of the shoulder" (see note 10 above).

12. K. L. Cameron, M. L. Duffey, T. M. DeBerardino, P. D. Stoneman, C. J. Jones, and B. D. Owens, "Association of generalized joint hypermobility with a history of glenohumeral joint instability," *Journal of Athletic Training* 45, no. 3 (2010): 253–8.

13. Cameron, Duffey, DeBerardino, Stoneman, Jones, and Owens, "Association of generalized joint hypermobility with a history of glenohumeral joint instability" (see note 12 above).

14. Wilk, Arrigo, and Andrews, "Current concepts: the stabilizing structures of the glenohumeral joint" (see note 2 above).

15. S. J. Snyder, R. P. Karzel, W. Del Pizzo, R. D. Ferkel, and M. J. Friedman, "SLAP lesions of the shoulder," *Arthroscopy* 6, no. 4 (1996): 274–9.

16. D. J. Magee, *Orthopedic Physical Assessment*, 5th Edition (St. Louis, MO: Saunders Elsevier, 2008).

17. Magee, *Orthopedic Physical Assessment* (see note 16 above).

18.   K. D. Johnson, K. M. Kim, B. K. Yu, S. A. Saliba, and T. L. Grindstaff, "Reliability of thoracic spine rotation range-of-motion measurements in healthy adults," *Journal of Athletic Training* 47, no. 1 (2012): 52–60; K. D. Johnson and T. L. Grindstaff, "Thoracic rotation measurement techniques: clinical commentary," *North American Journal of Sports Physical Therapy* 5, no. 4 (2010): 252–6.

19.   R. J. Emery and A. B. Mullaji, "Glenohumeral joint instability in normal adolescents: incidence and significance," *Journal of Bone and Joint Surgery, British Volume* 73-B, no. 3 (1991): 406–8; Magee, *Orthopedic Physical Assessment* (see note 16 above).

20.   Emery and Mullaji, "Glenohumeral joint instability in normal adolescents" (see note 19 above).

21.   E. Itoi, T. Kido, A. Sano, M. Urayama, and K. Sato, "Which is more useful, the 'full can test' or the 'empty can test,' in detecting the torn supraspinatus tendon?" *American Journal of Sports Medicine* 27, no. 1 (1997): 65–8.

22.   K. D. Johnson and T. L. Grindstaff, "Thoracic region self-mobilization: a clinical suggestion," *International Journal of Sports Physical Therapy* 7, no. 2 (2012): 252–6.

23.   C. Beardsley and J. Škarabot, "Effects of self-myofascial release: a systematic review," *Journal of Bodywork and Movement Therapies* 19, no. 4 (2015): 747–58; S. W. Cheatham, M. J. Kolber, M. Cain, and M. Lee, "The effects of self-myofascial release using a foam roll or roller massager on joint range of motion, muscle recovery, and performance: a systematic review," *International Journal of Sports Physical Therapy* 10, no. 6 (2015): 827–38.

24.   K. O'Sullivan, S. McAuliffe, and N. Deburca, "The effects of eccentric training on lower limb flexibility: a systematic review," *British Journal of Sports Medicine* 46, no. 12 (2012): 838–45.

25.   N. N. Mahieu, P. McNair, A. Cools, C. D'Haen, K. Vandermeulen, and E. Witvrouw, "Effect of eccentric training on the plantar flexor muscle-tendon tissue properties," *Medicine & Science in Sports & Exercise* 40, no. 1 (2008): 117–23; R. T. Nelson and W. D. Brandy, "Eccentric training and static stretching improve hamstring flexibility of high school males," *Journal of Athletic Training* 39, no. 3 (2004): 254–8.

26.   J. D. Borstad and P. M. Ludewig, "Comparison of three stretches for the pectoralis minor muscle," *Journal of Shoulder and Elbow Surgery* 15, no. 3 (2006): 324–30.

27.   C. B. Chant, R. Litchfield, S. Griffin, and L. M. Thain, "Humeral head retroversion in competitive baseball players and its relationship to glenohumeral rotation range of motion," *Journal of Orthopaedic & Sports Physical Therapy* 37, no. 9 (2007): 514–20; T. Mihata, H. Hirai, A. Hasegawa, K. Fukunishi, C. Watanabe, Y. Fujisawa, T. Kawakami, et al., "Relationship between humeral retroversion and career of pitching in elementary and junior high schools," *Orthopaedic Journal of Sports Medicine* 5, no. 7 suppl 6 (2017): 2325967117S00371.

28.   "5 reasons why I don't use the sleeper stretch and why you shouldn't either," MikeReinold.com, accessed June 1, 2019, https://mikereinold.com/why-i-dont-use-the-sleeper-stretch/.

29.   P. McClure, J. Balaicuis, D. Heiland, M. E. Broersma, C. K. Thorndike, and A. Wood, "A randomized controlled comparison of stretching procedures for posterior shoulder tightness," *Journal of Orthopaedic & Sports Physical Therapy* 37, no. 3 (2007): 108–14.

30.   M. M. Reinold, K. E. Wilk, G. S. Fleisig, N. Zheng, S. W. Barrentine, T. Chmielewski, R. C. Cody, G. G. Jameson, and J. R. Andrews, "Electromyographic analysis of the rotator cuff and deltoid musculature during common shoulder external rotation exercises," *Journal of Orthopaedic & Sports Physical Therapy* 34, no. 7 (2004): 385–94; M. M. Reinold, R. Escamilla, and K. E. Wilk, "Current concepts in the scientific and clinical rationale behind exercises for glenohumeral and scapulothoracic musculature," *Journal of Orthopaedic & Sports Physical Therapy* 39, no. 2 (2009): 105–17.

31.   Reinold, Wilk, Fleisig, et al., "Electromyographic analysis of the rotator cuff and deltoid musculature" (see note 30 above).

32.   R. A. McCabe, "Surface electromyographic analysis of the lower trapezius muscle during exercises performed below ninety degrees of shoulder elevation in healthy subjects," *North American Journal of Sports Physical Therapy* 2, no. 1 (2007): 23–43.

33. McCabe, "Surface electromyographic analysis of the lower trapezius muscle" (see note 32 above).

34. Reinold, Escamilla, and Wilk, "Current concepts in the scientific and clinical rationale behind exercises for glenohumeral and scapulothoracic musculature" (see note 30 above).

35. A. T. Ernst and R. L. Jensen, "Rotator cuff activation during the Olympic snatch under various loading conditions," in *Proceedings of XXXIII Congress of the International Society of Biomechanics in Sports*, eds. F. Colloud, M. Domalian, and T. Monnet (2015), 670–3.

36. Reinold, Escamilla, and Wilk, "Current concepts in the scientific and clinical rationale behind exercises for glenohumeral and scapulothoracic musculature" (see note 30 above); J. B. Myers, M. R. Pasquale, K. G. Laudner, T. C. Sell, J. P. Bradley, and S. M. Lephart, "On-the-field resistance-tubing exercises for throwers: an electromyographic analysis," *Journal of Athletic Training* 40, no. 1 (2005): 15–22.

37. Reinold, Escamilla, and Wilk, "Current concepts in the scientific and clinical rationale behind exercises for glenohumeral and scapulothoracic musculature" (see note 30 above).

38. J. B. Myers and S. M. Lephart, "The role of the sensorimotor system in the athletic shoulder," *Journal of Athletic Training* 35, no. 3 (2000): 351–63.

39. K. E. Wilk, L. C. Marcina, and M. M. Reinold, "Non-operative rehabilitation for traumatic and atraumatic glenohumeral instability," *North American Journal of Sports Physical Therapy* 1, no. 1 (2006): 16–31.

40. M. M. Reinold, T. J. Gill, K. E. Wilk, and J. R. Andrews, "Current concepts in the evaluation and treatment of the shoulder in overhead throwing athletes, part 2: injury prevention and treatment," *Sports Health* 2, no. 2 (2010): 101–15.

41. F. W. Jobe and D. R. Moynes, "Delineation of diagnostic criteria and a rehabilitation program for rotator cuff injuries," *American Journal of Sports Medicine* 10, no. 6 (1982): 336–9.

42. N. K. Poppen and P. S. Walker, "Forces at the glenohumeral joint in abduction," *Clinical Orthopaedics and Related Research* 135 (1978): 165–70.

43. C. A. Thigpen, D. A. Padua, N. Morgan, C. Kreps, and S. C. Karas, "Scapular kinematics during supraspinatus rehabilitation exercise: a comparison of full-can versus empty-can techniques," *American Journal of Sports Medicine* 34, no. 4 (2006): 644–52.

44. S. W. Alpert, M. M. Pink, F. W. Jobe, P. J. McMahon, and W. Mathiyakom, "Electromyographic analysis of deltoid and rotator cuff function under varying loads and speeds," *Journal of Shoulder and Elbow Surgery* 9, no. 1 (2000): 47–58; A. Dark, K. A. Ginn, and M. Halaki, "Shoulder muscle recruitment patterns during commonly used rotator cuff exercise: an electromyographic study," *Physical Therapy* 87, no. 8 (2007): 1039–46.

45. D. H. Hardwick, J. A. Beebe, M. K. McDonnell, and C. E. Lang, "A comparison of serratus anterior muscle activation during a wall slide exercise and other traditional exercises," *Journal of Orthopaedic & Sports Physical Therapy* 36, no. 12 (2006): 903–10.

46. M. J. Decker, R. A. Hintermeister, K. J. Faber, and R. J. Hawkins, "Serratus anterior muscle activity during selected rehabilitation exercises," *American Journal of Sports Medicine* 27, no. 6 (1999): 784–91.

47. Decker, Hintermeister, Faber, and Hawkins, "Serratus anterior muscle activity during selected rehabilitation exercises" (see note 46 above).

48. R. A. Ekstrom, R. A. Donatelli, and G. L. Soderberg, "Surface electromyographic analysis of exercises for the trapezius and serratus anterior muscles," *Journal of Orthopaedic & Sports Physical Therapy* 33, no. 5 (2003): 247–58.

49. Ekstrom, Donatelli, and Soderberg, "Surface electromyographic analysis of exercises for the trapezius and serratus anterior muscles" (see note 48 above); Decker, Hintermeister, Faber, and Hawkins, "Serratus anterior muscle activity during selected rehabilitation exercises" (see note 46 above).

50. Ekstrom, Donatelli, and Soderberg, "Surface electromyographic analysis of exercises for the trapezius and serratus anterior muscles" (see note 48 above).

51. J. B. Mosely, Jr., F. W. Jobe, M. Pink, J. Perry, and J. Tibone, "EMG analysis of the scapular muscles during a shoulder rehabilitation program," *American Journal of Sports Medicine* 20, no. 2 (1992): 128–34.

52. Hardwick, Beebe, McDonnell, and Lang, "A comparison of serratus anterior muscle activation during a wall slide exercise and other traditional exercises" (see note 45 above); Ekstrom, Donatelli, and Soderberg, "Surface electromyographic analysis of exercises for the trapezius and serratus anterior muscles" (see note 48 above); Mosely, Jr., Jobe, Pink, Perry, and Tibone, "EMG analysis of the scapular muscles during a shoulder rehabilitation program" (see note 51 above); Decker, Hintermeister, Faber, and Hawkins, "Serratus anterior muscle activity during selected rehabilitation exercises" (see note 46 above).

CHAPTER 5

ELBOW PAIN

Elbow injuries are often difficult to diagnose and treat. Many educated clinicians find that elbow injuries can be confusing, and the treatment can be somewhat complicated. If you look at the research, the elbow almost always ranks as one of the top injured joints among strength athletes like weightlifters and powerlifters.[1]

However, despite these injuries being so common, you can scour research journals and the internet for days and fail to find a consensus among medical and rehab professionals on the best approach to their management and treatment.

Why is it so difficult to understand elbow injuries? Let's start by discussing the anatomy of the elbow joint.

Elbow Injury Anatomy 101

Most medical doctors are taught that the elbow is a simple hinge joint that opens and closes like a metal bracket attaching a door to its frame. To the casual observer, this may seem accurate, but there's much more to the elbow than meets the eye. Unlike the hinging motion of the knee that occurs between the femur and tibia, the elbow joint contains three bones, the humerus and the radius and ulna of the forearm, which connect to form three small joints.

ELBOW JOINT BONY ANATOMY

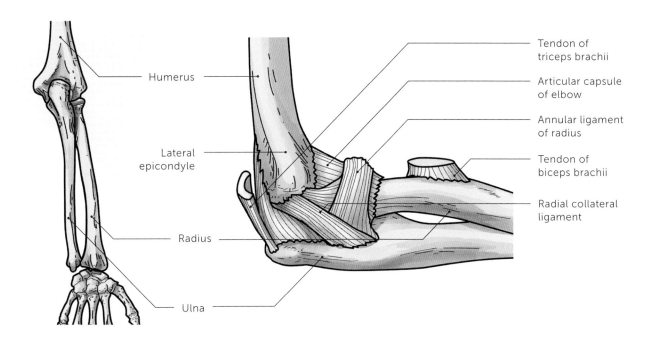

Humerus

Lateral epicondyle

Radius

Ulna

Tendon of triceps brachii

Articular capsule of elbow

Annular ligament of radius

Tendon of biceps brachii

Radial collateral ligament

Making things even more complicated are 16 small muscles that cross these joints. They work together to bend and straighten the elbow as well as rotate the forearm (the motion of pronation and supination).[2] As you're starting to see, the elbow is much more than a simple hinge joint.

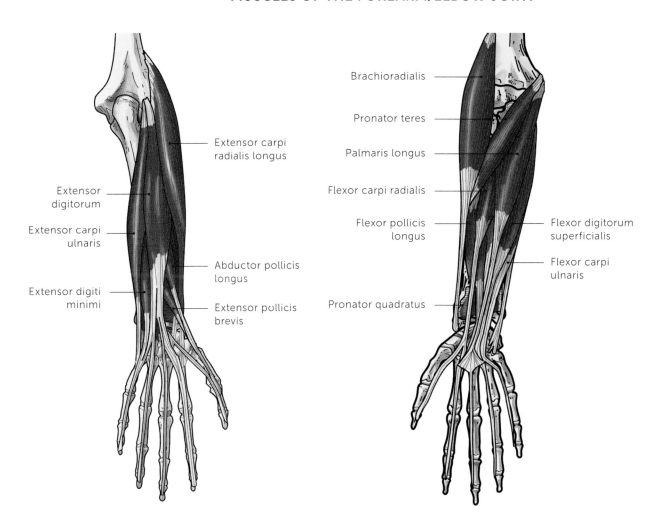

Extensor carpi radialis longus

Extensor digitorum

Extensor carpi ulnaris

Extensor digiti minimi

Abductor pollicis longus

Extensor pollicis brevis

Brachioradialis

Pronator teres

Palmaris longus

Flexor carpi radialis

Flexor pollicis longus

Pronator quadratus

Flexor digitorum superficialis

Flexor carpi ulnaris

To perform a proper screening of a pained elbow, we need to go through a small checklist:

- Where is the pain located?

- Is the pain due to nerve irritation?

- What reproduces the pain in that location?

The first thing I do when evaluating an athlete with elbow pain is to distinguish exactly where their symptoms present. While the rehab plan never focuses solely on the specific site of pain, pinpointing where the symptoms are felt can give us insight into the injury mechanism and lead us to the most efficient path for fixing it.

Lateral Elbow

Let's start with the lateral elbow. The bony nub on the outside of your elbow (the lateral epicondyle) is the common attachment site for your forearm extensor muscles. Historically, pain in this area has been referred to as "tennis elbow" or lateral epicondylitis. However, in recent years, many experts have recommended moving away from these two terms for a few reasons.

LATERAL ELBOW ANATOMY

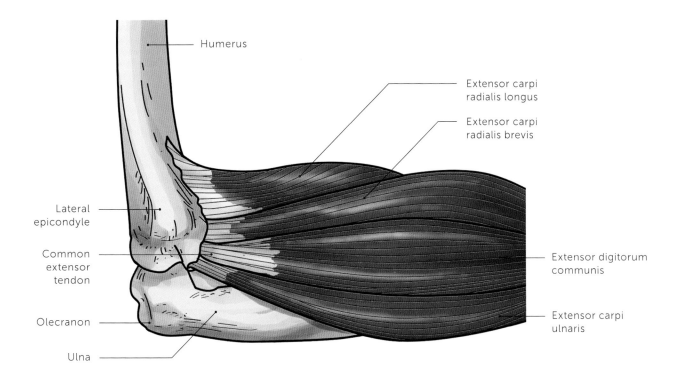

Humerus

Extensor carpi
radialis longus

Extensor carpi
radialis brevis

Lateral
epicondyle

Common
extensor
tendon

Extensor digitorum
communis

Extensor carpi
ulnaris

Olecranon

Ulna

First, inflammation (which the *–itis* ending of the word *tendinitis* refers to) has not been found in many cases of lateral elbow pain.[3] Second, many people develop this injury without ever having played tennis! Instead, pain in this area is now generally referred to as lateral epicondylalgia. The pain is often attributed to tendinopathy, degrading overuse of the tissues similar to a patellar or quad tendon injury.

Injury to this part of the elbow often brings out tenderness when the spot just below the lateral epicondyle (where the large extensor tendons of the forearm run and insert) is poked. Gripping activities also often re-create pain, especially when using a palm-down grip or doing a lift that requires rotating the hand from palm-down to palm-up, such as a biceps curl.[4]

Many people are confused by the notion that gripping movements can re-create pain at the lateral elbow. Isn't gripping performed by the forearm flexor muscles on the opposite side of the arm? The answer is yes.

The muscles on the anterior side of the forearm have the ability to flex the wrist (such as performing a wrist curl) *and* flex the fingers (making a fist). However, to flex the fingers to grip an object like a barbell without simultaneous wrist movement, something interesting has to happen. Basically, the extensor muscles on the back side of the forearm have to turn on in order to stop the wrist from flexing excessively. If the wrist flexors fired and the extensor muscles stayed silent, any gripping activity would be difficult because the wrist would be curled into extreme flexion.[5] This means the harder you grip, the more load you place on the common extensor tendon that originates on the lateral elbow.

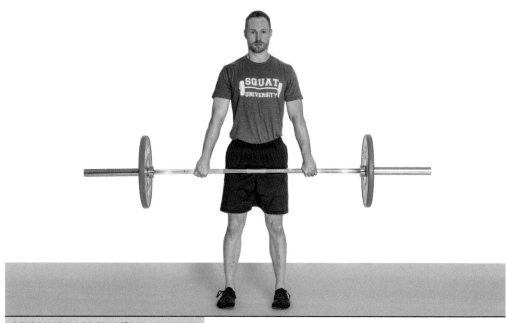

GRIPPING BARBELL HELD AT WAIST

Medial Elbow

Shifting to the other side of the elbow, we find another bony nub called the *medial epicondyle,* which is the common attachment site for a number of the forearm flexor muscles. Pain in this area is often referred to as "golfer's elbow" or medial epicondylitis, but, as with the lateral elbow, pain on the inside of the elbow is now generally referred to as medial epicondylalgia.

MEDIAL ELBOW ANATOMY

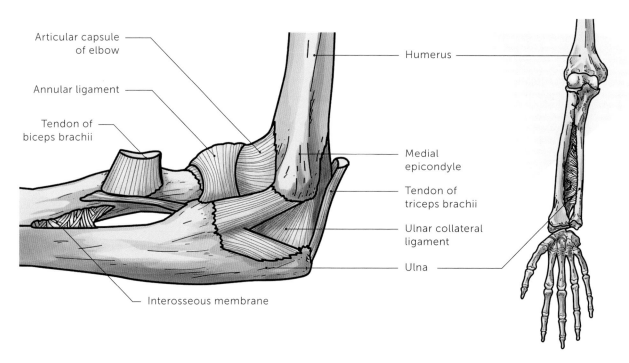

Articular capsule of elbow

Annular ligament

Tendon of biceps brachii

Interosseous membrane

Humerus

Medial epicondyle

Tendon of triceps brachii

Ulnar collateral ligament

Ulna

An overuse injury to this side of the elbow often creates tenderness in the tissues surrounding the medial epicondyle that is brought out and made worse when performing resisted wrist flexion (the motion of a heavy wrist curl) or stretching the wrist into extension.[6]

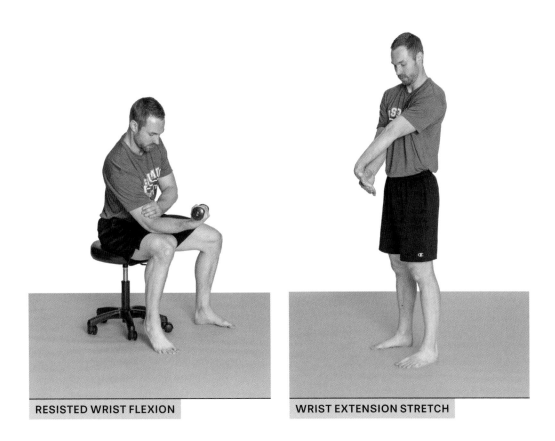

RESISTED WRIST FLEXION   **WRIST EXTENSION STRETCH**

Anterior and Posterior Elbow

While the sides of the elbow are the most common sites of pain for strength athletes, it is possible to injure the anterior and posterior aspects of the elbow. On the back side of the elbow, the three heads of the triceps converge to form a common tendon that inserts on the olecranon process. On the opposite side lie the attachments of the biceps, brachioradialis, and brachialis muscles.

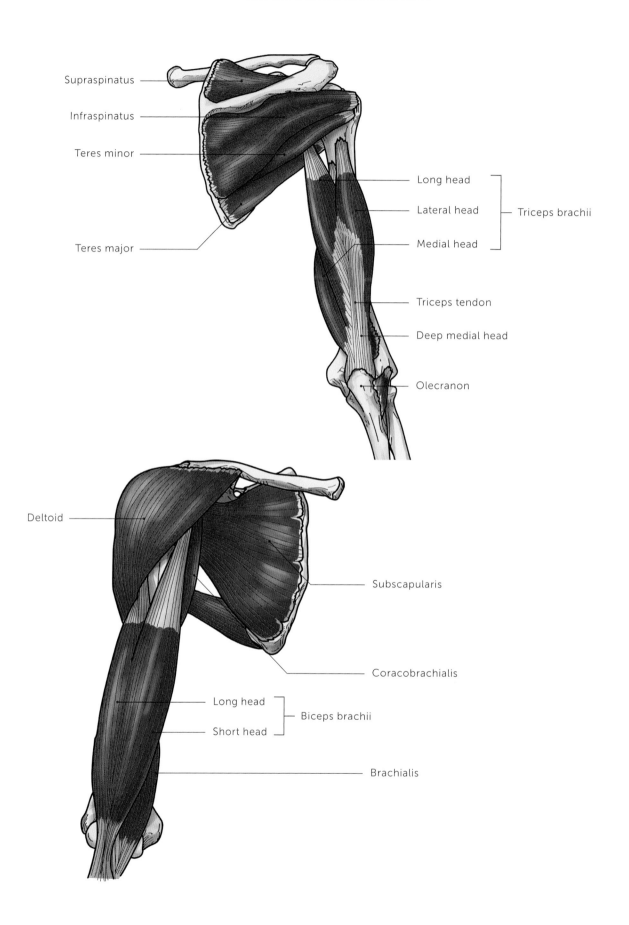

Supraspinatus

Infraspinatus

Teres minor

Teres major

Long head

Lateral head

Medial head

Triceps brachii

Triceps tendon

Deep medial head

Olecranon

Deltoid

Subscapularis

Coracobrachialis

Long head

Short head

Biceps brachii

Brachialis

Nerve Injuries

While most cases of elbow pain in strength athletes are due to repetitive overuse of soft tissues (muscles and tendons), an injury to one of the several nerves that span the arm can also cause symptoms. Excessive compression or stretching of any of these nerves can create pain in the elbow (often mimicking medial or lateral epicondylalgia), a burning sensation, and radiating numbness/tingling down the length of the forearm and possibly into the hand.[7]

NERVES OF UPPER ARM

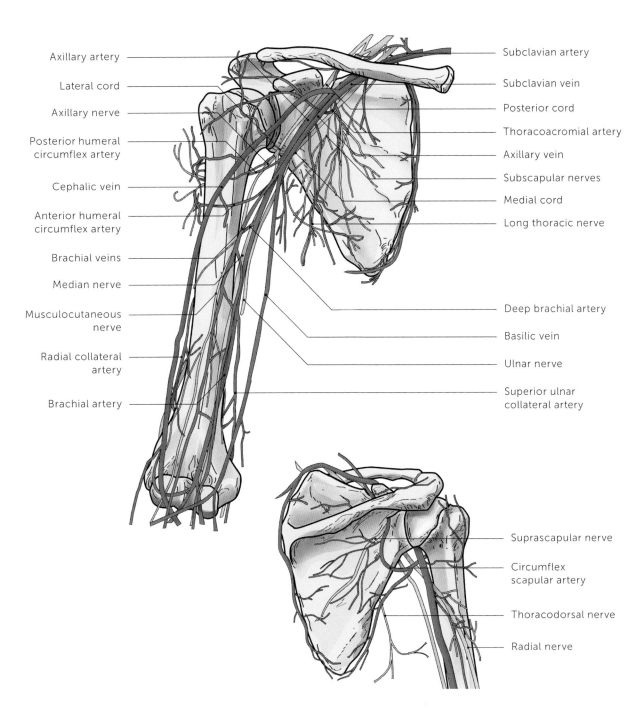

Axillary artery

Lateral cord

Axillary nerve

Posterior humeral circumflex artery

Cephalic vein

Anterior humeral circumflex artery

Brachial veins

Median nerve

Musculocutaneous nerve

Radial collateral artery

Brachial artery

Subclavian artery

Subclavian vein

Posterior cord

Thoracoacromial artery

Axillary vein

Subscapular nerves

Medial cord

Long thoracic nerve

Deep brachial artery

Basilic vein

Ulnar nerve

Superior ulnar collateral artery

Suprascapular nerve

Circumflex scapular artery

Thoracodorsal nerve

Radial nerve

How to Screen Your Elbow Pain

After you've identified where your elbow pain symptoms are located, it's time to try to pinpoint the potential causes. You can use two methods to determine the cause of your pain: nerve screening and kinetic chain screening.

Nerve Pain Screening

If you think you are experiencing any of the symptoms described in the preceding section, it is important to screen your cervical spine to make sure those symptoms aren't stemming from your neck. Start by moving your head as far as possible in every direction. Look up and down, look to the left and right, and tilt your head from side to side.

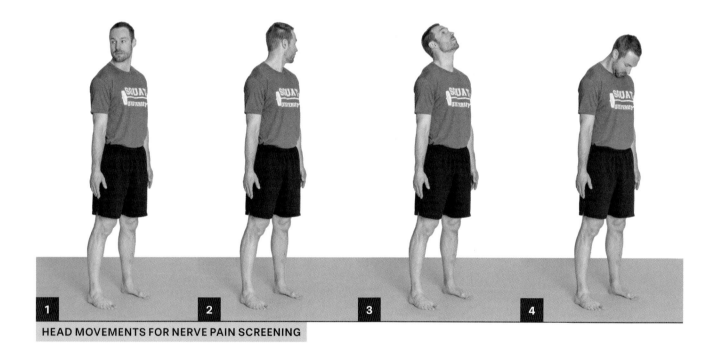

HEAD MOVEMENTS FOR NERVE PAIN SCREENING

Also look over each shoulder at an angle (creating extension, rotation, and a little side bending of your neck) and press down on your head slightly with your opposite-side hand. If any of these movements re-create pain in your elbow, I recommend that you see a medical doctor or other rehabilitation specialist for an evaluation. If you do not notice any changes in your symptoms when doing these neck movements, try these next few screens to determine which nerve may be the source of your pain.

Ulnar Nerve

Start with the ulnar nerve that runs along the inside of your elbow. Because of the surrounding anatomy, the ulnar nerve is susceptible to excessive compression, friction, and stretching. As the nerve runs down the arm, it passes through a small tunnel called the *cubital tunnel*. When you bend your elbow, this tunnel narrows by up to 55 percent of its original size, increasing the incidence of compression and eventual injury.[8]

ULNAR NERVE ANATOMY

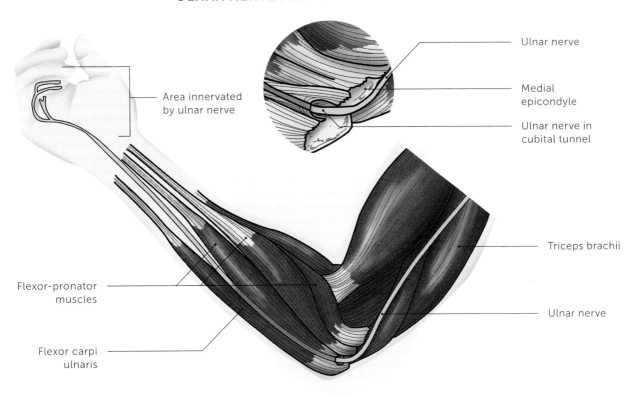

Area innervated by ulnar nerve

Ulnar nerve

Medial epicondyle

Ulnar nerve in cubital tunnel

Triceps brachii

Ulnar nerve

Flexor-pronator muscles

Flexor carpi ulnaris

Symptoms of a compression injury to the ulnar nerve at the elbow (called *cubital tunnel syndrome*) include aching and numbness on the inside of the forearm that may extend to the fourth and fifth fingers or shoot up the arm into the biceps region.[9] Movements that pull the elbow into repeated flexion, such as bench presses, pull-ups, and receiving the barbell in the front rack position during a clean, or even sleeping on your side with your elbow bent, can re-create these symptoms. Over time, irritation to this nerve can even progress to the point where your grip strength becomes limited.

Here's how to test if your medial elbow pain is possibly due to an injury of the ulnar nerve. With your wrist in a straight "neutral" position, bend your elbow as much as you can, as if doing a biceps curl, and hold this posture for one minute. You can also take the thumb of your pain-free arm and push hard into the inside of your elbow, just above the medial epicondyle. This over-pressure will compress the ulnar nerve that runs underneath. If either of these tests reproduces your symptoms, it is positive for an injury to the ulnar nerve.[10]

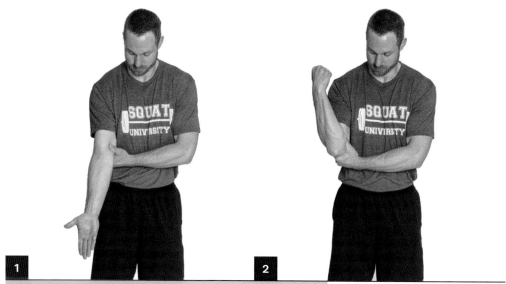

ULNAR NERVE TEST (BICEPS CURL WITH OVER-PRESSURE)

Radial Nerve

Another nerve that can become injured and create elbow pain is the radial nerve. As this nerve runs down the lateral arm and crosses the elbow joint, it moves through a small passageway between tissues called the *radial tunnel*. Just like the ulnar nerve on the opposite side of the elbow, the radial nerve can become compressed and pinched in this area, leading to what is called *radial tunnel syndrome*. Entrapment of the radial nerve often mimics lateral epicondylalgia, causing a deep aching or burning pain that can extend from the lateral elbow into the hand.[11]

RADIAL NERVE ANATOMY AT ELBOW

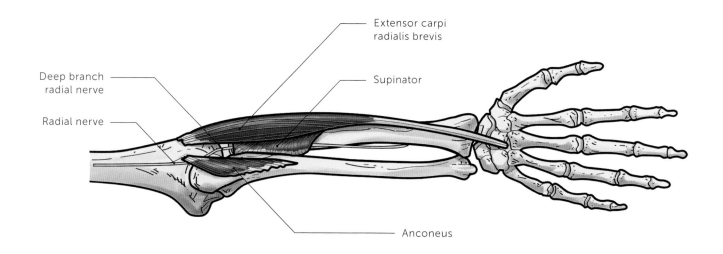

Deep branch radial nerve

Radial nerve

Extensor carpi radialis brevis

Supinator

Anconeus

If you have lateral elbow pain, try this test. Start by taking the hand of your pain-free arm and placing it on the opposite shoulder. Pull down slightly on your shoulder to try to keep it from shrugging upward during the next portion of the test.

With your symptomatic arm hanging by your side, fully straighten your elbow and turn your hand behind you with the palm facing up. Next, make a fist with your fingers clasped over your thumb as if performing a hook grip and curl your wrist slightly, bringing your fist toward your forearm. If this motion doesn't create pain, slowly raise your arm out to the side. A positive test will reproduce your lateral elbow pain, and either shrugging your shoulder or tilting your head toward your opposite arm will modify the intensity of that pain.[12]

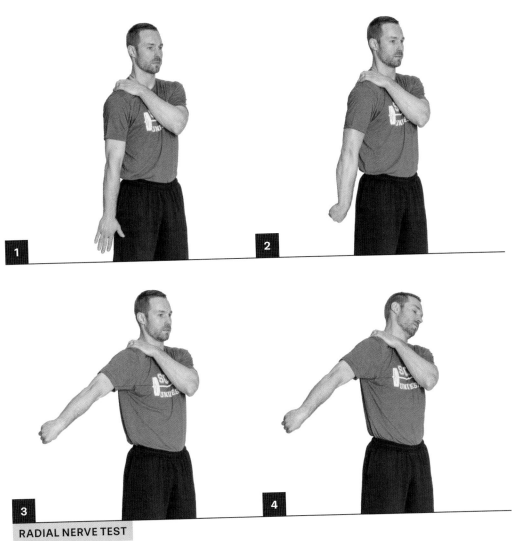

RADIAL NERVE TEST

As you can see, several injuries can take place at the elbow joint. After going over the basic anatomy of the elbow and the sites where injuries commonly present, we can dive into why pain develops in the first place. To better understand the cause of your pain, you have to take a step back and look at your whole body.

Kinetic Chain Screening

Most elbow injuries that occur in the weight room (such as a dislocated elbow) are not catastrophes. They result from wear-and-tear stresses on the body that accumulate over time. These stresses are influenced by the following factors:

- Mobility (the ability to move and control your body into optimal positions)
- Stability (the ability to maintain position and limit unwanted joint motion)
- Position/technique

Lifting weights places force (called *load*) on your tissues and joints. When proper loading schemes are carried out with ideal technique and paired with sufficient recovery and rest, the body adapts and grows in its capacity to handle more and more load. Problems arise, however, when this balanced equation is thrown off due to an issue with any of these factors. When it comes to the elbow joint, poor lifting mechanics and limitations related to mobility and/or stability are often the culprit. For this reason, a thorough evaluation must look beyond the site of symptoms.

I often see frustrated patients who have gone through a lot of unsuccessful treatments because the rehabilitation professional treats only the site of pain, neglecting the shoulder girdle or failing to look at movement/activities that cause pain. When it comes to the elbow joint, failed treatment plans usually encompass exercises directed to the forearm muscles and "passive" treatments (ultrasound, tape application, or scraping techniques) to the site of pain. While it is not my goal to discredit any of the prior modes of rehab, we are missing the big picture if we don't take a step back and look into other possible contributing factors.

Do you remember the childhood song that goes, "The knee bone's connected to the thigh bone, the thigh bone's connected to the hip bone...," and so on? This innocent melody is something that many medical and rehabilitation professionals could learn from.

There's a saying, "A chain is only as strong as its weakest link." If one link breaks, the whole chain fails. If we look at the body as a linked system or "chain," it becomes easier to see how a problem at one joint could have a direct effect on another joint elsewhere in the body. By searching out "weak links" in areas other than the site of pain, we can uncover all of the contributing factors for why an injury occurred.

Regardless of where your elbow symptoms present, we must start this process by looking at the joints directly below and above the site of pain: the wrist and shoulder complex.

ELBOW PAIN KINETIC CHAIN

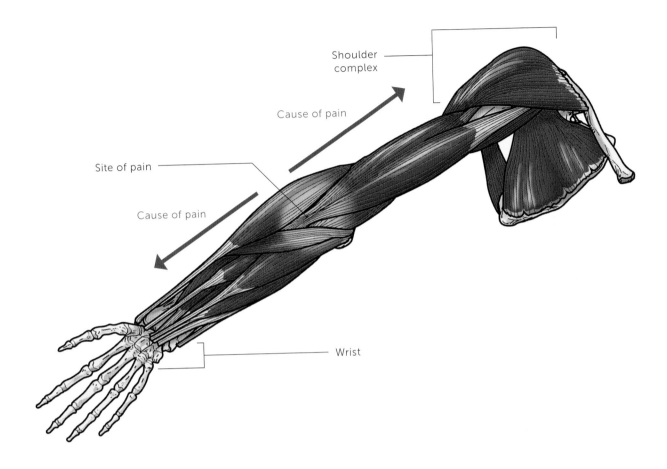

Mobility and Stability

Creating a stable platform for the barbell when performing a lift like the snatch, jerk, or overhead press requires a certain amount of wrist mobility. Think of the wrist position that a gymnast must assume to do a handstand. The extended wrist position is a requirement for creating a sufficient platform to bear weight, whether a gymnast is stabilizing their body weight in a handstand or a weightlifter is holding a barbell overhead. (Refer to the photos on the next page.) If an athlete is unable to position their wrists in an efficient weight-bearing position while pushing or pulling a barbell or dumbbell, the body is unable to function optimally.

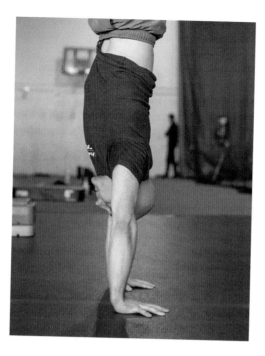

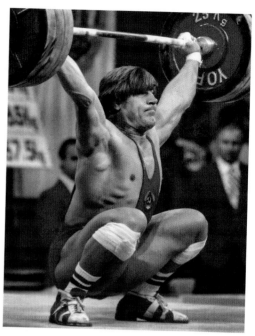

Gymnast wrist position in handstand.
© Dr. Dave Tilley

Weightlifter with barbell overhead and wrists extended.
David Rigert snatch,
© Bruce Klemens

Failure to sufficiently extend the wrists when lifting overhead can lead to excessive forces on smaller structures down the "chain" to make up for this lack of stability.[13] Over time, this increase in force can lead to injury at the elbow.

To screen your wrist mobility, press your palms together and pull them down as far as possible (prayer pose). Ideally, you want your wrists to move to a 90-degree "L" position. If you come up short, it could be due to stiff or short muscles in your forearms or limited wrist joint mobility—things I'll show you how to fix shortly!

The next step is to search upstream at the shoulder complex. This requires a thorough evaluation of shoulder strength/stability as well as mobility of the thoracic spine, lats, and pecs.

Numerous research studies have found a connection between weakness in the back and shoulder muscles and the development of elbow pain, especially lateral epicondylalgia.[14] Here's how this cascade of events could unwind. Take, for instance, someone performing the Olympic lifts. If the athlete lacks proper shoulder stability, their overhead positioning and control of the barbell during a snatch or clean and jerk will be affected. This less-than-ideal positioning and control can increase stability requirements in the muscles that surround the elbow joint (to keep the bar from falling to the ground), eventually leading to wear-and-tear injuries.

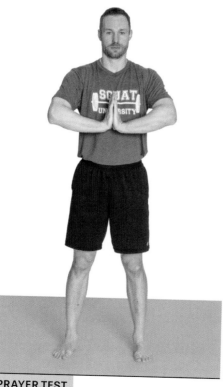

PRAYER TEST

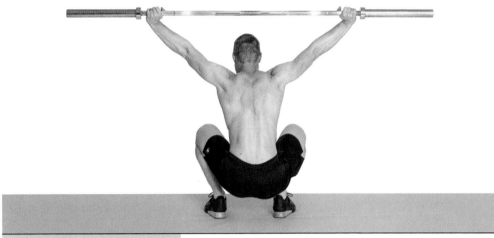

OVERHEAD SQUAT, BACK VIEW

In this instance, it wouldn't matter how much effort went into improving the strength of the overworked elbow musculature if the lack of stability at the shoulder was never addressed. It doesn't always take an expert clinician to remove the initial pain. Eliminate the offending activity (as many doctors will say, "Take two weeks off from barbell training"), prescribe some medication to ease the acute pain, sprinkle in a little light strengthening and stretching of the surrounding muscles, and—BAM!— you're feeling better. But was it a complete fix, or did you just get a window of temporary relief? I'll let you be the judge.

In this case, strength tests for shoulder external rotation with the arms by the sides and in an elevated position are helpful screening tools. With your elbows at your sides and bent to a 90-degree "L" position, try to prevent any movement of your arms as a friend tries to force your hands together. Then try the same test with your arm elevated, as if making a high five. Again, try to resist any movement as your friend attempts to push your hand forward in an effort to create shoulder internal rotation.

An inability to maintain the starting position without the hands collapsing inward when a force is applied clues us to take a closer look at the shoulder. To perform an in-depth screen on the rest of the shoulder complex, refer to pages 250 to 265 in the Shoulder Pain chapter.

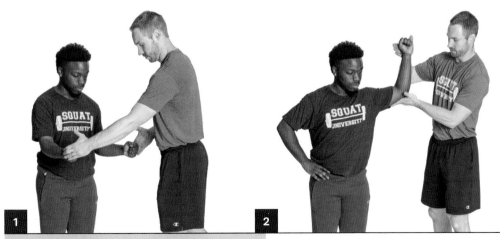

EXTERNAL ROTATION MANUAL MUSCLE TESTS

Position/Technique

Once you uncover mobility and/or stability deficits at joints above and/or below the site of pain, the next step is to evaluate your lifting technique. This is another area in which many in the medical community fall short in their injury evaluation process. You can perform all the strength and mobility tests you want and spend thousands on an MRI or a CT scan, but if you don't watch how someone moves, you'll never be able to create a complete analysis.

Let's return to the back squat example and look at how it could create pain in the medial elbow. While a slightly extended wrist position is optimal for creating a sufficient platform to stabilize the barbell overhead, grasping the bar with fully extended wrists can be problematic, especially in movements that require a full grip on the barbell. Take, for instance, an athlete performing a back squat who positions their elbows directly underneath the barbell. With their elbows held so low, their only option is to grab the bar with very extended wrists.

Fully extending your wrists like this stretches your forearm flexor muscles. In this lengthened position, the flexor muscles are unable to exert as much force (compared to a "neutral" straight wrist alignment), meaning that grip strength is automatically reduced.[15]

Trying to maintain a strong grip on the bar with your wrists fully extended increases your risk of overworking these muscles. Fatigue combined with repetitive training can set off a chain of events that culminates in wear and tear of the tendons

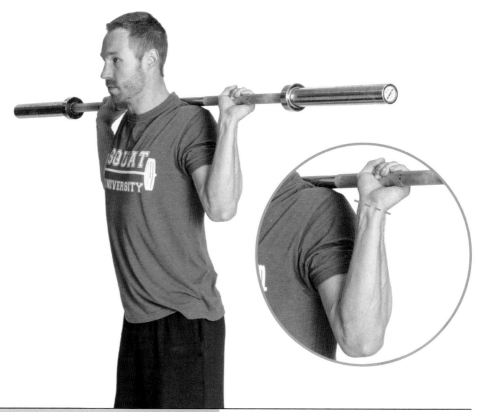

BACK SQUAT WITH OVEREXTENDED WRISTS

and the potential for developing medial elbow pain.[16] One of the first steps in the rehab process, therefore, is to correct the wrist alignment with some simple technique cues. Aligning the wrist in a more neutral position will take pressure off the medial elbow.

We must also factor in fatigue and how it affects movement quality during certain lifts. Take, for example, a powerlifter who is performing a high-volume day of bench training. If you've ever pushed yourself through a difficult workout, you know very well that fatigue during repetitive activity can produce changes in movement patterns. While your first set of lifts may look pristine, fatigue eventually sets in, and the quality of your reps starts to degrade.

Subtle alterations in lifting mechanics can have profound effects in how your body controls and produces force. For example, research has shown that performing bench presses to the point of significant fatigue leads to a change in technique, decreased strength in the surrounding muscles, and increased forces on the elbow joints.[17] Over time, substitutions in the way you move and subtle decreases in stability due to loss of strength make your body vulnerable to overuse injuries.[18]

For this reason, if you continue to lift while you work to fix your elbow pain, it would be wise to manipulate your programming to allow for adequate rest/recovery time and minimize the frequency of repetitive loading so that you can focus on reinforcing proper technique and movement quality.

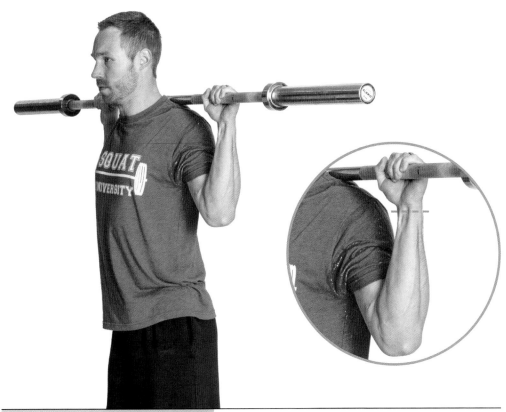

BACK SQUAT WITH NEUTRAL WRISTS

The Rebuilding Process

As you have come to realize by now, there are many different classifications of elbow pain. When we take into account the potential "weak links" above and below the site of pain (the shoulder and wrist), we find a number of scenarios for why pain could develop at the elbow. For this reason, there isn't a one-size-fits-all approach to rehabbing an injury to this joint. You must craft an individualized plan to address your specific elbow pain.

The Global Approach

If you did a thorough job during the screening process, you should have a fairly detailed list of your "weak links." This list will help guide your comprehensive approach to fixing the injury. (This is called taking a "global" approach, as opposed to a "local" approach that addresses only the site of symptoms.) With your list completed, review the Shoulder Pain chapter, and you'll find help for addressing each factor you've uncovered.

One of my favorite exercises that encompasses mobility, stability, and movement coordination at the shoulder complex is the paused scap pull-up. Start by hanging from a pull-up bar with a shoulder-width grip. Completely relax your upper body, letting your shoulder blades pull as far out to the sides of your back as possible. If you have stiffness in your lat muscles, this will bring out a gentle stretch up through the lateral armpit (where the muscle runs and attaches to the humerus).

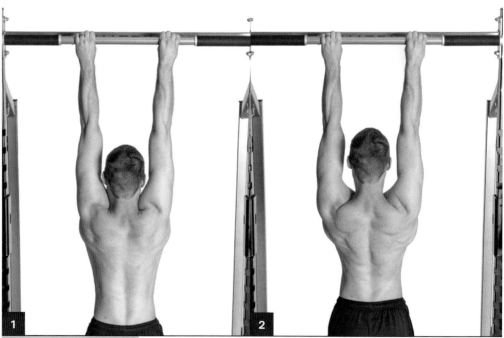

PAUSED SCAP PULL-UP

After holding this stretch for 5 to 10 seconds, engage your back muscles by moving your shoulder blades together and down. If you do this correctly, your elbows will remain locked into extension (only your shoulder blades will move as they pull together and down slightly). After holding this position for 5 seconds, relax back down into the extended hang position. Perform 2 or 3 sets of 5 repetitions. As your elbow pain decreases, you can eventually add in a full pull-up after the paused scapular retraction.

This sequence not only addresses lat flexibility but also teaches your body to properly coordinate movement of the upper body by first setting the shoulder blades into a stable position. Much like the concrete foundation that creates the stability for a house to stand, proper positioning and function of the shoulder blade are vital to the performance and long-term health of the elbow joint.

I also like to use the half-kneeling dumbbell or kettlebell press to windmill. While kneeling, hold a weight by your shoulder in a racked position. You can hold your opposite arm out to the side for balance or place it on your torso to give you some feedback for potential rib flaring during the pressing motion.

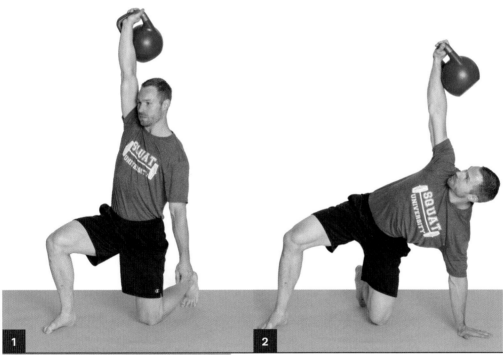

HALF-KNEELING KETTLEBELL WINDMILL

After you press the weight above your head, hold for a second and feel for the muscles on your posterior shoulder contracting to stabilize the joint. Your shoulder blade should be in a stacked alignment with your arm, elbow, and wrist without excessive shrugging in your upper trap muscles.

Next, slowly tip your torso laterally toward the ground while keeping your hand pointed directly toward the sky. This mimics the top-down sequence of a Turkish kettlebell get-up. As you pause in this bottom position, feel for your shoulder blade pulling in toward your spine and the surrounding muscles working hard to stabilize your arm. Finally, slowly rotate back up to the start position, making sure to limit excessive shrugging of your shoulder blade, before lowering the weight back to the front rack position. Perform 2 or 3 sets of 3 to 5 repetitions.

Improving scapular and shoulder joint stability through exercises like this that target the muscles of the shoulder girdle (the trapezius, rhomboids, rotator cuff, and posterior deltoid, for example) has been shown in research to be a fundamental component in eliminating many symptoms of elbow pain.[19]

The Local Approach

While I cannot overstate how important it is to take a global approach to addressing elbow pain, a few local exercises and rehab techniques can be helpful additions to a comprehensive treatment plan. These include forearm strengthening, banded joint mobilization (specifically for lateral elbow pain), soft tissue mobilization, and nerve gliding.

Isolated Strengthening

Many cases of medial and lateral elbow pain respond well to forearm strengthening.[20] It comes down to choosing the most efficient method of strengthening to fit your injury.

As discussed earlier, recent research has classified lateral elbow pain as tendinopathy. Isometric exercises (muscle contraction without joint movement) have been shown to be very effective in treating these kinds of injuries in the lower body, such as the use of the Spanish squat for patellar tendinopathy.[21] While more research is needed on the effectiveness of isometrics in upper-body tendon injuries, I have found them to be quite helpful in many cases of lateral elbow pain.[22]

For this reason, if you have very inflamed symptoms at the lateral elbow, try isometric holds and see if they help modify your pain. Position your arm over the edge of a table (or across your thigh, as shown) and hold a light dumbbell in slight wrist extension for 30 to 45 seconds for 4 or 5 reps.

If this exercise is right for your body, these holds should be completely pain-free by the second or third repetition and cause fatigue only in the extensor muscles of your forearm. If the exercise is too easy with the weight you're using, increase the weight until you find the hold difficult to perform for a full 45 seconds but can still perform it pain-free.

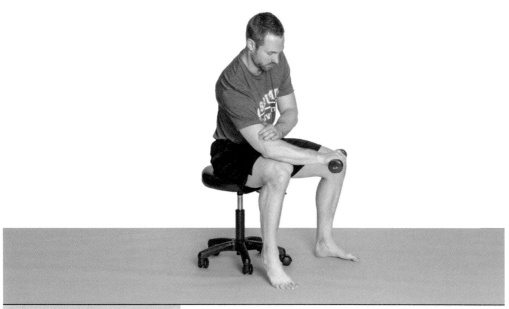

WRIST EXTENSION ISOMETRIC

While isometrics can be helpful for decreasing pain levels, you must eventually move to more traditional strength exercises with movement. Wrist curls—into extension for lateral elbow pain or into flexion for medial elbow pain—are the simplest to start with. Perform 10 to 15 repetitions with a 3-second concentric raise and a 3-second eccentric lower at a weight you can tolerate for 3 or 4 sets without increasing pain.[23] Tendon injuries often have a delayed response to loading, so make sure the difficulty of the forearm strengthening isn't leading to more pain the next day! As your strength and pain tolerance improve, increase the weight.

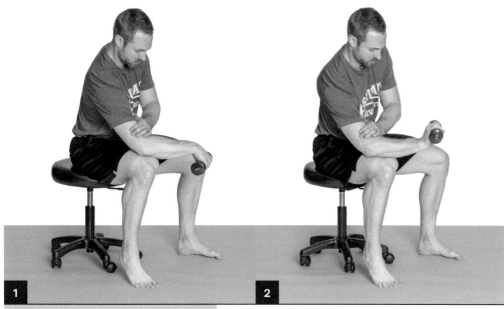

WRIST EXTENSION WITH MOVEMENT

Isolated strength work can also be progressed to more functional movements with carries. The amount of load placed on the wrist extensor muscles during either a single-arm "suitcase" or a double-arm "farmer" carry (due to the neutral wrist position) will be more easily tolerated during the early rehab process for those dealing with lateral elbow pain than the overhand pronated position needed for a front-loaded barbell lift like a deadlift.

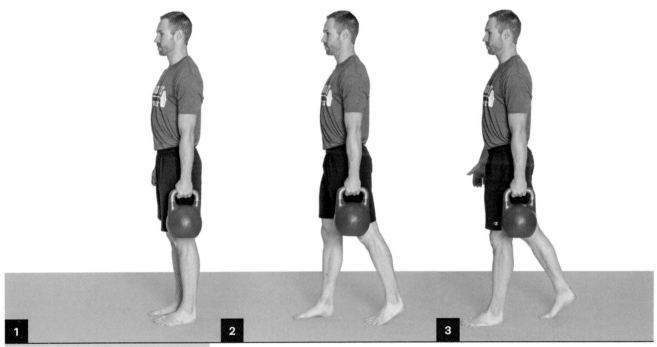

SUITCASE CARRY WITH KETTLEBELL

If you are dealing with lateral elbow pain, you must eventually return to strengthening your wrist extensors in the overhand grip position. An exercise I first saw performed by elite powerlifter Blaine Sumner for this purpose is a rack hold. Start with a barbell positioned around hip height in a squat rack. Grip the middle of the barbell with one hand. Brace your core and tense all the muscles from your shoulder down to your hand, and then lift the barbell a few inches from the rack. Hold the barbell for 10 seconds before setting it back down; that's one rep. This exercise should be loaded to the point where the tenth rep is very fatiguing but does not bring out any prior symptoms of pain.

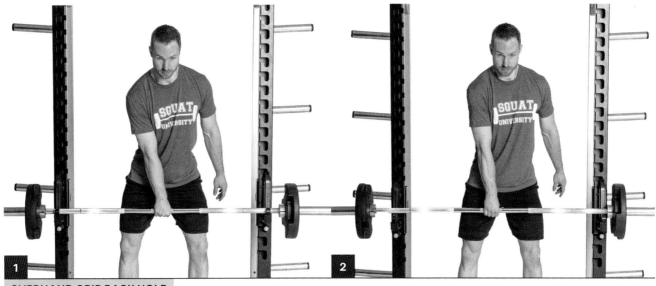

OVERHAND GRIP RACK HOLD

Banded Joint Mobilization with Movement

For some people, elbow pain can be modified with a joint mobilization exercise. A technique called *mobilization with movement* (MWM), developed by physiotherapist Brian Mulligan, is thought to help correct for a positional fault (a problem in alignment and/or movement) of the elbow joint.[24] This technique can be especially helpful for those who experience lateral elbow pain when making a fist, grabbing an object and rotating the hand over and back, and/or performing other gripping activities.

To perform the mobilization, place a thick band (between 2 and 4 inches wide) across your forearm just below the crease of your elbow. Lie on your back with your arm by your side, palm down, so that the band is pulling laterally at a 90-degree angle away from your body.

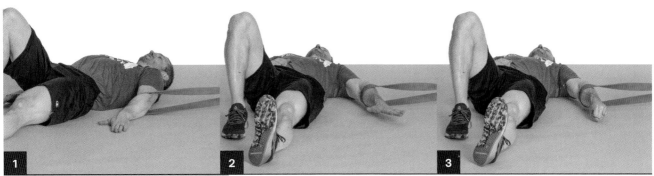

LATERAL BANDED JOINT MOBILIZATION

With constant tension from the band attempting to pull your arm to the side (creating a lateral joint glide of the elbow joint), perform 10 to 20 repetitions of clenching and relaxing your fist. You can also hold a small dumbbell in your hand and rotate it back and forth. Make sure to keep your entire arm (other than your hand) flat on the ground.

If this exercise is right for your injury and you perform it correctly with enough tension in the band, the pain you experience when gripping or moving your hand while holding an object should be instantly eliminated or greatly reduced during and directly after finishing.[25] If you do not find significant pain relief from this mobilization, don't waste your time performing it because it is likely not right for you.

Soft Tissue Mobilization

Soft tissue mobilization can be a helpful addition to treatment for almost any type of elbow pain.[26] Two useful tools are a small ball (lacrosse or tennis ball) and a barbell.

If you are dealing with medial or lateral elbow pain, slowly work the ball between the top of a table or bench and your forearm. Roll it around and seek out spots of tissue that feel tender. Once you've arrived at a tender area, pause for a few seconds before pumping your wrist up and down for a minute or so. This active release technique can help improve tissue and joint mobility.

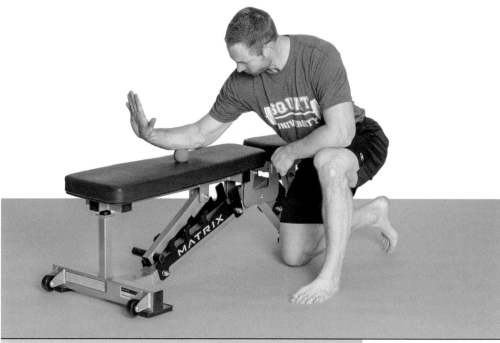

LACROSSE BALL SOFT TISSUE MOBILIZATION ON WRIST FLEXORS

If you lack wrist extension, try retesting your wrist mobility after doing this soft tissue mobilization. You may experience some short-term increases in wrist range of motion.

If you are dealing with symptoms in your posterior elbow or lower triceps, place a barbell in a rack and throw your arm over the top. (I first saw this mobilization done by physical therapist Kelly Starrett.) Pull down on your arm as you slowly glide your triceps up and down the barbell. Just like the prior exercise with the ball, pause on areas of tenderness before moving your elbow up and down for a minute. Some athletes might notice improved symptoms directly after doing the barbell soft tissue mobilization.

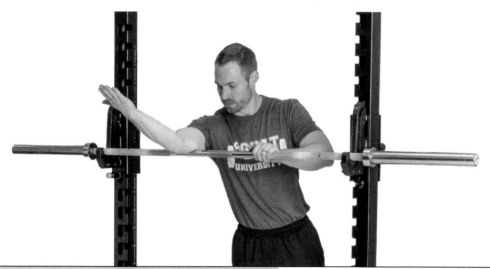

BARBELL SOFT TISSUE MOBILIZATION ON TRICEPS

Nerve Gliding

If you found that nerve testing reproduced your pain, a helpful technique to decrease your symptoms is a nerve glide. Nerve mobilization techniques fall into one of two categories, aiming to either stretch or slide the nerve (relative to the surrounding tissues).[27]

Gliding techniques that stretch the nerve, called *nerve tensioning*, temporarily increase tension and pressure in the surrounding sheath and may make symptoms worse in some people. On the other hand, "sliders" that move the nerve place significantly less tension on the structure and are therefore less aggressive in mobilizing the nerve in a way that will not increase symptoms.[28] The overall goals of using nerve mobilization techniques are to reduce swelling in and around the nerve, increase blood circulation, and help restore the natural movement capabilities and mobility of the nerve, which in turn decreases symptoms.[29]

To perform an ulnar nerve slider, as shown on the next page, start with your arm out to the side with your elbow straight and your wrist slightly extended (palm up and fingers pointed toward the ground). Next, simultaneously bend your elbow as you pull your arm in front of your body. Keep your wrist in the same extended position during the entire movement. Hold this position for a second before slowly moving back to the start position.[30]

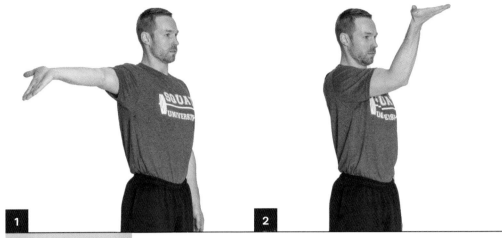

ULNAR NERVE SLIDER

To perform a radial nerve slider, start in the same testing position. Use your opposite-side hand to hold your shoulder down. With your arm hanging by your side, fully straighten your elbow and turn your hand behind you with the palm facing up. Next, make a fist with your fingers clasped over your thumb as if performing a hook grip and curl your wrist slightly, bringing your fist toward your forearm. Then raise your arm to the side while you follow your hand with your eyes. Move only to the point where you feel slight tension in your elbow, and then return to the start position.

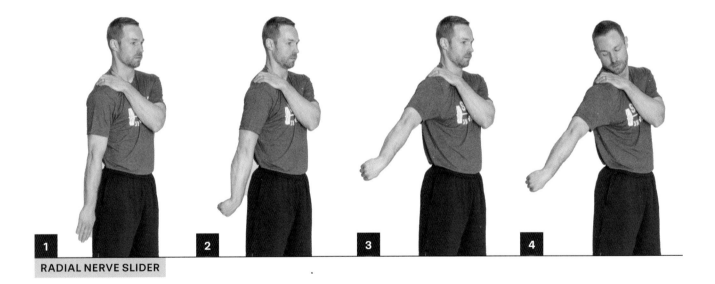

RADIAL NERVE SLIDER

Make sure you do only a few sliders at a time because overstressing the nerve, even with a less aggravating slider technique, could potentially increase your symptoms. Also limit any excessive stretching of the wrist flexor muscles; doing so may irritate the nerve and intensify your symptoms.

If these mobilizations help decrease your symptoms, I recommend performing them every few hours throughout the day.

Final Thoughts on Elbow Rehabilitation

As you have come to learn, there is no one-size-fits-all approach to fixing elbow pain. However, a thorough screening process like the one outlined in this chapter can help you develop a program tailored to your body, allowing you to be that much more efficient in addressing your symptoms.

Unfortunately, there is no quick fix. Treatment will almost certainly take more time than you would like, but have patience. Nothing complicated was ever solved quickly, and the elbow is a much more complicated joint than many people realize.

If at any time during this process you experience symptoms that limit your ability to fully straighten your elbow, feel your elbow getting "stuck" during movement, feel a painful popping or clicking sensation, or have neck pain, I highly recommend seeing a medical doctor or other rehabilitation professional.

Notes

1. U. Aasa, I. Svartholm, F. Andersson, and L. Berglund, "Injuries among weightlifters and power-lifters: a systematic review," *British Journal of Sports Medicine* 51 (2017): 211–20.

2. M. Stroyan and K. E. Wilk, "The functional anatomy of the elbow complex," *Journal of Orthopaedic & Sports Physical Therapy* 17, no. 6 (1993): 279–88; C. M. Hall and L. T. Brody, *Therapeutic Exercise: Moving Toward Function*, 2nd Edition (Philadelphia: Lippincott Williams & Wilkins, 2005).

3. E. Waugh, "Lateral epicondylalgia or epicondylitis: what's in a name," *Journal of Orthopaedic & Sports Physical Therapy* 35, no. 4 (2005): 200–2.

4. L. M. Bissert and B. Vicenzino, "Physiotherapy management of lateral epicondylalgia," *Journal of Physiotherapy* 61, no. 4 (2015): 174–81; S. Dimitrios, "Lateral elbow tendinopathy: evidence of physiotherapy management," *World Journal of Orthopedics* 7, no. 8 (2016): 463–6; C. M. Kaczmarek, "Lateral elbow tendinosis: implications for a weight training population," *Strength and Conditioning Journal* 30, no. 2 (2008): 35–40.

5. Hall and Brody, *Therapeutic Exercise* (see note 2 above).

6. Hall and Brody, *Therapeutic Exercise* (see note 2 above).

7. Hall and Brody, *Therapeutic Exercise* (see note 2 above).

8. M. R. Safran, "Elbow injuries in athletes: a review," *Clinical Orthopaedics* 310 (1995): 257–77; C. B. Novak, G. W. Lee, S. E. Mackinnon, and L. Lay, "Proactive testing for cubital tunnel syndrome," *Journal of Hand Surgery* 19, no. 5 (1994): 817–20; M. F. Macnicol, "Extraneural pressures affecting the ulnar nerve at the elbow," *Hand* 14, no. 1 (1982): 5–11.

9. Hall and Brody, *Therapeutic Exercise* (see note 2 above).

10. Novak, Lee, Mackinnon, and Lay, "Proactive testing for cubital tunnel syndrome" (see note 8 above).

11. R. A. Ekstrom and K. Holden, "Examination of and intervention for a patient with chronic lateral elbow pain with signs of nerve entrapment," *Physical Therapy* 82, no. 11 (2002): 1077–86.

12. B. K. Coombes, L. Bisset, and B. Vicenzino, "Bilateral cervical dysfunction in patients with unilateral lateral epicondylalgia without concomitant cervical or upper limb symptoms: a cross-sectional case-control study," *Journal of Manipulative and Physiological Therapeutics* 37, no. 2 (2014): 79–86; B. K. Coombes, L. Bisset, and B. Vicenzino, "Management of lateral elbow tendinopathy: one size does not fit all," *Journal of Orthopaedic & Sports Physical Therapy* 45, no. 11 (2015): 938–49.

13. C. M. Kaczmarek, "Lateral elbow tendinosis: implications for a weight training population," *Strength and Conditioning Journal* 30, no. 2 (2008): 35–40.

14. O. Alizadehkhaiyat, A. C. Fisher, G. J. Kemp, K. Vishwanathan, and S. P. Frostick, "Upper limb muscle imbalance in tennis elbow: a functional and electromyographic assessment," *Journal of Orthopaedic Research* 25, no. 12 (2007): 1651–7; A. M. Lucado, M. J. Kolber, M. S. Cheng, and J. L. Echternach, Sr., "Upper extremity strength characteristics in female recreational tennis players with and without lateral epicondylalgia," *Journal of Orthopaedic & Sports Physical Therapy* 42, no. 12 (2012): 1025–31; J. M. Day, H. Bush, A. J. Nitz, and T. L. Uhl, "Scapular muscle performance in individuals with lateral epicondylalgia," *Journal of Orthopaedic & Sports Physical Therapy* 45, no. 5 (2015): 414–24.

15. V. B. Parvatikar and P. B. Mukkannavar, "Comparative study of grip strength in different positions of shoulder and elbow with wrist in neutral and extension positions," *Journal of Exercise Science & Physiotherapy* 5, no. 2 (2009): 67–75.

16. Hall and Brody, *Therapeutic Exercise* (see note 2 above).

17. Y. P. Huang, Y. L. Chou, F. C. Chen, R. T. Wang, M. J. Huang, and P. P. H. Chou, "Elbow joint fatigue and bench-press training," *Journal of Athletic Training* 49, no. 3 (2014): 317–21.

18. Hall and Brody, *Therapeutic Exercise* (see note 2 above).

19. J. B. Bhatt, R. Glaser, A. Chavez, and E. Yung, "Middle and lower trapezius strengthening for the management of lateral epicondylalgia: a case report," *Journal of Orthopaedic & Sports Physical Therapy* 43, no. 11 (2013): 841–7.

20. Hall and Brody, *Therapeutic Exercise* (see note 2 above); Coombes, Bisset, and Vicenzino, "Management of lateral elbow tendinopathy" (see note 12 above); J. Raman, J. C. MacDermid, and R. Grewal, "Effectiveness of different methods of resistance exercises in lateral epicondylosis—a systematic review," *Journal of Hand Therapy* 25, no. 1 (2012): 5–25; T. F. Tyler, S. J. Nicholas, B. M. Schmitt, M. Mullaney, and D. E. Hogan, "Clinical outcomes of the addition of eccentrics for rehabilitation of previously failed treatments for golfers elbow," *International Journal of Sports Physical Therapy* 9, no. 3 (2004): 365–70.

21. E. Rio, C. Purdam, M. Girdwood, and J. Cook, "Isometric exercise to reduce pain in patellar tendinopathy in-season: is it effective 'on the road'?" *Clinical Journal of Sports Medicine* 29, no. 3 (2019): 1–5.

22. J. Y. Park, H. K. Park, J. H. Choi, E. S. Moon, B. S. Kim, W. S. Kim, and K. S. Oh, "Prospective evaluation of the effectiveness of a home-based program of isometric strengthening exercises: 12-month follow-up," *Clinics in Orthopedic Surgery* 2, no. 3 (2010): 173–8.

23. K. Starrett and G. Cordoza, *Becoming a Supple Leopard: The Ultimate Guide to Resolving Pain, Preventing Injury, and Optimizing Athletic Performance,* 2nd Edition (Las Vegas: Victory Belt Publishing Inc., 2015).

24. Coombes, Bisset, and Vicenzino, "Management of lateral elbow tendinopathy" (see note 12 above).

25. A. Amro, I. Diener, W. O. Bdair, I. M. Hameda, A. I. Shalabi, and D. I. Ilyyan, "The effects of Mulligan mobilisation with movement and taping techniques on pain, grip strength, and function in patients with lateral epicondylitis," *Hong Kong Physiotherapy Journal* 28, no. 1 (2010): 19–23; W. Hing, R. Bigelow, and T. Bremner, "Mulligan's mobilisation with movement: a review of the tenets and prescription of MWMs," *New Zealand Journal of Physiotherapy* 36, no. 3 (2008): 144–64.

26. Hing, Bigelow, and Bremner, "Mulligan's mobilisation with movement: a review of the tenets and prescription of MWMs" (see note 25 above); J. H. Abbott, C. E. Patla, and R. H. Jensen, "The initial effects of an elbow mobilization with movement technique on grip strength in subjects with lateral epicondylalgia," *Manual Therapy* 6, no. 3 (2001): 163–9; Coombes, Bisset, and Vicenzino, "Management of lateral elbow tendinopathy" (see note 12 above).

27. M. W. Coppieters and D. S. Butler, "Do 'sliders' slide and 'tensioners' tension? An analysis of neurodynamic techniques and considerations regarding their application," *Manual Therapy* 13, no. 3 (2008): 213–21.

28. Coppieters and Butler, "Do 'sliders' slide and 'tensioners' tension?" (see note 27 above).

29. M. W. Coppieters, K. E. Bartholomeeusen, and K. H. Stappaerts, "Incorporating nerve-gliding techniques in the conservative treatment of cubital tunnel syndrome," *Journal of Manipulative and Physiological Therapeutics* 27, no. 9 (2004): 560–8; D. Oskay, A. Meric, N. Kirdi, T. Firat, C. Ayhan, and G. Leblebicioglu, "Neurodynamic mobilization in conservative treatment of cubital tunnel syndrome: long-term follow-up of 7 cases," *Journal of Manipulative and Physiological Therapeutics* 33, no. 2 (2010): 156–63; V. Arumugam, S. Selvam, and J. C. MacDermid, "Radial nerve mobilization reduces lateral elbow pain and provides short-term relief in computer users," *Open Orthopaedics Journal* 8 (2014): 368–71.

30. Coppieters and Butler, "Do 'sliders' slide and 'tensioners' tension?" (see note 27 above).

CHAPTER 6

ANKLE PAIN

One of the most common ankle injuries among CrossFitters, weightlifters, and powerlifters is not the classic sprained ankle. Instead, it is an injury to the Achilles tendon. So, even though many possible injuries can occur at the ankle joint, this chapter is going to focus on the Achilles tendon.

How does someone develop Achilles tendon pain? To answer this question, we first have to discuss a little anatomy.

Achilles Tendon Injury Anatomy 101

A tendon is a thick, fibrous band of tissue that connects muscle to bone. The Achilles tendon connects the two calf muscles (larger gastrocnemius and smaller soleus) to the back of the heel (calcaneus bone). It is covered by a thin sheath called the *peritendon* that helps it move freely against the surrounding tissues. Structurally, the Achilles is similar to the patellar tendon of the knee in that every time you walk, run, or jump, it acts to absorb, store, and then release energy like a spring.

ACHILLES TENDON ANATOMY

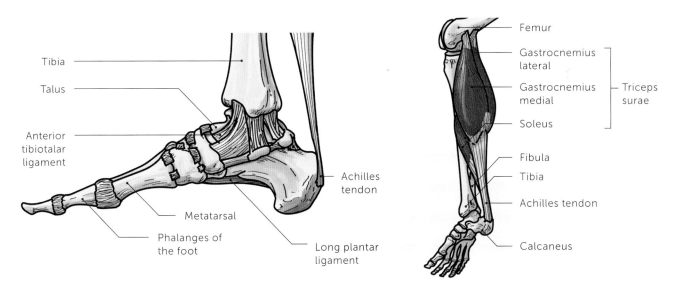

Every day, the tissues of your body—muscles, tendons, and even bones—are in a constant process of fluctuation. Every time you place a stress on your body, like when you work out, portions of your tissues are degraded and then regenerated. Over time, this natural replenishing process builds strength.

In your tendons, this process is largely controlled by small cells called *tenocytes* that are dispersed among aligned fibers called *collagen* (type 1 collagen, to be exact). Tenocyte cells react to the forces and loads placed on the tendon and adapt the cellular makeup of the tissue accordingly (called the *extracellular matrix*). Depending on several factors, such as how intensely you have trained, the medications you take, and whether you have diabetes, your body will have adapted your Achilles tendons to a certain set point of strength called the *load tolerance level*.

Training loads placed on the tendons that do not severely exceed this set point create a cellular response in the tendons (that can actually be seen by ultrasound) that will return to normal in two to three days given proper recovery methods; this is the normal time frame for the adaptation "replenishment" process to take place.[1] However, if the load is too extreme or if there is inadequate recovery in your training program, the balance is disrupted, and the process tips from being adaptive to pathological. A spark is lit, and the injury process begins.

The Continuum of Tendon Pathology

Before we get into how to treat tendon injuries, let's dive a little deeper into how the injury process occurs. The most practical way to understand this comes from the Continuum of Tendon Pathology developed by renowned expert Jill Cook.[2] As I explained in the Knee Pain chapter, this model describes a continuum with three overlapping stages of injury:

1. Reactive tendinopathy

2. Tendon disrepair

3. Degenerative tendinopathy

Progression from one stage to the next is met with a decreasing ability to recover to the prior healthy state.

THE CONTINUUM MODEL

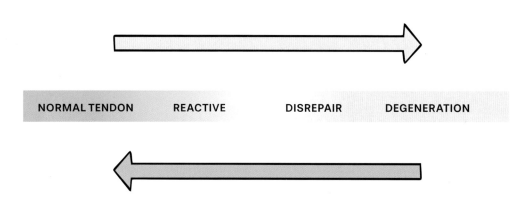

NORMAL TENDON   REACTIVE   DISREPAIR   DEGENERATION

Cook's model is fairly new and goes against the way many in the medical community view chronic tendon injuries. Contrary to what your doctor may have told you, the term *tendinitis* isn't technically correct (the ending *–itis* refers to inflammation); newer studies have shown that there is no inflammation in affected tendons![3] For this reason, the term *tendinopathy* is a better description of any tendon injury.[4]

As mentioned before, when exposed to an overload of any nature, the cells that make up the tendon react with a short-term exaggerated response known as *reactive tendinopathy.* Specifically, small proteins called *proteoglycans* flood the extracellular matrix, causing the tendon to become swollen and painful. Again, this swelling is not caused by inflammation.[5]

This response can be sparked in a few ways:

- The first is acute overload in one specific training session or a group of sessions that were much more intense than normal. In this scenario, the tendon experiences loads much higher than it can currently tolerate.

- Reactive tendinopathy can also occur upon returning to relatively "normal" training after an extended break, such as a weeklong vacation or a period of recovery from an unrelated injury. In this scenario, the time away from the gym leads to an adaptive lowering of the tendon's load capacity. Jumping quickly back into "normal" training causes an overload and sparks the exaggerated cellular response.

- Overload can even occur due to something as simple as a change in footwear—a shoe that provides less support, has stiffer soles, or has a lower heel than your previous pair.

There is no set amount of weight or number of reps of any drill that will trigger this injury response; it comes down purely to whether an individual's tendon "load tolerance" has been exceeded. Elite athletes place more load on their tendons during their day-in-and-day-out training compared to amateurs in the same sports, yet injury prevalence is not higher for elite athletes. Their tendons have adapted to heavy training loads through good recovery methods combined with excellent programming/training regimens.

Now, here's the good thing: reactive tendinopathy is reversible if properly managed. If you remove the trigger that caused the overload and allow the tendon to heal with proper rehabilitation principles (which we'll talk about shortly), the tendon is likely to return to its normal healthy self within a few weeks.

However, if the excessive load is not removed and you continue to train through the tendon pain, the injury will progress to the next stage, which Cook calls disrepair. In response to the continued overload, more and more proteoglycans flood the extracellular matrix, drawing in water, which eventually starts to disrupt the architectural struts (collagen) that make up the tendon. If this overload is not halted, the disorganized collagen starts to break down even more and eventually dies off as the injury enters the third stage, degeneration.

Unfortunately, it is very difficult to distinguish whether a tendon is in disrepair. To make matters worse, you may not even know that your tendon has slipped into the third stage because the degenerated part doesn't elicit pain.

Figuring Out Which Stage of Injury the Tendon Is In

Researchers like Cook have found that tendon pain is primarily a symptom of the reactive (first) stage. For this reason, if you are experiencing pain in your Achilles, you can characterize your injury using an even simpler two-stage model of either "reactive" or "reactive on disrepair/degeneration" tendinopathy.[6] Let me explain.

Let's say this is the first time you've felt Achilles tendon pain. The day after a really difficult training session, your Achilles hurts so bad you're forced to limp. Because this is an acute (brand-new) episode of tendon pain, you're likely experiencing the initial stage of "reactive" tendinopathy.

Or maybe this is not the first time you've felt Achilles tendon pain. You had a small flare-up last year and another a few months ago. You took a few weeks off, and the pain eventually went away, but it keeps coming back. Due to the chronic nature of these symptoms, you are likely experiencing a case of "reactive on disrepair/ degeneration" tendinopathy.

NORMAL, REACTIVE, AND REACTIVE ON DEGENERATION

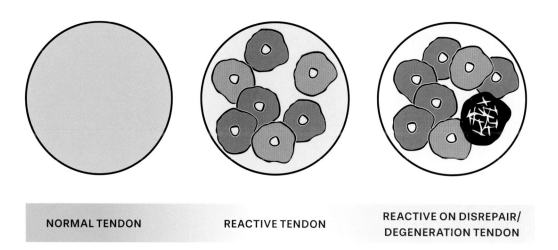

| NORMAL TENDON | REACTIVE TENDON | REACTIVE ON DISREPAIR/ DEGENERATION TENDON |

When the tendon experiences continued episodes of overload, degradation can begin, but the entire tendon doesn't just die off. If you looked deep into the tendon, you'd notice small "islands" of degenerated collagen tissue dispersed amid healthy tendon tissue. These islands of degenerated tissue are unable to bear any load. They usually lose tensile strength and springlike capacity, which renders them "mechanically deaf," as Cook says.

Think of the islands of degenerated Achilles tendon tissue as holes in donuts. They are surrounded by healthy tissue. Research has shown that the body will actually adapt and grow more normal tendon tissue around these dead spots in an effort to recover lost strength.[7]

NORMAL TENDON WITH DEGENERATION ISLAND

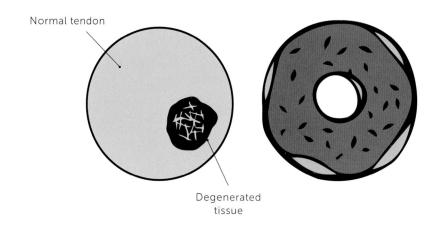

Normal tendon

Degenerated tissue

As mentioned previously, these "holes" in the tendon do not create any pain.[8] Not until the surrounding healthy tissue becomes overloaded and slips into a reactive phase (in the same way that a perfectly healthy tendon would) does pain develop in a degenerated tendon. This is why someone could have a very degenerated tendon rupture without having any pain symptoms.[9]

Some good ways to differentiate between "reactive" and "reactive on disrepair/degeneration" tendon pain (other than a history of symptoms) are the intensity of the pain, the exact mechanism that set off the injury, and how long recovery takes. For example, a true "reactive" tendon is very painful and swollen. It is sparked by a severe overload (such as running a half marathon for the first time or an extremely difficult training session filled with a ton of plyometric exercises). On the other hand, a "reactive on disrepair/degeneration" tendon can be sparked by much less dramatic activity overload and often isn't accompanied by as much swelling. Pain from this form of tendinopathy can resolve in as little as a few days with proper rest, whereas pain in true "reactive" tendons can take anywhere from four to eight weeks to dissipate.[10] Understanding which stage your symptoms indicate will dramatically affect how you attempt to manage the injury.

Classifications of Achilles Tendon Injuries

Overload causes tendons to spark into reactive mode and become painful. Simple enough, right? Unfortunately, the Achilles tendon is a little more complicated. The Achilles tendon complex can become overloaded and injured in a few ways, all of which have slightly different symptoms and require different approaches to fix.[11]

Mid-tendon

A mid-tendon injury is caused by an overload in tensile load (a pulling force similar to stretching a rubber band). Your Achilles tendon acts like a spring when you run and perform multiple jumps. As you land, it stretches under load and quickly releases power to propel your body up and away. This rapid recoil force production is called the *stretch shortening cycle* (SSC) and is the foundation of plyometric training.

ACHILLES TENDON ANATOMY

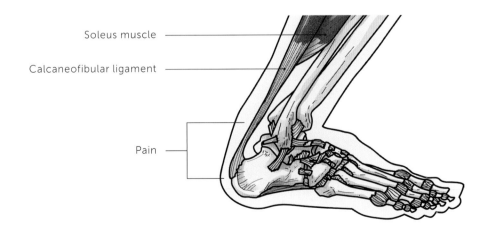

Soleus muscle

Calcaneofibular ligament

Pain

If the adapted load tolerance set point is exceeded due to too much volume or intensity of training, the reactive phase can be sparked. For this reason, it is common to see mid-tendon Achilles injuries in athletes who perform intense periods of plyometric movements in training or competition, such as runners, basketball players, and volleyball players.

Insertional

Unlike a mid-tendon injury, insertional tendinopathy is localized to the point where the tendon attaches to the heel bone. This area may be swollen and appear more pronounced upon examination. While a mid-tendon injury is believed to be largely due to an overload of tensile loads, insertional tendinopathies are largely a combination of tensile loads and compression.

ACHILLES TENDON ANATOMY

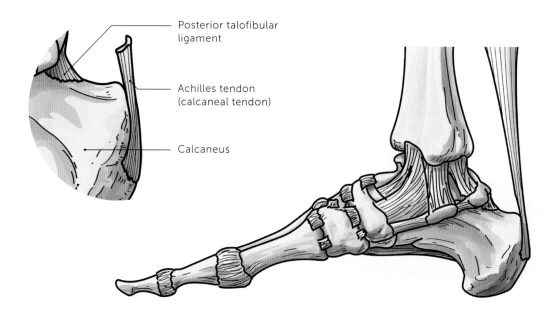

Posterior talofibular ligament

Achilles tendon (calcaneal tendon)

Calcaneus

The amount of compression placed on the Achilles tendon against the calcaneus bone depends on the position of the ankle. Activities that load the Achilles but keep the ankle in a plantarflexed position, such as repetitive hopping on the toes, are not likely to bring out pain. On the other hand, activities that involve loading the ankle in dorsiflexion (squatting, lunging, running up hills or on soft surfaces like a sandy beach, or even walking barefoot) will bring out pain as the shin is pulled into a more angled position, compressing the Achilles against the heel bone.[12] Interestingly enough, stretching the calf muscles in an attempt to relieve the symptoms of insertional tendinopathy will only cause more pain as the ankle is pulled into dorsiflexion, creating more compression.

Peritendon

This type of injury is not a true tendinopathy like the prior two. The injury is not to the tendon itself but to the thin sheath that surrounds it, called the *peritendon.* Pain is created by constant friction of the Achilles tendon against the peritendon during continuous low-load ankle movement rather than an overload of force.

PERITENDON ANATOMY

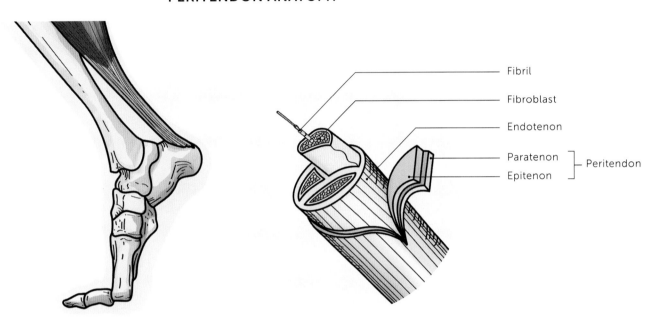

For example, the peritendon can become injured during a long bike ride or after rowing a long distance. A major diagnostic sign is a cracking or popping sound/sensation called *crepitus* that occurs as the tendon fails to move smoothly within the thickened peritendon.[13] Left untreated, this injury can become debilitating.

How to Screen Your Achilles Tendon Pain

The first priority during a physical examination for Achilles tendon pain is to make sure there hasn't been a complete rupture of the tendon. The calf squeeze test is an easy way to do so.[14]

To perform the calf squeeze test (not pictured), lie on your stomach with your feet hanging freely over the edge of a bed or bench. Have a friend squeeze your calf muscle and see what happens to your foot. If the foot moves when the calf is squeezed, the Achilles tendon is intact, and you can move on to the next step, which is to diagnose the type of tendinopathy you are experiencing. If the foot does not move at all when the calf is squeezed, it would be a good idea to follow up with a medical professional for additional testing.

The next step in the testing process is fairly simple. You don't need an expensive MRI machine. All you need to do is review how the pain started and where you're experiencing symptoms and then evaluate how your Achilles tendon responds to loading.

Load Testing

True Achilles tendinopathy symptoms manifest either at the insertion or in the mid-tendon and are provoked by load.[15] While both are related to overload, the mechanism of overload differs. Here's how to test your hypothesis. During each test, grade your pain on a scale of 0 to 10, 0 being no pain and 10 being the worst pain you can imagine.

Start with a double-leg heel raise while standing on flat ground, followed by a single-leg heel raise. If you do not feel pain, perform the same actions with your heels hanging off a plate or step. This time, allow your heels to sink below the ledge after performing the initial heel raise. If you had no pain on flat ground but you do have pain with the heel-dropped version, you probably have insertional Achilles tendinopathy.

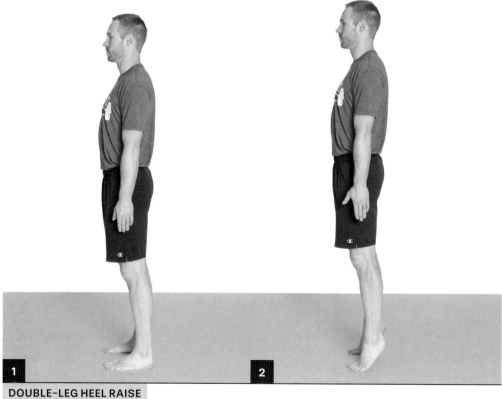

DOUBLE-LEG HEEL RAISE

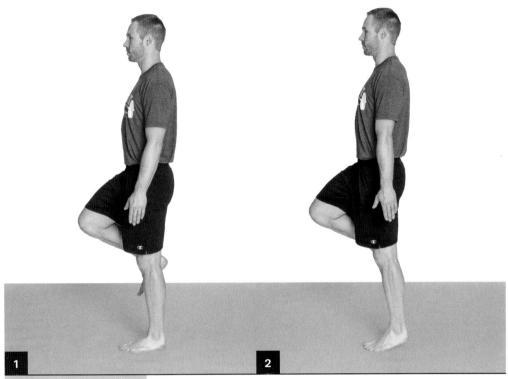

SINGLE-LEG HEEL RAISE

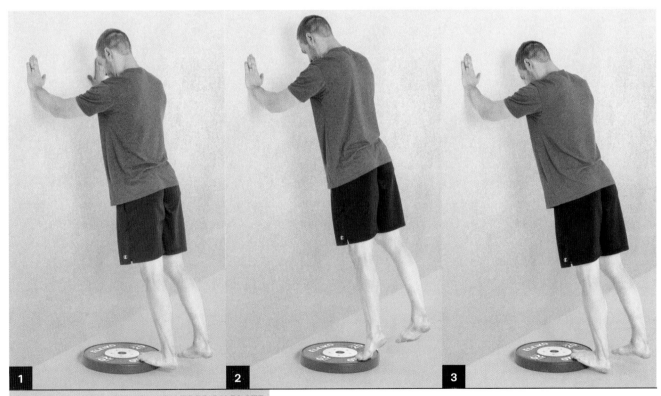

SINGLE-LEG HEEL RAISE WITH TOES ON PLATE

On the other hand, if you do have pain with the heel raise on flat ground and your pain is located between 1 and 3 inches above the calcaneus, you are likely dealing with mid-tendon Achilles tendinopathy. Try performing multiple jumps or hops. If this repetitive higher-load motion creates more pain than a slow, controlled heel raise, you can bet it's mid-tendon Achilles tendinopathy. The location of the pain and when the pain occurs during testing can help differentiate between mid-tendon and insertional Achilles tendinopathy.

Someone with a peritendon injury will respond to these loading tests very differently. While a person with a mid-tendon injury will have more pain as the load is increased from a slow heel raise to a faster hop, a peritendon injury may present in the opposite manner: a slow heel raise could cause more pain as the ankle is controlled through a larger range of motion, contributing to more friction of the peritendon.

The main takeaway here is that diagnosing a tendinopathy doesn't require a pricey MRI. In fact, looking at an MRI may lead your diagnosis astray because it is common to see abnormal signs of tendon degeneration in those without symptoms of pain![16] A doctor may be able to detect tendon pathology by your imaging, but the image alone doesn't necessarily explain any symptoms you're having.

Poking and prodding around the tendon to see if it hurts is not enough to diagnose tendinopathy, either. You must assess the functional capacity of the tendon with load testing. If it really is a tendinopathy injury, the results of the tests I've suggested will tell you so. Keep in mind that if your tendon is very reactive, you may have pain with all of the prior tests regardless of whether your injury is insertional or mid-tendon.

Other Helpful Tests

Testing ankle mobility should be a part of the screening process when dealing with an injury to this area. When the gastroc and/or soleus muscles are stiff or short, there is less range of motion to absorb load during activities like landing from a jump, which places the Achilles tendon under greater strain.[17] Limited ankle mobility can be a risk factor for mid-tendon Achilles tendinopathy because the tendon has less range to absorb load; therefore, the tendon has to take more load more quickly.[18] With insertional Achilles tendinopathy, less dorsiflexion may place less compression on the insertion. Therefore, poor dorsiflexion mobility is more of a risk factor for mid-tendon Achilles tendinopathy than for insertional tendinopathy.

The 5-inch wall test is a simple screen that you can perform on your own.[19] Kneel by a wall and place your toes 5 inches from its base. Drive your knee straight forward over your toes, attempting to touch the wall without letting your heel pop up off the ground.

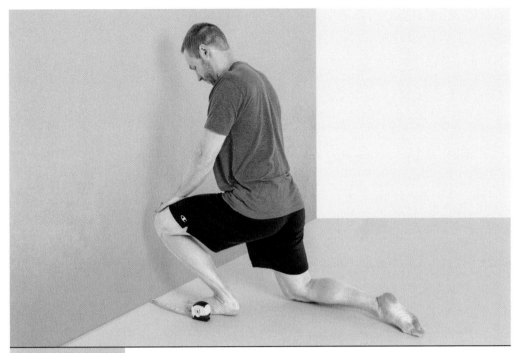

5-INCH WALL TEST

Were you able to touch the wall with your knee, or did your heel pull up off the ground? If you fail the 5-inch wall test, you have uncovered a weak link in ankle mobility that needs to be addressed.

Although not supported by strong research, these other factors *may* influence Achilles tendinopathy:

- **Biomechanical dysfunction**
  - » Poor double-leg or single-leg squat
  - » Poor jumping/landing mechanics
  - » Poor/inefficient running mechanics (forefoot striker or low steps per minute)
- **Weak hip muscles (glute max and glute medius)**

Final Thoughts on Screening

Achilles tendon pain is no simple injury. The tendon complex is engineered to absorb high levels of load and will adapt over time and become stronger if trained appropriately. However, this adaptation process is slow, and overload can easily occur in athletes in almost any sport.

Understanding how this injury starts and progresses will empower you to manage the symptoms better and return to the sports and activities you love. In the next part of this chapter, we will go over how to fix your Achilles tendon pain.

The Rebuilding Process

Step 1: The Balancing Act

As you have learned, when a tendon enters the first "reactive" stage of injury, pain is due to one simple mechanism: overload. The pain you're experiencing started because you placed too much load on your Achilles tendon and surpassed its load tolerance level. This overload may have occurred due to one specific workout (for example, 200 box jumps as a part of a CrossFit class), or it may have accumulated over a number of sessions (such as a basketball player who usually trains two or three times a week being thrust into training two or three times a day during a week-long camp). Regardless of the cause, the first step in decreasing symptoms is to take a step back from what caused the pain in the first place.

Now, when most people think "rest," they automatically think about taking weeks away from the gym, sitting on the couch, and bingeing their favorite TV show. Complete rest is often the first piece of advice most medical doctors give to patients complaining of tendon pain. However, this is the *last thing* you want to do. You never want to rest a tendon completely!

The strength of your tendons follows the simple motto "If you don't use it, you lose it."[20] Taking away all loading and only resting for a few weeks sets you up for the pain to return. As mentioned earlier, the injury occurred because your training surpassed your current load tolerance level. If you take the next few weeks off, your body will adapt, and the tolerance level of your tendon will drop even further (because minimal load is being placed on it), making it easier to overload whenever you do return.

On the flip side, if you continue to push through pain and load a painful tendon too much, the injury will only get worse; eventually, structural changes can take place in the tissues. Load management is the most important factor in recovering from a tendon injury. This is a difficult balancing act and a reason why so many people develop chronic tendon injuries.

Start by making a list of which movements, volumes, and intensities of exercise aggravate your symptoms. Make a separate list of exercises that you tolerate well without pain while performing them or the day after. Knowing exactly what brings out your symptoms will empower you to make the right adjustments for healing to take place.

Movements that create high loads and use the tendon as a spring—jumping or sprinting activities, for example—increase cell signaling and can create the over-response that sparked the pain. Therefore, if jump-roping double-unders, running hills, box jumps, and other movements from your first list cause symptoms, take those out of your training for the time being and replace them with low-load "tendon-friendly" modes of exercise from your second list (squatting, deadlifts, rowing, etc.). Make sure to recognize the depth to which you can squat without pain. Deep squatting may aggravate symptoms because the forward shin position can increase load on the tendon. You will gradually reintroduce these aggravating exercises into your training as your tendon heals and adapts to tolerate greater loads.

If you are an elite athlete preparing for an important competition and you have no desire to step back from training to address your injuries, you must make a change to your training program (along with adding some of the exercises discussed later). The pain you're experiencing is your tendon telling you that it is not tolerating the loads you are placing on it. It is there for a reason. Listen to it. Try changing one variable in your training program and see how your tendon responds. For example, if you currently train seven days a week, decrease the frequency by dropping one session. If you can't sacrifice one day of training, you must make a change to either the amount of high-intensity loads or the total volume of your training. Regardless of which variable you choose, change only one factor at a time and wait to see how your body responds. Everyone will be slightly different; there is no golden rule.

Should You Stretch?

Stretching the calf muscles can be a helpful addition to many rehab programs to improve ankle mobility and allow for better quality movement. For example, limited ankle mobility due to stiff and tight tissues of the gastroc/soleus can create compensations "up the chain" at the knee, hip, and low back. To focus your calf stretch on the larger gastroc muscle, you want to keep your knees relatively straight. Bending your knees takes slack off the gastroc muscle and allows you to focus your stretch on the smaller underlying soleus.

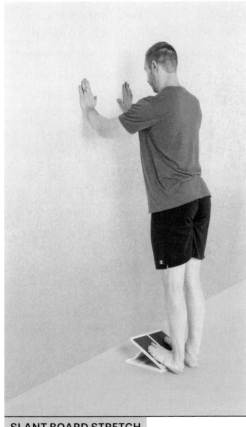

SLANT BOARD STRETCH

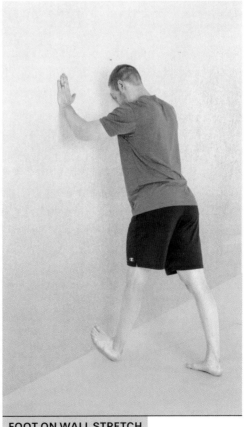

FOOT ON WALL STRETCH

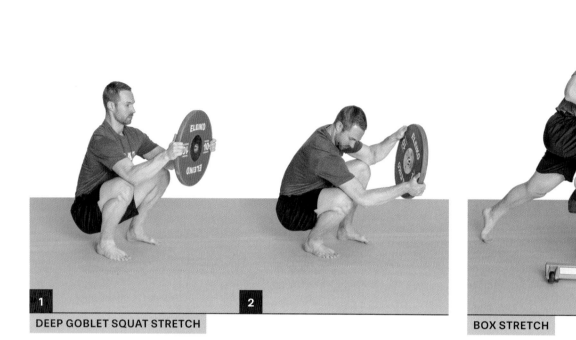

DEEP GOBLET SQUAT STRETCH

BOX STRETCH

Despite what you may have learned elsewhere, you do not want to stretch an Achilles tendon injury! No matter what form of tendinopathy you are experiencing, stretching should *not* be a part of your rehabilitation program. As previously mentioned, insertional Achilles tendinopathy injuries occur due to high levels of compressive load on the tendon against the calcaneus bone. Stretching your calf muscles will only add more compression (and lead to more pain) in the injured area.[21]

The initial goal of rehab for a peritendon injury is to limit excessive movement of the ankle (and therefore friction of the tendon against the peritendon). Stretching would only create more movement and potential for more friction.

While there is less cause for concern for those dealing with a mid-tendon tendinopathy injury, research has not shown any benefit whatsoever to stretching. This is one reason why the commonly prescribed night splints that maintain a constant stretch as you sleep are not an effective treatment for tendinopathy.

Mobilization Exercises

Instead of stretching, if you have limited ankle mobility, you can safely perform soft tissue mobilization to your calf muscles with a foam roller or massage stick. Foam rolling has been shown to improve ankle mobility without placing harmful compressive loads on the Achilles tendon.[22]

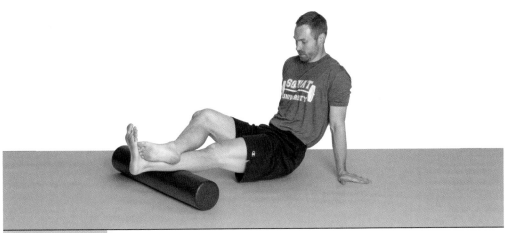

FOAM ROLL CALF

If you have limited ankle mobility due to a joint restriction (felt as a pinch or blocked sensation at the front of the ankle during the 5-inch wall test), banded joint mobilizations can be performed safely with any form of Achilles tendinopathy. Assume a kneeling position with a resistance band loop over the top of your foot (directly over the talus bone).

ANKLE ANATOMY

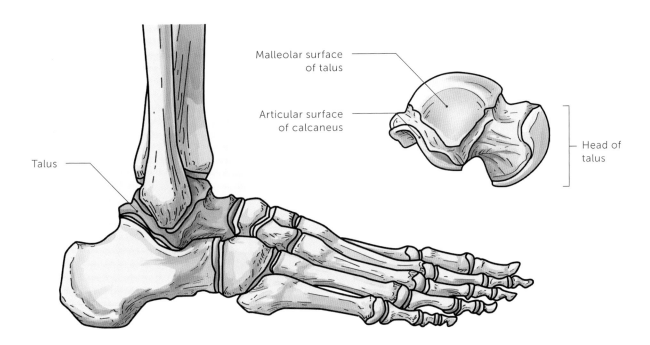

Malleolar surface of talus

Articular surface of calcaneus

Head of talus

Talus

With your foot firmly planted, drive your knee over your toes and hold for a few seconds before returning to the start position. The posterior and downward pull of the band against the talus while you drive your knee forward will help restore the natural movement of the ankle joint.[23] Perform 20 repetitions before rechecking your mobility to make sure you were successful at bringing out a change.

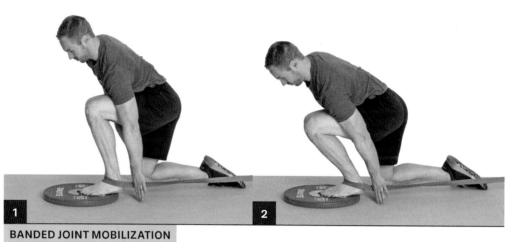

BANDED JOINT MOBILIZATION

Adding a Heel Raise Insert

A heel raise insert for your shoe can be very helpful for certain types of Achilles tendinopathy. For example, adding a heel lift of 1 to 1½ inches will move your foot into a small amount of plantarflexion and decrease compression of the tendon against the calcaneus.[24] This can unload harmful levels of compression for those dealing with insertional tendinopathy.

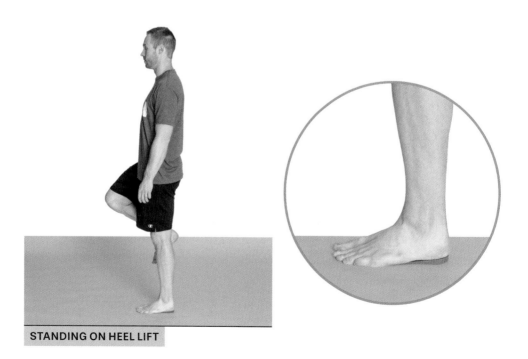

STANDING ON HEEL LIFT

A heel lift can also be helpful if you are dealing with a peritendon injury. Adding the insert will decrease the amount of movement of the ankle during activity.

There is even some evidence to suggest that a heel raise insert may be helpful for those experiencing pain in the mid-tendon region. A less common form of tendinopathy can occur when the plantaris muscle (a smaller muscle whose tendon runs near the Achilles) stiffens and places excessive shearing or compressive loads on the Achilles.[25] For this reason, adding a heel lift could potentially decrease compression and therefore lessen pain.

While a heel raise insert can be very helpful for some people, an orthotic insert is not. Research has shown that inserts that aim to prevent foot pronation are not effective for reducing symptoms or improving function in those with Achilles tendinopathy.[26]

"Passive" Treatments

I have had many patients seek my help after failed treatments under the care of other rehabilitation professionals. What they had gone through often revolved around some kind of passive treatment. A "passive" treatment is something that is done *to you*, whereas as an "active" treatment is something in which you physically participate. Passive treatments include

- Ice
- Electrotherapy
- Dry needling
- Ultrasound
- Iontophoresis (a process of delivering medication through an electrical current or ultrasound device)
- Scraping techniques with various tools made of metal, hard plastic, or bone

These "treatments" are often ineffective and misused in the care of Achilles tendinopathy. They do nothing to address the cause of injury and have limited long-term effectiveness.

Ultrasound in particular is a common physical therapy modality used to treat tendon injuries. However, if you look at the research, you will find very little evidence of its effectiveness! In fact, a 2001 systematic review (a study of many studies) stated, "Ultrasound is no more beneficial than placebo ultrasound for treatment of people with pain or soft tissue injury."[27]

Many rehabilitation practitioners use scraping techniques (called *instrument-assisted soft tissue mobilization,* or IASTM) incorrectly on the painful tendon with the idea that they are stimulating collagen growth and bringing more vascularity (blood flow) to the area to promote healing. The first idea (stimulating collagen growth) has never been proven in a degenerated tendon, and the second (more vascularity) is counterintuitive, as most injured tendons have already grown more blood vessels![28]

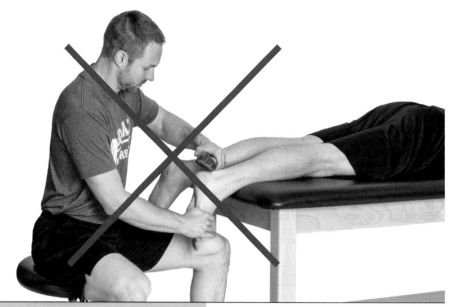

DON'T: SCRAPING TOOL ON ACHILLES TENDON

The only way this technique could be perceived as beneficial when applied to the tendon is in creating a possible short-term decrease in pain. This change in symptoms would be due to a change in how the surrounding nerves are working (called *neurapraxia*), however; there would be little physical change to the tendon tissues themselves.

Performing scraping techniques on an already angered and reactive tendon often does more harm than good and increases the level of irritation. If you want to employ IASTM, it should be directed to your calf muscles and *not* to the tendon itself.

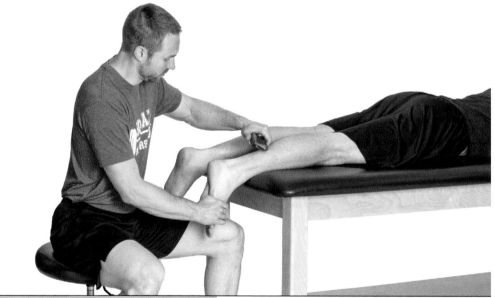

DO: SCRAPING TOOL ON CALF MUSCLES

Step 2: The Rehab Plan

Exercise is the best treatment for any type of tendon pain, period. If a doctor or other medical practitioner recommends injections or other "passive" treatments like electrotherapy or scraping techniques as the main mode of treatment, you have sought help from the wrong person. While passive treatments may decrease your pain in the short term, they will not be helpful in the long term because they do not address why your tendon became injured in the first place. You must strengthen the tendon and improve its ability to tolerate load.

There is no one-size-fits-all recipe for treating tendinopathy. The program must be tailored to how your pain presents, your injury and training history, and your goals.

Phase 1: Decreasing Pain with Isometrics

The first step in rehabilitating almost every tendon injury is isometrics, which are exercises in which the muscle contracts but the joint does not move. Early on, pain can make it difficult to load a very reactive tendon with classic strength exercises. Isometrics can be a great intervention, as their main objective is to decrease pain!

The body often responds to pain by inhibiting neural output (called *cortical inhibition*). Think about it like this: If your body experiences pain every time you perform a jump, your brain will eventually say, "Stop it!" This is why a person who has been dealing with tendon pain for a long time will eventually see decreases in their performance. Heavy isometric exercises have been shown to alter this trajectory.

Research shows that isometrics have the potential to decrease tendon pain for upwards of 45 minutes afterward and can improve a person's strength thereafter by decreasing cortical inhibition. Isometrics allow you to express your strength by accessing more motor units that were previously "turned off" due to pain. These benefits (less pain and decreased inhibition) come from only heavy and long-duration (45-second) isometrics; they have not been seen after classic strength exercises.[29]

Performing isometrics should be relatively pain-free. While you may have a little pain at the start, it should decrease significantly by the third or fourth repetition.

An isometric for the Achilles tendon is a partial heel raise performed while standing. In this position, you activate both calf muscles (the gastroc and soleus) and place the most load on the tendon. Performing a seated heel raise isometric places emphasis on the deeper soleus muscle because the gastroc will be in a shortened position with the knees bent at 90 degrees. If you have a high level of pain, a seated soleus press might be a better option initially.

The way you perform your standing heel raise isometric will depend on your current level of strength. For example, the simplest isometric for the Achilles tendon is a double-leg bodyweight heel raise (photo A on the next page). If this exercise is too easy, perform it while holding a weight in your hand (B). Stronger athletes might need a single-leg heel raise (C) or even a single-leg heel raise with a weight in hand (D). Try each variation to find out which is difficult for you to perform 5 sets for a 45-second hold. Initially, you should perform these exercises two or three times a day with at most a 2-minute rest after each hold.

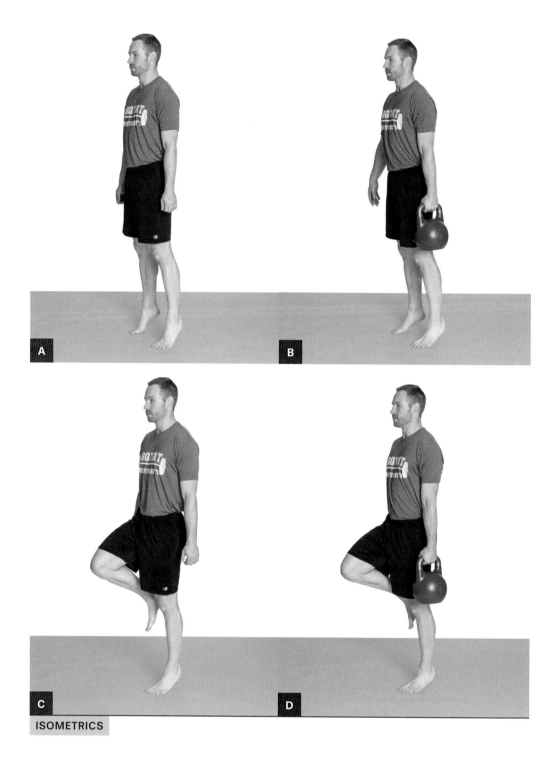

ISOMETRICS

For isometric exercises to be effective, they must be difficult to perform. This is where most people come up short. Research shows that you must find a load that contracts your muscle(s) to 70 percent of its maximum capabilities. While there is no way to self-test precisely for this level, you can estimate it by finding the intensity and load combination that makes an isometric exercise difficult to hold for 45 seconds. If you finish your 45-second heel raise (either double or single leg) and think, "I could have held that for at least for 30 seconds more," you don't have enough load on your tendon. Grab a weight and try again!

Isometrics are used for every kind of Achilles tendinopathy, including a peritendon injury. While adding a heel raise insert to your shoe is the first step in dealing with the pain from a peritendon injury, you still need to place some load on your muscles and tendon as you recover. Only resting a peritendon injury decreases the load tolerance capacity of the tendon, and you risk a mid-tendon or insertional tendinopathy injury when you resume your normal training.

Isometrics are only a starting point for the rehab plan. While they can help you feel better by decreasing your pain and increasing your strength, they are not the only exercises you should do. Eventually, you need to transition to the next phase of the plan. Once your pain levels are at or below a 3 out of 10 in intensity, it's time to start isotonic strength exercises.

Phase 2: Improving Strength with Isotonics

The goal of any tendinopathy rehabilitation plan is to increase the load-bearing capacity of the tendon. No matter whether you had a first-time "reactive" injury or a "reactive-on-degeneration" injury, you must eventually move past isometric exercises and start using traditional strength exercises to accomplish this goal.

Most exercises you see performed in the gym have two phases: eccentric and concentric. The eccentric phase of a movement is the lowering portion where the muscle fibers are lengthened under tension. In the concentric phase, the muscle fibers are shortened under tension. If we look at the standing heel raise, for example, the gastroc and soleus muscles shorten as you rise onto your toes (concentric phase) and lengthen as you descend to the start position (eccentric phase).

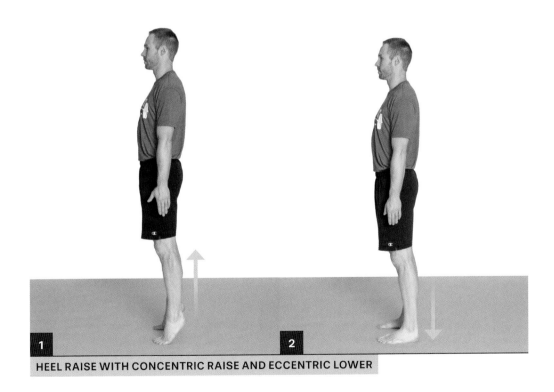

HEEL RAISE WITH CONCENTRIC RAISE AND ECCENTRIC LOWER

In the early days of tendinopathy research, rehabilitation professionals prescribed eccentric exercises as an integral part of a rehab program.[30] For an Achilles tendon injury, this would have consisted of performing a heel raise where you assisted yourself to the top portion with your uninjured leg, shifted all of your body weight onto the injured side, and then slowly lowered into the bottom position on the injured leg alone. No concentric phase was performed, so to perform the next repetition, you would assist yourself back to the top position with your noninjured side.

Initial research on the use of an eccentric-only rehabilitation did show good results, and many subjects were able to return to their pre-injury activity levels.[31] However, our bodies use both eccentric and concentric muscle actions. Focusing strength efforts on only one portion of a movement does not strengthen it in a way that will carry over functionally to the activities you perform throughout the day and in training. Your muscles aren't performing *only* eccentric contractions when you sprint down a track. It's not that eccentrics don't work, but why ignore the other half of the movement?

In the early 2000s, research began to emerge on the use of heavy slow resistance (HSR) training in the rehabilitation of tendon injuries. HSR describes traditional exercises performed slowly with both concentric and eccentric muscle contractions, called *isotonic movements*. The initial research showed these heavy and slow exercises were just as effective as eccentric-only exercises in the rehab of tendinopathy.[32] They are excellent at building load tolerance during this phase of rehabilitation without using the tendon as a spring, which would overload the current capabilities of the tissues and exacerbate symptoms. As soon as your pain has decreased to a 3 out of 10 during normal day-to-day function, I recommend starting HSR exercises.

HSR exercises should target both the gastroc and the soleus muscles. The soleus is highly active during running; therefore, seated heel raises are a great option for those whose training programs involve running.

To sufficiently target the soleus muscle and place enough load on the muscle/tendon, you need to place a weight on top of your leg during the seated heel raise. Placing a weight plate or dumbbell across the length of your femur is not enough, however, because the majority of the load would be spread across your thigh. Instead, you need to place the weight directly over your shin (tibia).

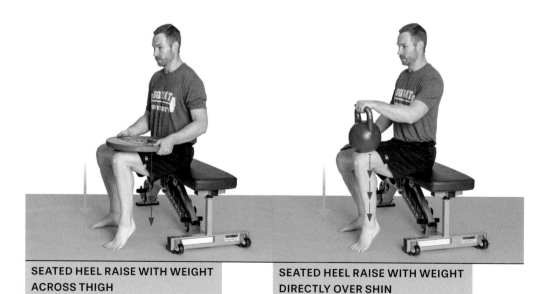

SEATED HEEL RAISE WITH WEIGHT ACROSS THIGH

SEATED HEEL RAISE WITH WEIGHT DIRECTLY OVER SHIN

The right way to load the seated heel raise will vary from person to person. Start with a heavy dumbbell stacked vertically over your knee. If the weight you choose is not sufficient to cause the desired fatigue in the muscles after the fourth set of 10 repetitions, either increase the weight of the dumbbell or place a barbell across your knees, as shown below. The barbell can then be loaded to increase the load for your individual needs.

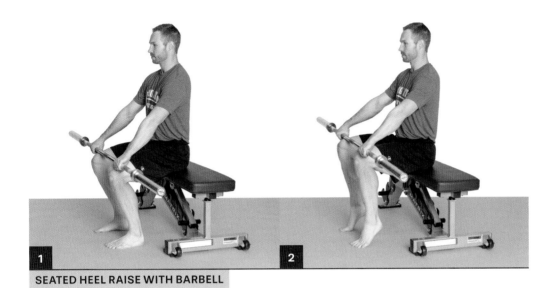

SEATED HEEL RAISE WITH BARBELL

To target the gastroc muscle, try performing standing heel raises while holding a weight. Once you find double-leg heel raises easy, you can progress to single-leg heel raises. Do both seated and standing heel raises at a very slow tempo (with a three-second eccentric lower and a three-second concentric ascent) with as much weight as you can tolerate while maintaining good technique.

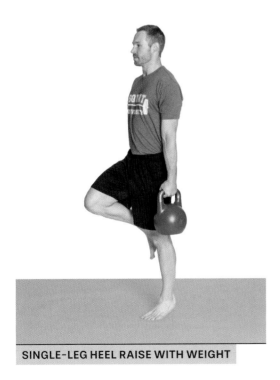

SINGLE-LEG HEEL RAISE WITH WEIGHT

To really benefit from HSR exercises, you must perform them slow and heavy! Sounds simple enough, right?

The "slow" portion of HSR refers to the tempo at which the exercise is performed. Ideally, you should take three seconds in the eccentric phase and three seconds in the concentric phase, meaning each rep takes six seconds to complete.[33] The "heavy" portion of HSR refers to the intensity of the exercise, or how much weight is being used. This is where most rehabilitation professionals come up short because they are afraid to load the injured tendon. Don't be! Remember, a degenerated tendon has more "healthy" tissue than a normal tendon.[34]

When you're starting the HSR phase of the rehab plan, start with 4 sets of 15 repetitions every other day. (On your off-days, continue to perform the isometrics from phase 1.) Perform your isometric exercises before any HSR because the cortical inhibition benefits derived from the isometrics will enable you to access more motor units and a greater strength stimulus.

The weight with which you choose to perform the exercise should be light enough that you can control each repetition with good technique but heavy enough that, after completing your fourth set, you are too fatigued to perform a fifth.[35] If you get done with your fourth set and feel like you have enough energy for another, add more weight!

Research on the use of HSR with tendinopathy has recommended performing these strength exercises for 4 sets of 15 repetitions for a week before increasing the weight and dropping the volume to 4 sets of 12 reps for the next 2 weeks.[36] Eventually, progress to 4 sets of 10 reps, followed by 4 sets of 8 and then 6 reps for 2 to 3 weeks each.

Phase 3: Recovering "the Spring" with Plyometrics

Along with the HSR component of strengthening the muscles/Achilles tendon complex, you also need to increase the ability of the tendon to absorb and store loads. The highest loads placed on the Achilles tendon occur when it is used as a spring, utilizing what is called the *stretch-shortening cycle* (SSC).

Powerful movements like running and repetitive jumping use the Achilles to store and then release energy to generate large amounts of power. Exercises that emphasize the storage of loads, such as jumping from a box and landing, are a bridge to eventually returning to the full energy storage *and* release capabilities of the tendon.

Start by performing a depth drop. Stand on a small box—maybe 6 to 8 inches in height. (In the photos I'm using a stack of bumper plates.) Step off and land with both feet in a mini squat position. Don't land with stiff joints; instead, make sure to absorb the force of the impact. Begin with 3 sets of 10 landings. Once you find that your body is responding well to the 8-inch height, move to a taller box (12 to 14 inches). Once you've mastered double-leg landings and they feel good, you can progress to single-leg landings.

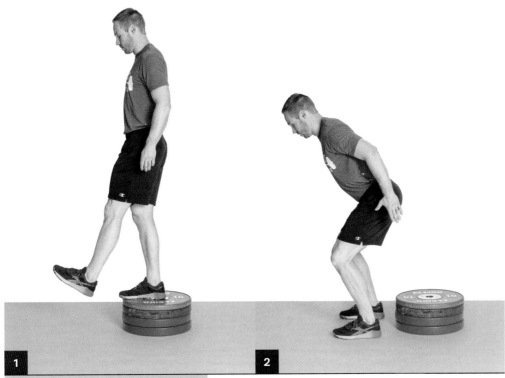

DEPTH DROP OFF STACK OF PLATES

Before starting plyometrics, where the tendon is used as a spring to store and release energy, you must see profound changes in muscle strength. The strength of the injured leg should be equal to that of the noninjured leg before you attempt plyometrics. Those who have been experiencing chronic Achilles tendon pain may have developed noticeable differences in muscle size (calf atrophy of the injured leg); however, muscle size will take much longer to normalize than strength and therefore is not the best predictor of when to return to plyometric loads.[37]

A great way to assess your strength is to perform the load testing protocol from pages 350 to 352. Perform 20 double-leg heel raises followed by 20 single-leg heel raises. Look and feel for how easy it is to perform the movement on each leg. Is it the same? Did you have any pain?

Next, perform a faster, more explosive movement like a single-leg hop on each leg. In the initial phase of injury, this movement was likely painful and hard to perform on the injured leg. If you are ready to move on to the plyometric phase of rehab, you must have the ability to control your body well without pain during slow movements like the single-leg heel raise and during high-load functional movements like the single-leg hop.

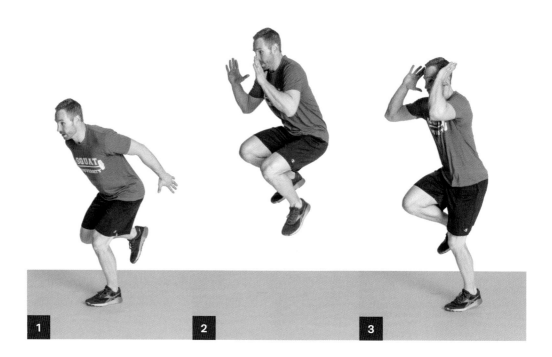

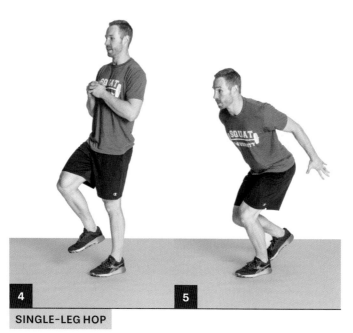

SINGLE-LEG HOP

The goal of this phase of rehab is to start using the tendon as a spring again and see how it responds. An example of an entry-level plyometric is the double-leg pogo hop. Simply perform repetitive small jumps only a few inches off the ground, like bouncing on a pogo stick. Start with 30 to 50 reps before resting for a few minutes, and perform 3 or 4 sets. If you can perform pogo hops without pain, try a few light jogs (1-minute duration maximum).

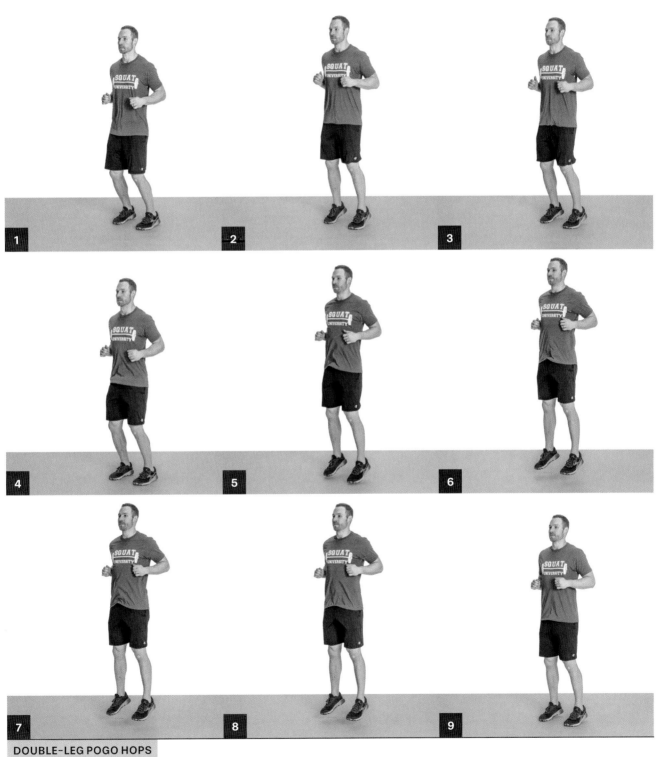

DOUBLE-LEG POGO HOPS

Notice how your Achilles tendon responds to the loading during the exercise and over the next 24 hours. If you feel great while doing the exercise and you do not have any increase in tendon pain or stiffness the following day, increase the load in the next training session. For the first few weeks, increase the volume of your loading by adding more jumps per set or doing longer runs to help build your tendon's capacity.

Recording every aspect of your plyometric program will allow you to progress and build this capacity as efficiently as possible. For example, Athlete A and Athlete B both performed 3 sets of 30 pogo hops and 3 sets of 1-minute jogs on the first day.

- Athlete A woke up feeling great the next morning, so they were cleared to progress to 3 sets of 50 pogo hops in the next session while keeping the running the same.

- Athlete B, however, woke up with a slight increase in Achilles tendon pain. For this reason, Athlete B's plan would need to be modified for the next plyometric session (by dropping the volume on either the hops or the jogs).

Make sure to increase only one variable per training session, whether it's adding or taking away volume or intensity. If you change too many variables at one time, you won't be able to determine whether it was a change in volume or a change in intensity that was too much for your tendon to handle.

Start with two or three sessions a week of light plyometric exercises (one session every three days). At this stage of rehabilitation, the Achilles tendon cannot take daily plyometric loads without getting angry. For this reason, structure your weekly training by mixing in HSR days between plyometric sessions. If your tendon continues to respond well to the increases in plyometric loading every third day, you can continue to add more volume or start to increase the intensity.

Eventually, you'll be able to progress to medium-level plyometric exercises, including squat jumps, jump-roping, and double-leg jumps for distance. If you are a runner (or your sport involves running), adding acceleration and deceleration drills along with cutting/change-of-direction activities may be a good option at this time.

After a few weeks of progressing these drills, you can move to even higher-level plyometric activities, including single-leg pogo hops, double-under jump-roping, and sprinting mixed with agility drills and longer distance runs. For anyone participating in Olympic lifts like the snatch and clean, I recommend waiting until this stage to reinitiate the full lifts because the explosive nature of the movements coupled with a loaded barbell may be too much for the tendon to handle before now.

In time, you can start manipulating the frequency of loading by performing plyometrics every two days instead of three. As always, see how your Achilles tendon responds and adjust accordingly.

There is no perfect recipe for progressing through this plyometric stage. Everyone will respond differently, and you need to find which loads work best for your body.

Final Thoughts on Rehabilitation

The rehabilitation process for an Achilles tendon injury can be boiled down to one simple sentence: "Err on the side of caution." If you're reading this chapter, you are undoubtedly trying to find the quickest and most efficient way to fix your ankle pain and return to the activities you love. I urge you to take it slow and have patience. Depending on the severity of your injury, this process could take weeks or months.

   If at any time you feel like you are not progressing well when trying to work through this process on your own, I strongly recommend contacting a rehabilitation professional to help you through it.

Notes

1.   S. D. Rosengarten, J. L. Cook, A. L. Bryant, J. T. Cordy, J. Daffy, and S. I. Dock, "Australian football players' Achilles tendons respond to game loads within 2 days: an ultrasound tissue characterization (UTC) study," *British Journal of Sports Medicine* 49 (2015): 183–7.

2.   J. L. Cook, E. Rio, C. R. Purdam, and S. I. Docking, "Revisiting the continuum model of tendon pathology: what is its merit in clinical practice and research?" *British Journal of Sports Medicine* 50, no. 19 (2016): 1187–91.

3.   K. M. Khan, J. L. Cook, P. Kannus, N. Maffulli, and S. F. Bonar, "Time to abandon the 'tendinitis' myth: painful, overuse tendon conditions have non-inflammatory pathology," *British Medical Journal* 324, no. 7338 (2002): 626–7.

4.   N. Maffulli, K. M. Khan, and G. Puddu, "Overuse tendon conditions: time to change a confusing terminology," *Arthroscopy* 14, no. 8 (1998): 840–3.

5.   Khan, Cook, Kannus, Maffulli, and Bonar, "Time to abandon the 'tendinitis' myth" (see note 3 above).

6.   Cook, Rio, Purdam, and Docking, "Revisiting the continuum model of tendon pathology" (see note 2 above).

7.   S. I. Docking, M. A. Girdwood, J. Cook, L. V. Fortington, and E. Rio, "Reduced levels of aligned fibrillar structure are not associated with Achilles and patellar tendon symptoms," *Clinical Journal of Sports Medicine* (published online ahead of print, July 31, 2018).

8.   Cook, Rio, Purdam, and Docking, "Revisiting the continuum model of tendon pathology" (see note 2 above).

9.   E. K. Rio, R. F. Ellis, J. M. Henry, V. R. Falconer, Z. S. Kiss, M. A. Girdwood, J. L. Cook, and J. E. Gaida, "Don't assume the control group is normal—people with asymptomatic tendon pathology have higher pressure pain thresholds," *Pain Medicine* 19, no. 11 (2018): 2267–73.

10.   J. Cook, podcast interview, November 5, 2018.

11.   H. Alfredson and J. Cook, "A treatment algorithm for managing Achilles tendinopathy: new treatment options," *British Journal of Sports Medicine* 41, no. 4 (2007): 211–6; J. L. Cook, D. Stasinopoulos, and J. M. Brismée, "Insertional and mid-substance Achilles tendinopathies: eccentric training is not for everyone—updated evidence of non-surgical management," *Journal of Manual & Manipulative Therapy* 26, no. 3 (2018): 119–22; S. I. Docking, C. C. Ooi, and D. Connell, "Tendinopathy: is imaging telling us the entire story?" *Journal of Orthopaedic & Sports Physical Therapy* 45, no. 11 (2015): 842–52.

12.   J. L. Cook and C. Purdam, "Is compressive load a factor in the development of tendinopathy?" *British Journal of Sports Medicine* 46, no. 3 (2012): 163–8.

13.   N. L. Reynolds and T. W. Worrell, "Chronic Achilles peritendinitis: etiology, pathophysiology, and treatment," *Journal of Orthopaedic & Sports Physical Therapy* 13, no. 4 (1991): 171–6.

14. N. Maffulli, "The clinical diagnosis of subcutaneous tear of the Achilles tendon. A prospective study in 174 patients," *American Journal of Sports Medicine* 26, no. 2 (1998): 266–70.

15. A. Kountouris and J. Cook, "Rehabilitation of Achilles and patellar tendinopathies," *Best Practice & Research Clinical Rheumatology* 21, no. 2 (2007): 295–316.

16. S. I. Docking, E. Rio, J. Cook, D. Carey, and L. Fortington, "Quantification of Achilles and patellar tendon structure on imaging does not enhance ability to predict self-reported symptoms beyond grey-scale ultrasound and previous history," *Journal of Science and Medicine in Sport* 22, no. 2 (2019): 145–50.

17. Reynolds and Worrell, "Chronic Achilles peritendinitis" (see note 13 above).

18. J. Cook, podcast interview, November 5, 2018.

19. K. Bennell, R. Talbot, H. Wajswelner, W. Techovanich, and D. Kelly, "Intra-rater and inter-rater reliability of a weight-bearing lunge measure of ankle dorsiflexion," *Australian Journal of Physiotherapy* 44, no. 3 (1998): 175–80; "Ankle mobility exercises to improve dorsiflexion," MikeReinold.com, accessed April 30, 2020, https://mikereinold.com/ankle-mobility-exercises-to-improve-dorsiflexion/.

20. K. Kubo, H. Akima, J. Ushiyama, I. Tabata, H. Fukuoka, H. Kanehisa, and T. Fukunaga, "Effects of 20 days of bed rest on the viscoelastic properties of tendon structures in lower limb muscles," *British Journal of Sports Medicine* 38, no. 3 (2004): 324–30.

21. Cook and Purdam, "Is compressive load a factor in the development of tendinopathy?" (see note 12 above).

22. S. Kelly and C. Beardsley, "Specific and cross-over effects of foam rolling on ankle dorsiflexion range of motion," *International Journal of Sports Physical Therapy* 11, no. 4 (2016): 544–51; C. Beardsley and J. Škarabot, "Effects of self-myofascial release: a systematic review," *Journal of Bodywork and Movement Therapies* 19, no. 4 (2015): 747–58.

23. B. Vicenzino, M. Branjerdporn, P. Teys, and K. Jordan, "Initial changes in posterior talar glide and dorsiflexion of the ankle after mobilization with movement in individuals with recurrent ankle sprain," *Manual Therapy* 9, no. 2 (2004): 77–82; A. Reid, T. B. Birmingham, and G. Alcock, "Efficacy of mobilization with movement for patients with limited dorsiflexion after ankle sprain: a crossover trial," *Physiotherapy Canada* 59, no. 3 (2007): 166–72.

24. C. Ganderton, J. Cook, S. Docking, and E. Rio, "Achilles tendinopathy: understanding the key concepts to improve clinical management," *Australasian Musculoskeletal Medicine* 19, no. 2 (2015): 12–8.

25. Cook and Purdam, "Is compressive load a factor in the development of tendinopathy?" (see note 12 above).

26. S. E. Munteanu, L. A. Scott, D. R. Bonanno, K. B. Landrof, T. Pizzari, J. L. Cook, and H. B. Menz, "Effectiveness of customized foot orthoses for Achilles tendinopathy: a randomised controlled trial," *British Journal of Sports Medicine* 49, no. 15 (2015): 989–94.

27. V. J. Robertson and K. G. Baker, "A review of therapeutic ultrasound: effectiveness studies," *Physical Therapy* 81, no. 7 (2001): 1339–50.

28. Cook, Rio, Purdam, and Docking, "Revisiting the continuum model of tendon pathology" (see note 2 above).

29. E. Rio, D. Kidgell, C. Purdam, J. Gaida, G. L. Moseley, A. J. Pearce, and J. Cook, "Isometric exercise induces analgesia and reduces inhibition in patellar tendinopathy," *British Journal of Sports Medicine* 49, no. 19 (2015): 1277–83.

30. S. Curwin and W. D. Stanish, *Tendinitis: Its Etiology and Treatment* (Lexington, Mass.: Collamore Press, 1984); H. Alfredson, T. Pietilä, P. Jonsson, and R. Lorentzon, "Heavy-load eccentric calf muscle training for the treatment of chronic Achilles tendinosis," *American Journal of Sports Medicine* 26, no. 3 (1998): 360–6.

31. Alfredson, Pietilä, Jonsson, and Lorentzon, "Heavy-load eccentric calf muscle training for the treatment of chronic Achilles tendinosis" (see note 30 above).

32. M. Kongsgaard, V. Kovanen, P. Aagaard, S. Doessing, P. Hansen, A. H. Laursen, N. C. Kaldau, M. Kjaer, and S. R. Magnusson, "Corticosteroid injections, eccentric decline squat training and heavy slow resistance training in patellar tendinopathy," *Scandinavian Journal of Medicine & Science in Sports* 19, no. 6 (2009): 790–802; P. Malliaras, J. Cook, C. Purdam, and E. Rio, "Patellar tendinopathy: clinical diagnosis, load management, and advice for challenging case presentations," *Journal of Orthopaedic & Sports Physical Therapy* 45, no. 11 (2015): 887–98.

33. Kongsgaard et al., "Corticosteroid injections, eccentric decline squat training and heavy slow resistance training in patellar tendinopathy" (see note 32 above).

34. Docking, Girdwood, Cook, Fortington, and Rio, "Reduced levels of aligned fibrillar structure are not associated with Achilles and patellar tendon symptoms" (see note 7 above).

35. J. Cook, podcast interview, November 5, 2018.

36. Kongsgaard et al., "Corticosteroid injections, eccentric decline squat training and heavy slow resistance training in patellar tendinopathy" (see note 32 above).

37. J. Cook, podcast interview, November 5, 2018.

CHAPTER 7

DON'T ICE; WALK IT OFF!

The focus of this book is the step-by-step guide to resolving pain and building a strong foundation to enhance your future performance. However, a book about the process of rebuilding your body would not be complete without a discussion of one of the most common methods for treating pain in the world today: ice.

What I'm going to say in this final chapter may shock you. It may even anger you. The statement I'm going to make flies in the face of what many in the medical field have been preaching for decades, but it's something *you* need to hear:

You need to *stop* using ice on injuries and sore muscles.

Now, before you throw up your hands in disbelief and yell at the top of your lungs about how ridiculous that statement is, hear me out. Ice does *not* do what you think it does. It does not aid the process of healing from injury; in fact, an overwhelming amount of research shows that it does the opposite! Other than temporarily numbing pain, ice *delays* healing and recovery. But before you take my word for it, let's take a deep dive into the history of icing and why its use became conventional "wisdom."

From a young age, we're taught that if something hurts, you put ice on it. If you sprain your ankle at soccer practice, wrapping a bag of ice around the injured area is the first step toward feeling better. We do this because we're told that icing helps reduce harmful inflammation and swelling and even kick-starts the recovery process after an intense workout.

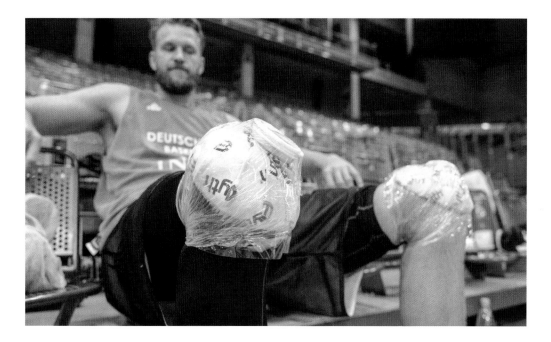

Icing after games is all too common among elite athletes.
© Harald Tittel/dpa/ Alamy Live News
Image ID: W88F0E

It's not uncommon to see the best athletes in the world doing post-game inter-views with bags of ice wrapped around their knees or shoulders. With a simple online search, you can easily find photos of Michael Jordan with ice on both knees. With so many professional athletes like MJ using ice after their practices and games on TV for all of us to see, it's understandable that we all wanted to use ice as well! As the saying goes, we all wanted to "be like Mike."

As a competitive weightlifter, I commonly used ice on my sore knees and back after intense training sessions. I was told that this was a normal part of being a strength athlete. I would even jump into an ice bath after an intense squat session to help kick-start the recovery process...or at least that's what I thought I was doing.

In the rehabilitation world, physical therapists, athletic trainers, and chiropractors use ice in clinics and training rooms around the globe every day. Early in my career as a physical therapist, it wasn't uncommon for every one of my patients to get a cold pack wrapped tightly around their injury after their rehab session.

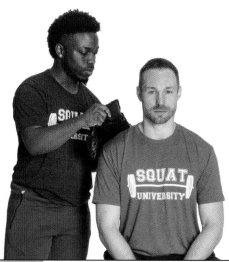

However, the field that has been using ice the longest is medicine. Articles dating back to the early 1940s explain that medical doctors would commonly use ice to help decrease infection rates, block pain, and reduce the rate of patients dying on the operating table during amputation surgeries.[1] Ice slows cellular metabolism, which allowed surgeons to keep as much muscle tissue alive as possible. While icing was originally intended to preserve severed limbs and decrease complications in the operating room, it eventually sneaked its way into being used for all injuries.

In 1978, Harvard physician Gabe Mirkin coined the term RICE (Rest, Ice, Compression, Elevation) for the recommended treatment for sports injuries in his landmark *The Sports Medicine Book*.[2] Since then, the medical community has used this protocol religiously for the treatment of acute injuries.

Now, if you ask a medical doctor today *why* they recommend ice for a common ankle sprain or backache, they'll likely say that it alleviates pain, reduces inflammation, and restricts swelling. In fact, this is why some surgeons insist that their patients use ice for *months on end* after surgery.

If literally *everyone* is using ice, how could it be so wrong?

There is no denying that ice provides temporary pain relief. Slap an ice pack on an area of your body that hurts, and you're going to feel better instantly. In fact, if you look at the scientific research on the use of ice (called *cryotherapy*), pain reduction is the number one benefit! But here's the deal: Just because the pain is decreased does *not* mean that you're fixing the injury. In fact, you're doing more harm than good.

What may blow your mind is that Dr. Mirkin withdrew his endorsement of the RICE protocol (which he invented!) in the foreword to the second edition of Gary Reinl's groundbreaking book *Iced! The Illusionary Treatment Option* in 2013. He wrote: "Subsequent research shows that ice can actually delay recovery. Mild movement helps tissue to heal faster, and the application of cold suppresses the immune responses that start and hasten recovery. Icing does help suppress pain, but athletes are usually far more interested in returning as quickly as possible to the playing field. So, today, RICE is not the preferred treatment for an acute athletic injury."[3]

I hope I've caught your attention. Let's dive into how ice actually affects the body.

Inflammation and Swelling

We've always been told that inflammation and swelling are bad things that we need to stop as soon as possible. I'm here to tell you that they are *not* bad things. In fact, inflammation and swelling are *normal responses to injury.*

Inflammation: The First Stage of the Healing Process

Ask a bunch of medical professionals what the three phases of healing are, and they'll all tell you the same thing: inflammation, repair, and remodel. Don't believe me? Check any medical textbook, and you'll find this answer. Inflammation is the first stage of the healing process, no matter the location or severity of the injury. If it is a normal response to injury, then why do we want to prevent it?

When an injury such as a sprained ankle occurs, inflammatory cells called *white blood cells* rush to the site to kick-start the healing process. Specifically, tiny cells called *neutrophils* are deployed to destroy bacteria (if there is an open wound), and others called *macrophages* remove the tissue cells damaged by the initial trauma. Macrophages are like Pac-Man chomping down all those tiny dots—in this case, the cells that died due to the initial trauma. At the same time, these cells release an anabolic hormone called *insulin-like growth factor 1* (IGF-1) into the surrounding area to spark the next phase of the healing process: muscle repair and regeneration.

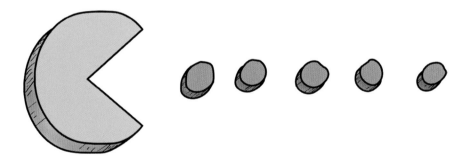

Plain and simple, healing *requires* inflammation. It isn't a bad thing at all; it is an essential biological response to injury. Although chronic levels of systemic inflammation clearly play a role in certain diseases, such as autoimmune disorders like rheumatoid arthritis and lupus, localized inflammation is extremely beneficial to muscle regeneration directly after an acute muscle injury. In fact, a lack of inflammation blunts the healing process and contributes to poor muscle regeneration![4] This "blunting" of the healing process occurs when you use ice.

Placing ice on an injured area essentially puts a roadblock in front of the white blood cells trying to get to the area. You think you're helping the healing process by placing a bag of ice on your body, but you're actually delaying its start by preventing your body from doing what it *wants* and *needs* to do.[5]

Think about it like this: A car accident just occurred, and debris (shattered glass, shards of metal, and so on) is scattered all over the road. 9-1-1 has been called, and emergency vehicles are on the way. All of a sudden, a barricade is set up in the middle of the highway, putting an immediate halt to all incoming traffic.

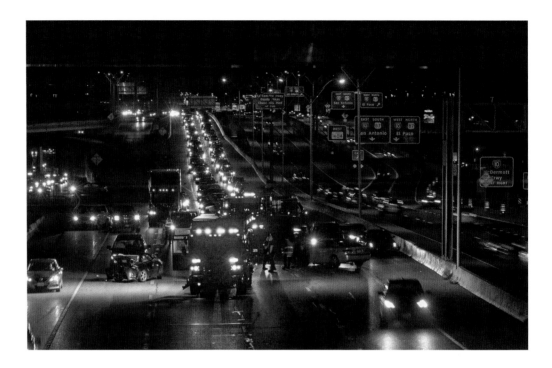

Like a barricade preventing emergency vehicles from getting to the scene of a car accident, icing keeps white blood cells from getting to damaged tissue in order to clean it up.
Editorial credit: Moab Republic / Shutterstock.com

What do you think is going to happen to the people involved in the accident and the mess strewn over the highway? Like the barricade that keeps the emergency vehicles from getting to the scene, ice prevents the ever-important white blood cells, whose sole purpose is to clean up damaged tissue (akin to the debris on the road), from arriving on time *and* delays the production of IGF-1, whose job is to spark muscle repair and regeneration. Pressing the pause button on this process by applying ice restricts blood flow to the injured site and prevents the essential inflammatory cells from doing their job—sometimes for long after the cold pack or ice bag has been removed.[6]

What About Swelling? Isn't Ice Good for That?

If you ask any medical doctor why they use ice for swelling, they'll likely tell you that "excessive" swelling can lead to increased pain and decreased range of motion and lengthen recovery time. This is true. If swelling in a joint is allowed to persist, it can have negative effects. However, swelling in itself isn't good or bad; it's simply the end of the inflammatory cycle. It's what we do about it that makes all the difference.

You see, following an injury, the blood vessels that surround the damaged tissue "open up" to allow inflammatory cells to arrive. This rush of cells out of the small blood vessels and into the damaged site also pulls additional fluid into the surrounding tissue. We call this accumulation of fluid "swelling."

Swelling occurs for a reason, however. The accumulating fluid contains the waste by-product of the damaged tissue. The firefighters, police officers, and ambulance have arrived at the site to clear the debris, and they need a way to remove it from the roadway. Unfortunately, the fluid that now contains waste can't leave the same way it came in (through the circulatory system); it has to be evacuated through an intricate network of vessels called the *lymphatic system.*

Your body has a few different pathways to move fluid from place to place. One is the circulatory system composed of arteries and veins, which pumps blood cells and fluid to and from your heart. This continuous transport system works day and night, both when you're moving around and when you're resting.

The lymphatic system is another tubelike system that runs throughout the body, except it doesn't have an "engine" like the heart to transport fluids. The lymphatic system is completely passive, which means you have to make it work. When you contract your muscles, you squeeze the lymphatic vessels deep inside your body, and the fluid within is forced to move. (Think about this like a cow being milked.)

CIRCULATORY SYSTEM VERSUS LYMPHATIC SYSTEM

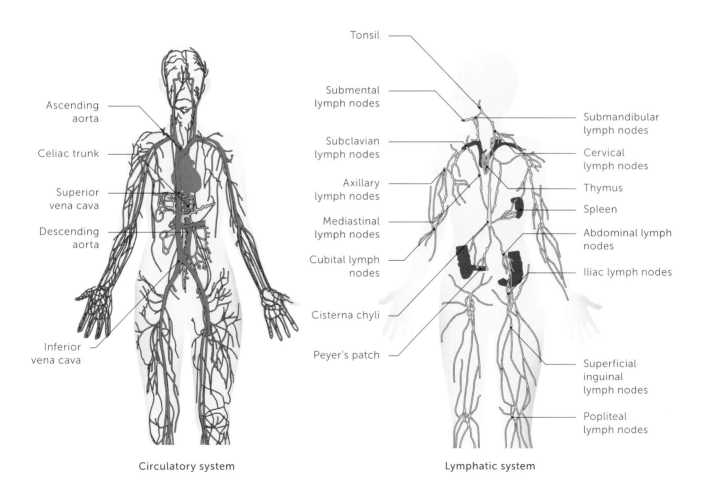

Circulatory system

Lymphatic system

Swelling is merely the buildup of waste around an injured area that needs to be evacuated via the lymphatic system. It is a natural response to injury that becomes a problem only when the waste-filled fluid is allowed to accumulate. When you see an athlete whose lower leg has ballooned two to three sizes the day after an ankle sprain, the issue isn't a swelling problem; it's an evacuation problem.

Ice does *not* facilitate clearance of swelling through the passive lymphatic system. While resting and icing may feel good in the short term, that approach actually traps debris around the injury and stunts the natural healing process!

But What About the Science? There Has to Be Research to Back Up the Use of Ice!

Wrong. Scientific research does *not* support the use of ice.

For example, a 2011 study looked into the effects of ice after a muscle injury.[7] One group received ice for 20 minutes following the injury; the other did not. The injuries were then closely followed for the next 28 days. The results were not what you might think.

During the initial few hours after injury, it is common to see macrophages (the "cleanup crew") flood the area. The researchers found several within the damaged muscle fibers of the "no icing" group; however, those who had been given ice showed almost no sign of macrophages.

Three days post-injury, the "no icing" group already showed signs of regenerating muscle cells. Yet in the icing group, these cells were nowhere to be found. After four days, regenerated muscle cells were found in both groups, but those in the "no-icing" group were significantly larger than those in the icing group. At 28 days post-injury, the regenerating muscle of the "no icing" group was 65 percent larger than that of the icing group!

In addition, the researchers found *significantly* more scarring in the icing group compared to the untreated "no icing" muscles. The authors of the study concluded, "Judging from these findings, it might be better to avoid icing, although it has been widely used in sports medicine." Despite conventional "wisdom" telling us that ice is a good idea, research shows that icing delays muscle repair after injury and gives us direct evidence that icing can lead to increased scarring!

To make matters even worse, the way ice is used has the potential to decrease muscle strength and size. Remember the common RICE (Rest, Ice, Compression, Elevation) protocol? When most people have an injury, they wrap a bag of ice tightly around the painful joint or muscle and stop moving. They do so because they've always been told that moving the injured area will cause further damage. However, immobilizing an injury does more harm than good!

When you stop moving for an extended period, your body responds by shutting down the essential processes that regulate muscle mass. Studies have estimated that we can lose 0.5 percent of muscle per day and up to 5 percent in a week.[8] This shrinkage in muscle size (called *disuse atrophy*) is one of the major complications following severe injuries and those that require surgery.

But what about directly after surgery? There has to be evidence that ice is helpful after that...right?

Wrong. Studies on the use of ice to promote healing after surgery have shown little to no benefit at all! In 2005, researchers conducted a meta-analysis (a study of all available studies) on the use of cryotherapy directly after ACL reconstruction surgery.[9] They concluded that the only benefit was lowering pain. Icing did not improve how much a person could move their knee or lead to any decrease in swelling.

Swelling is no doubt a significant concern after any surgery, especially surgeries in the lower body, such as an ACL reconstruction. Swelling that builds in and around an injured area and remains can lead to a cascade of problems—decreased mobility, blunted strength, increased pain, and more.[10] But remember, icing does *not* help facilitate the pumping action of the "passive" lymphatic system, which is the *only* way to remove swelling.

Gary Reinl gave me a great analogy for this concept that I want to share with you. If you knew it was going to snow 2 inches every hour for the next 12 hours, what would you do? You'd likely open your front door and sweep off a small amount of snow every hour. If you procrastinate and wait until the snow has stopped falling, you'll open the door to find 24 inches accumulated. Imagine how much more difficult it is to shovel 2 feet of snow all at once!

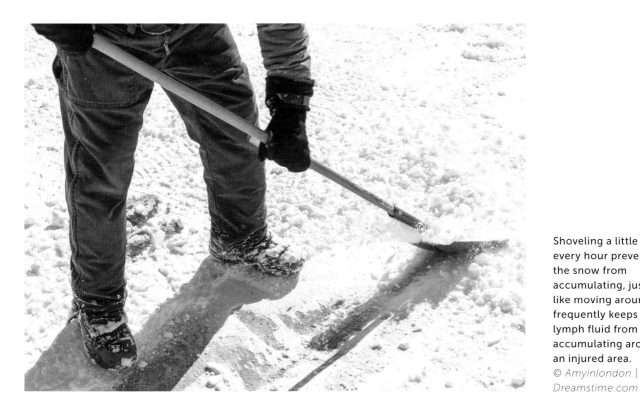

Shoveling a little bit every hour prevents the snow from accumulating, just like moving around frequently keeps lymph fluid from accumulating around an injured area.
© Amyinlondon | Dreamstime.com

Similarly, swelling accumulates around an injured area because you stop moving! It's not because there is "excessive swelling" but rather because you aren't doing anything to facilitate lymphatic drainage to pull it away. Instead of using ice to try to block swelling from accumulating in the first place (which clearly has detrimental effects), you need to be proactive and work on improving the evacuation of the fluid and waste that does accumulate. No matter whether you sustained a minor injury like a sprained ankle or you just got out of surgery to repair a torn meniscus, you need to turn your attention to evacuating swelling, not preventing it.

But how do you facilitate this evacuation?

You move.

Using Muscle Contraction to Reduce Swelling and Facilitate Healing

Remember when you would fall as a child and your mom or dad would yell, "Walk it off!" It's quite possible that your parent was right all along about keeping it moving after getting injured. Too quickly we instruct athletes to shut it down completely after an ankle or knee injury. Keep in mind that moving too much and too aggressively may make things worse; I am merely proposing that you consider kicking off the healing process with light movement and active recovery methods.

Exercises performed in a relatively pain-free manner not only accelerate the removal of swelling through muscle contraction but also optimize the healing process without causing further damage. Moving the injured area may seem counterintuitive, but it's actually the best thing to do! Loading damaged tissue with proper exercises as soon as possible after injury accelerates the healing of muscle and bone.[11] The last thing you want to do is wait around to see how you feel tomorrow or the next day.

Performing pain-free exercise following injury has countless benefits. To start, muscle contraction enhances the inflammation process by improving macrophage function (the cleanup crew) and allowing these essential white blood cells to remove damaged cells.[12] It also boosts muscle repair and regeneration and limits the formation of scar tissue through activation of stem cells (called *satellite cells*).[13]

After injury, the goal of movement is to facilitate healing without causing additional damage. Exercise too intensely and place too much load on your body, and you're only going to make the injury worse. This is why it's not a good idea to perform heavy back squats one day after spraining your ankle or attempt to run four weeks after ACL reconstruction surgery.

Loading the body in a pain-free manner allows you to find the crossroads between efficient and safe recovery. One of the safest muscle contractions for acute injuries and post-op cases is isometrics. *Isometric* describes the action of muscle contraction without joint movement. Try this: First straighten your knee. Then squeeze your quad muscle as hard as you can for 10 seconds. You just completed an isometric contraction for this muscle group! In the early rehabilitation stage following ACL reconstruction surgery (one to four weeks post-op), I often prescribe isometric quad sets to my patients to restore quad strength, decrease pain, and—guess what?—evacuate swelling.

The smallest amount of muscle contraction can help remove swelling through the passive lymphatic system, prevent disuse atrophy by increasing muscle protein synthesis (helping you preserve muscle mass while you recover), and reduce pain. This is why simple exercises like ankle pumps (repeatedly moving your toes toward and away from your head) can be so helpful for athletes directly after sustaining an ankle sprain.

As the pain decreases, the load should be increased to facilitate optimal healing. For someone with knee pain, for example, this may mean progressing bodyweight squats from partial depth to full depth and eventually adding a weighted barbell.

Using NMES to Facilitate Healing When Movement Is Limited

People always ask, "What about those who cannot physically contract their muscles because of significant weakness or for whom weight-bearing exercises are limited due to post-op surgical precautions?"

While voluntary exercise is undoubtedly the most effective way to preserve muscle mass, reduce swelling, and kick-start the healing process after injury, neuromuscular electrical stimulation (NMES) devices come in a close second. NMES devices work by stimulating muscle contraction through electricity. Place the electrode pads on your quad, turn up the intensity, and suddenly your muscles begin to contract all by themselves!

NMES devices have multiple uses that can be helpful for an athlete recovering from injury. One of the best-known uses is to reduce swelling.[14] By stimulating involuntary muscle contraction, NMES devices help pump excess fluid/waste out of the injured area through the passive lymphatic system and dilate blood vessels to bring in nutrients and white blood cells to enhance the healing process. Because swelling buildup can create pain and lead to muscle atrophy (as most people don't want to move a painful area of the body), NMES can decrease symptoms and prevent loss of muscle mass in the early stages of recovery.[15] In fact, research has shown that a single NMES session can increase muscle protein synthesis by 27 percent.[16]

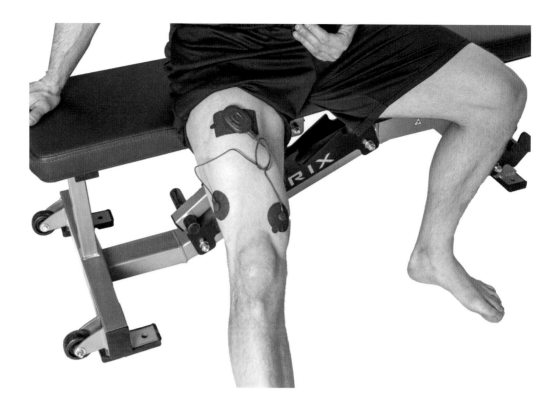

A neuromus-
cular electrical
stimulation
(NMES) device.

The other great feature of NMES devices is their ability to eliminate pain through sensory modification. This allows an athlete recovering from severe injury or surgery to manage pain safely without having to rely on narcotics. Simply put, after injury, we want to promote movement (even if it's as little as stimulated muscle contractions through the use of an E-stim device) to optimize healing and safely return to the sports we love.

Icing After Workouts

So I've touched on how ice can hinder the natural healing process after minor and major injuries, but what about using ice after an intense workout?

Elite athletes around the world are always searching for the best techniques to accelerate recovery and gain an edge on the competition. In this quest, many swear by jumping in an ice bath or strapping some ice packs across their legs after heavy training. I've known many weightlifters who claim that ice baths are the only recovery technique that allows them to get through a high-volume squat cycle. But what does the science say?

During a hard workout, your muscles sustain tiny amounts of damage. This "trauma" sparks inflammation, similar to what happens after an acute injury, like a sprained ankle. The rush of inflammatory cells to the site of "damage" helps kick-start recovery by eliminating damaged cells and then recruiting stem cells from the surrounding tissues to assist in repairing and regenerating new muscle cells.

If you comb through the available science on the use of ice after intense workouts, the main finding is that ice baths decrease the perception of muscle soreness by changing how the body senses pain.[17] As far as the effect of ice baths on recovery of performance in the next training session, the research is split. Some studies show that a 5- to 10-minute plunge can boost performance during the next training session, while others say it has no effect. A few even say that it can be detrimental.[18]

Here's my opinion: Periodic use of ice baths may assist some athletes who need to recover quickly between same-day training sessions and competitions. In general, however, you should avoid the regular use of ice baths because the continued use of ice can be harmful to the natural adaptation process for developing muscle strength and hypertrophy. Let me explain why.

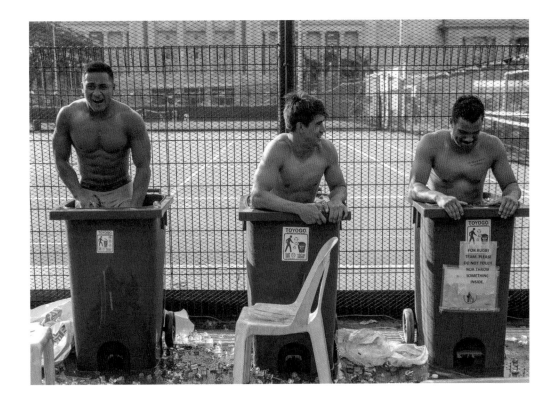

The research on the benefits of using ice baths after training is not conclusive.
© Olaf Schuelke / Alamy Stock Photo
Image ID: KGKH1E

Muscle soreness and muscle fatigue are not the same thing. While you may *feel* less soreness after icing, you're not necessarily recovering any faster physiologically. Remember, there is a reason for soreness. It is a normal reaction to intense training, just like the inflammation cycle is a normal response to injury. However, the more accustomed an athlete is to a particular style and intensity of training, the quicker they recover between sessions, and the less soreness they feel.

This is why, the day after a high-volume squat session, you feel so sore you can barely stand up from a chair. However, two weeks into the same training cycle, you don't feel nearly as sore following similar workouts. Your body adapts to the training stimulus; this is known as the *repeated bout effect*. This is why a majority of the research on elite athletes has shown ice baths *not* to help with recovery and performance.[19]

In fact, multiple research studies have shown that icing interferes with the normal adaptive response to exercise that helps us recover and gain strength. Here is a direct quote from one such article: "These data suggest that topical cooling, a commonly used clinical intervention, seems to not improve but rather delay recovery from eccentric exercise-induced muscle damage."[20]

Unless you're looking for an instantaneous bounce-back on the day of a competition, you should be very cautious of the long-term effects of ice on recovery. When you take time to look at the science, you can see that using ice after a workout has the long-term potential to stunt muscle growth and strength gains.[21]

Instead of reaching for that ice pack or jumping into a tub filled with ice, I recommend using an active recovery approach. Go for a 10-minute walk, perform a light workout of bodyweight squats, or even go for a swim or bike ride—basically, get off the couch and do any nonfatiguing exercise that gets your body moving and your blood pumping.

If you're extremely sore the day after an intense workout, I recommended performing a few minutes of soft tissue mobilization. Research has shown that a few minutes of rolling on a foam roller or small ball (such as a lacrosse or tennis ball) can significantly reduce delayed-onset muscle soreness (DOMS).[22]

If you don't have time to get in a light workout or you're feeling a little under the weather, try using an NMES device like the Marc Pro, Powerdot, or Complex. These devices mimic the muscle pump of active movement. The use of such a device delivers nonfatiguing muscle contraction without effort that will enhance lymphatic drainage to remove cellular waste that accumulates after heavy training and increase blood flow to stimulate the recovery and repair process.[23]

Final Thoughts on Icing

If you still aren't convinced that the benefits of icing have been overblown and that icing is flat-out wrong in many cases, I offer you one last piece of evidence.

Every year, a group of experts in the treatment of acute injuries gather to comb over the current scientific literature and establish position statements for the National Athletic Trainers' Association (NATA). In 2013, the group released a statement on the recommended treatment for ankle sprains, an injury commonly addressed with the RICE protocol.[24]

After evaluating all of the available scientific literature on possible treatments for ankle sprains, the experts assigned ratings from best ("A") to worst ("C"). Do you know which rating icing got? A big fat "C." The NATA team even wrote that "strong clinical evidence for advocating cryotherapy is limited."

Do you know which treatment was assigned an "A" rating? Functional rehabilitation! With this position statement, the profession that sees a majority of acute injuries among athletes acknowledges that icing is *not* as good as we all once thought; rather, the best form of treatment is moving and loading the injured area through rehabilitation exercises.

At the end of the day, our approach to treating injuries and soreness after training is quite simple. We want to get the good stuff (white blood cells) in and the bad stuff (swelling that includes cellular debris from the damaged tissue) out. I hope you can see that this process is not optimized by using ice.

Notes

1. F. M. Massie, "Refrigeration anesthesia for amputation," *Annals of Surgery* 123, no. 5 (1946): 937–47.

2. G. Mirkin and M. Hoffman, *The Sports Medicine Book* (Boston: Little Brown & Co., 1978).

3. G. Reinl, *Iced! The Illusionary Treatment Option*, 2nd Edition (Henderson, NV: Gary Reinl, 2014).

4. H. Lu, D. Huang, N. Saederup, I. F. Charo, R. M. Ransohoff, and L. Zhou, "Macrophages recruited via CCR2 produce insulin-like growth factor-1 to repair acute skeletal muscle injury," *FASEB Journal* 25, no. 1 (2011): 358–69; M. Summan, G. L. Warren, R. R. Mercer, R. Chapman, T. Hulderman, N. Van Rooijen, and P. P. Simeonova, "Macrophages and skeletal muscle regeneration: a clodronate-containing liposome depletion study," *American Journal of Physiology—Regulatory, Integrative, and Comparative Physiology* 290, no. 6 (2006): R1488–95; L. Pelosi, C. Giacinti, C. Nardis, G. Borsellino, E. Rizzuto, C. Nicoletti, F. Wannenes, and L. Battistini, "Local expression of IGF-1 accelerates muscle regeneration by rapidly modulating inflammatory cytokines and chemokines," *FASEB Journal* 21, no. 7 (2007): 1393–402; D. P. Singh, Z. B. Lonbani, M. A. Woodruff, T. P. Parker, and R. Steck, "Effects of topical icing on inflammation, angiogenesis, revascularization, and myofiber regeneration in skeletal muscle following contusion injury," *Frontiers in Physiology* 8 (2017): 93; R. Takagi, N. Fujita, T. Arakawa, S. Kawada, N. Ishii, and A. Miki, "Influence of icing on muscle regeneration after crush injury to skeletal muscles in rats," *Journal of Applied Physiology* 110, no. 2 (2011): 382–8.

5. P. M. Tiidus, "Alternative treatments for muscle injury: massage, cryotherapy, and hyperbaric oxygen," *Current Reviews in Musculoskeletal Medicine* 8, no. 2 (2015): 162–7.

6. S. Khoshnevis, N. K. Kraik, and K. R. Diller, "Cold-induced vasoconstriction may persist long after cooling ends: an evaluation of multiple cryotherapy units," *Knee Surgery, Sports Traumatology, Arthroscopy* 23, no. 9 (2015): 2475–83.

7. Takagi, Fujita, Arakawa, Kawada, Ishii, and Miki, "Influence of icing on muscle regeneration after crush injury to skeletal muscles in rats" (see note 4 above).

8. M. L. Dirks, B. T. Wall, and L. C. J. van Loon, "Interventional strategies to combat muscle disuse atrophy in humans: focus on neuromuscular electrical stimulation and dietary protein," *Journal of Applied Physiology* 125, no. 3 (2018): 850–61.

9. M. C. Raynor, R. Pietrobon, U. Guller, and L. D. Higgins, "Cryotherapy after ACL reconstruction: a meta-analysis," *Journal of Knee Surgery* 18, no. 2 (2005): 123–9.

10. J. D. Spencer, K. C. Hayes, and I. J. Alexander, "Knee joint effusion and quadriceps reflex inhibition in man," *Archives of Physical Medicine and Rehabilitation* 65, no. 4 (1984): 171–7.

11. J. A. Buckwalter and A. J. Grodzinsky, "Loading of healing bone, fibrous tissue, and muscle: implications for orthopaedic practice," *Journal of the American Academy of Orthopaedic Surgery* 7, no. 5 (1999): 291–9.

12. E. M. Silveria, M. F. Rodrigues, M. S. Krause, D. R. Vianna, B. S. Almeida, J. S. Rossato, L. P. Oliveira, Jr., R. Curi, and P. I. H. de Bettencourt, Jr., "Acute exercise stimulates macrophage function: possible role of NF-kappaB pathways," *Cell Biochemistry & Function* 25, no. 1 (2007): 63–73.

13. E. Teixeira and J. A. Duarte, "Skeletal muscle loading changes its regenerative capacity," *Sports Medicine* 46, no. 6 (2016): 783–92; H. Richard-Bulteau, B. Serrurier, B. Cassous, S. Banzet, A. Peinnequin, X. Bigard, and N. Koulmann, "Recovery of skeletal muscle mass after extensive injury: positive effects of increased contractile activity," *American Journal of Physiology Cell Physiology* 294, no. 2 (2008): C467–76.

14. L. C. Burgess, T. K. Immins, I. Swain, and T. W. Wainwright, "Effectiveness of neuromuscular electrical stimulation for reducing oedema: a systematic review," *Journal of Rehabilitation Medicine* 51, no. 4 (2019): 237–43; T. W. Wainwright, L. C. Burgess, and R. G. Middleton, "Does neuromuscular electrical stimulation improve recovery following acute ankle sprain? A pilot randomised controlled trial," *Clinical Medicine Insights Arthritis and Musculoskeletal Disorders* 12 (2019): 1–6; Y. D. Choi and J. H. Lee, "Edema and pain reduction using transcutaneous electrical nerve stimulation treatment," *Journal of Physical Therapy Science* 28, no. 11 (2016): 3084–7.

15. Dirks, Wall, and van Loon, "Interventional strategies to combat muscle disuse atrophy in humans" (see note 8 above).

16. B. T. Wall, M. L. Dirks, L. B. Verdijk, T. Snijders, D. Hansen, P. Vranckx, N. A. Burd, P. Dendale, and L. J. C. van Loon, "Neuromuscular electrical stimulation increases muscle protein synthesis in elderly type 2 diabetic men," *American Journal of Physiology: Endocrinology and Metabolism* 303, no. 5 (2012): E614–23.

17. F. Crowther, R. Sealey, M. Crowe, A. Edwards, and S. Halson, "Influence of recovery strategies upon performance and perceptions following fatiguing exercise: a randomized controlled trial," *BMC Sports Science, Medicine and Rehabilitation* 9 (2017): 25; J. Leeder, C. Gissane, K. A. Van Someren, W. Gregson, and G. Howatson, "Cold water immersion and recovery from strenuous exercise: a meta-analysis," *British Journal of Sports Medicine* 46, no. 4 (2011): 233–40.

18. N. G. Versey, S. L. Halson, and B. T. Dawson, "Water immersion recovery for athletes: effect on exercise performance and practical recommendations," *Sports Medicine* 43, no. 11 (2013): 1101–30.

19. M. C. Stenson, M. R. Stenson, T. D. Matthews, and V. J. Paolone, "5000 meter run performance is not enhanced 24 hrs after an intense exercise bout and cold water immersion," *Journal of Sports Science & Medicine* 16, no. 2 (2017): 272–9.

20. C. Y. Tseng, J. P. Lee, Y. S, Tsai, S. D. Lee, C. L. Kao, T. C. Liu, C. H. Lai, M. B. Harris, and C. H. Kuo, "Topical cooling (icing) delays recovery from eccentric exercise–induced muscle damage," *Journal of Strength and Conditioning Research* 27, no. 5 (2013): 1354–61.

21. L. A. Roberts, T. Raastad, J. F. Markworth, V. C. Figueiredo, I. M. Egner, A. Shield, D. Cameron-Smith, et al., "Post-exercise cold water immersion attenuates acute anabolic signalling and long-term adaptations in muscle to strength training." *Journal of Physiology* 593, no. 18 (2015): 4285-301.

22. C. Beardsley and J. Škarabot, "Effects of self-myofascial release: a systematic review," *Journal of Bodywork and Movement Therapies* 19, no. 4 (2015): 747–58.

23. W. L. Westcott, T. Chen, F. B. Neric, N. DiNubile, A. Bowirrat, M. Madigan, B. W. Downs, et al., "The Marc Pro™ device improves muscle performance and recovery from concentric and eccentric exercise induced muscle fatigue in humans: a pilot study," *Journal of Exercise Physiology Online* 14, no. 2 (2011): 55–67; W. Westcott, D. Han, N. DiNubile, F. B. Neric, R. L. R. Loud, S. Whitehead, and K. Blum, "Effects of electrical stimulation using Marc Pro™ device during the recovery period on calf muscle strength and fatigue in adult fitness participants," *Journal of Exercise Physiology Online* 16, no. 2 (2013): 40–9.

24. T. W. Kaminski, J. Hertel, N. Amendola, C. L. Docherty, M. G. Dolan, J. T. Hopkins, E. Nussbaum, et al., "National Athletic Trainers' Association position statement: conservative management and prevention of ankle sprains in athletes," *Journal of Athletic Training* 48, no. 4 (2013): 528–45.

Acknowledgments

There is no way this book would have happened without the help of so many people.

First and foremost, I want to thank my amazing wife, Christine. You are my angel, and I wouldn't be half the man I am today without you in my life.

To my parents and my brothers, Brandon and Justin, I love you guys!

To Kevin Sonthana, it feels like just yesterday that we sat around and talked about the idea of writing *The Squat Bible.* None of this would have been possible without your help in teaching me how to write more clearly. You helped me co-author two amazing books that will help so many people, and for that I am forever grateful.

To Ryan Grout and Nate Varel, thank you for your friendship and for always allowing me to bounce my business ideas (some good and many bad) off of you.

To my team from Boost Physical Therapy & Sports Performance, I can't begin to tell you how much you mean to me. I will never forget the time I spent with you all in Kansas City. You were my second family for close to a decade, and there will always be a place in my heart for you.

A special thank you to Travis Neff for giving me the opportunity to start Squat University while working full-time as a young physical therapist. You trusted me and allowed me to follow my passions. For that I am forever grateful.

To the entire team at Victory Belt Publishing who helped make this book possible, including Glen Cordoza, Pam Mourouzis, Susan Lloyd, Justin-Aaron Velasco, and Lance Freimuth. It is truly amazing to see the pages I wrote on my MacBook transformed into such a beautiful book.

Lastly, I want to thank the many amazing teachers, professors, coaches, and clinicians who came before me, including Stuart McGill, Jill Cook, Shirley Sahrmann, Kelly Starrett, Chad Vaughn, Eric Cressey, Mike Reinold, and Gray Cook. If the words in this book do anything to help others around the world, it is only because I stand on the shoulders of giants like you.

Index

A

abdominal head, 260
abductor pollicis longus, 314
accommodating resistance, 93
acetabular retroversion, 122
acetabulum (hip socket), 43, 121, 130
Achilles tendon injury, 343–349
acromioclavicular ligament, 236
acromion, 235, 260
acromion process, 241
adduction, 141
adductor brevis, 128–129
adductor isometric, 154–155
adductor longus, 128–129, 197
adductor magnus, 128–129, 197
adductor manual muscle test, 146
adductor muscles, 128–129
age, as risk factor for hamstring strains, 139
Alekseyev, Vasily, 102
anatomy
    Achilles tendon injury, 343–349
    back, 19–35
    core, 64–66
    elbow, 313–319
    hip, 121–127
    knee, 171–184
    quads, 197
    shoulder, 235–250
    technique considerations for bodyweight squat based on, 164–165
Anatomy for Runners (Dicharry), 191
anconeus, 322
ankle mobility, testing, 45, 191–192
ankle pain
    about, 342

Achilles tendon injury
    anatomy, 343–349
    improving with plyometrics, 366–370
    rebuilding process for, 354–371
    screening, 349–353
annular ligament, 313, 316
anterior banded joint mobilization, 42–43
anterior elbow, 317–318
anterior humeral circumflex artery, 319
anterior sheath of rectus abdominis, 260
anterior tibiotalar ligament, 343
anteverted hip, 124–125, 127
arteries, 379
arthrogenic neuromuscular inhibition, 51
articular capsule of elbow, 316
articular surface of calcaneus, 357
articulate capsule of elbow, 313
ascending aorta, 379
assessing
    flexibility for hip pain, 144
    hip internal rotation, 143
    load for hip pain, 145–147, 164
    strength for hip pain, 145–147
    strength imbalance, 260–264
assisted hip airplane/tippy bird, 151
Atlas Stone lift, 28
axillary lymph nodes, 379
axillary nerve, 319
axillary vein, 319

B

back extension machine or Roman chair, for low back injury rehab, 102–103

back injuries
    disc bulges, 22–28
    facet injury, 31–32
    herniation, 22–28
    mechanism of, 34–35
    muscle pain, 34
    nerve pain, 34
    spondylolysis, 32–33
    vertebral end-plate fracture, 28–30
Back Mechanic (McGill), 20
back muscles, 260
back pain
    about, 14–15
    anatomy of injuries, 19–35
    cautionary exercises for low back injury rehab, 98–103
    classifying, 58–61
    core stability and, 62–66
    exercise modifications after, 90–94
    exercises for rehabbing, 80–90
    glutes and, 74–76
    guidelines for, 59–61
    hamstring stretches and, 104–111
    how it occurs, 20–22
    imaging abnormalities and, 16–18
    rebuilding process, 61–76
    rehab plan for, 76–90
    relationship with hip pain, 147
    screening, 36–57
    signs/symptoms of, 59–60
    stretching for, 73–74
    treatment plan for, 109
    triggers for, 37–38
    weightlifting belts, 95–98
back squat, 81
back squat with neutral wrists, 328–329

back squat with overextended wrists, 328
balance, improving, 208
balance and reach exercise, 208
ball into piriformis, 149
ball-and-socket joint, 121. *See also* hip pain
banded joint mobilization, 149–150, 335–336, 358
banded squat hold, as glute medius isometric, 156
banded "W," 288
bands
    banded joint mobilization, 149–150, 335–336, 358
    banded squat hold, as glute medius isometric, 156
    banded "W," 288
    full can with banded loop, 300
    hamstring stretch with, 105
bar on back spinal extension, 46
barbells
    barbell clean with twisted hips, 32
    barbell push press with extended spine, 33
    barbell RDL, 47, 103
    barbell soft tissue mobilization on triceps, 337
    barbell squat, 43
basilic vein, 319
Berra, Yogi, 38
biceps brachii, 235, 260, 318
biceps femoris, 137
biceps femoris short, 182
Big Three exercises, for core stability, 67–73
bird dog, for core stability, 71–73
bird dog quadruped, 72
body control, enhancing lower, 209–210
bodyweight squat
    with butt wink, 26
    with neutral spine, 26
    technique considerations based on anatomy, 164–165
bottoms-up kettlebell press, 295–296
box depth drop, 221
box lat stretch, 274
box squat, 216–218
braces, for knees, 226

brachial artery, 319
brachial veins, 319
brachialis, 235, 318
brachioradialis, 314
bridge
    for back pain rehab, 74–75
    for hip pain rehab, 157
Bulgarian split squat, 218–219
bursa sac, 130
bursitis, 132
butt wink
    about, 25, 26
    barbell squat with, 43
    illustrated, 44

C

calcaneofibular ligament, 347
calcaneus, 343, 348
Calhoon, Gregg, 171
cam impingement, 44
capsular distension arthrogram, 51
capsular ligament, 236
capsule, 236
cartilage, 174
cat-camel, 26, 67–68
celiac trunk, 379
cephalic vein, 319
cervical lymph nodes, 379
chain squat, 93–94
chest muscles, 260
chondromalacia, 174
Cho-Pat strap, 226
circumflex scapular artery, 319
cisterna chyli, 379
clavicle, 235, 260
clavicular head, 260
"closed chain" exercises, 197, 201
coccyx, 121
collagen, 23, 25, 343
compressive load intolerance, back pain and, 60
concentric contraction, 275
congenital, 245
conoid ligament, 236
Continuum of Tendon Pathology, 178–179, 344–345
Cook, Gray, 36, 162, 209
Cook, Jill, 178, 181, 344, 346
Copenhagen side plank, 155
coracoacromial ligament, 236
coracobrachialis, 235, 318

coracoclavicular ligament, 236
coracoid process, 257
core anatomy, 64–66
core stability
    exercises for, 76–90
    in rebuilding process for back pain, 62–66
corner pec stretch, 276–277
Craig's test, for hips, 127
crepitus, 349
Cressey, Eric, 138
cross-body stretch, 285
crunch, for core stability, 63
cryotherapy, 376
cubital tunnel, 321
cubital tunnel syndrome, 321
curl-up, for core stability, 68–69

D

deadlift
    with belt, 97
    from blocks, 83
    for core stability, 83–84
    deadlift start with moment arms, 83
    with neutral spine, 25
    with rounded spine, 25
decline board squat, for knee pain rehab, 215
deep brachial artery, 319
deep goblet squat stretch, 356
deep medial head, 318
deep receiving position snatch or clean, 124
deep squat with isometric hold, for back pain, 75–76
deep squat with plate stretch, for back pain, 76
deep squat with rotation, 271
deep trochanteric bursa, 132
degenerative tendinopathy, 178–182, 346–347
delamination, 24–25, 45
delayed-onset muscle soreness (DOMS), 386
deltoids, 235, 237, 260, 318
depth drop jump, 223
depth drop off stack of plates, 367
descending aorta, 379
Dicharry, Jay, *Anatomy for Runners,* 191
disc bulges, 17–18, 22–28

disc delamination, 24–25
DOMS (delayed-onset muscle soreness), 386
DonJoy Cross strap, 226
double-leg bridge
  about, 51–52
  for back pain, 74–75
  for reawakening glutes, 203
double-leg heel raise, 350
double-leg pogo hops, 369–370
double-leg squats with forward knee travel, 188
dry needling, 225
"duck walk," 125
dynamic forces, 238
dynamic load intolerance, back pain and, 60

E

eccentric curl-ups, 275
elbow pain
  about, 312–313
  injury anatomy, 313–319
  rebuilding process for, 330–339
  screening, 320–329
elite deadlift end pull, 84
elite powerlifter squatting, illustrated, 96
"empty can," 298–300
end plate, 28–30
endotenon, 349
epitenon, 349
equipment, 13
erector spinae, 64
E-stim, 383–384
extended bird dog, 72
extensibility, as a measure of elasticity, 106
extension, facet injury and, 31
extension intolerance, 59–60
extensor carpi radialis brevis, 314, 322
extensor carpi radialis longus, 314
extensor carpi ulnaris, 314
extensor digiti minimi, 314
extensor pollicis brevis, 314
external derotation test, 146
external impingement, 241–242
external oblique, 65, 66
external rotation, of hips, 125–127

external rotation manual muscle tests, 327
external rotation press, 289–290
external rotation test, 262–263

F

FABER test, 142–143
facet injury, 31–32
facets, 19
FADIR test, 142
femoral head, 121
femur, 121, 125, 130, 132, 172, 176, 177, 343
fibril, 349
fibula, 172, 176, 177, 343
fibular collateral ligament, 176, 182
fibularis longus, 182
first degree, for hamstring strain, 138
5-inch wall test, 45, 192, 352–353
flexed lumbar spine, 24
flexibility
  assessing for hamstrings, 109–111, 138
  assessing for hip pain, 144
  assessing for shoulders, 253–259
  of lats, 243, 272
flexion, facet injury and, 31
flexion intolerance, back pain and, 59
flexor carpi radialis, 314
flexor carpi ulnaris, 314, 321
flexor digitorum superficialis, 314
flexor pollicis longus, 314
foam roller
  foam roll calf, 357
  foam roller pec stretch, 277
  foam-roll lateral leg, 196
  for hip pain, 148–149
  for knee pain, 195–196
  for lats, 273
  prayer stretch with, 57, 267
  wall slide with, 307
foot on wall stretch, 355–356
force, 20
front squat, 81
Fry, Andrew, 171
full can test, 263–264, 298–300
full side plank, 71

G

gastrocnemius lateral, 343
gastrocnemius medial, 182, 343
GHD (glute ham developer), 102–103
Gift of Injury (McGill), 29
glenoid, 236
glenoid cavity, 247
glenoid fossa, 247
glenoid labrum, 241, 247
"global" approach, 330
glute ham developer (GHD), 102–103
glute medius isometric, 156
gluteal amnesia, 50–51
glutes, reawakening, 202–203
gluteus maximus, 66
gluteus medius, 132, 133, 134
gluteus minimus, 133, 134
goblet squat, 81
"golf ball," of the humerus, 237, 238
golfer's elbow, 316–317
gracilis, 128–129, 197
grades, of hamstring strains, 138
greater trochanter bursitis/glute medius strain, 132–135
greater trochanter of femur, 121
groin strain, 128–129
ground-up approach, for improving knee stability, 201–202

H

half-kneel kettlebell windmill, 331–332
half-prone angel, 278
hamstring tendinopathy, 136–137
hamstrings
  improving flexibility of, 109–111
  strains of, 138–139
  stretching for back pain, 104–111
Hawkins-Kennedy test, 284–285
head movements, for nerve pain screening, 320
head of femur, 130
head of humerus, 241, 247

heavy slow resistance (HSR)
  training
    about, 215
    for ankle rehab, 364–366
    testing, 219–220
heel drop test, 49–50
heel raise insert, 358–359
heel raise with barbell, 365
heel raise with concentric raise
  and eccentric lower, 363
herniation, 22–28, 131
hinge with box in front of knees,
  78–79
hinge with hands on thighs, 79
hinge with plate on hips, 79–80
hip airplane/tippy bird
  progression, 159–161
hip extension coordination, for
  back pain, 50–52
hip extension "reverse hyper"
  machine, for low back injury
  rehab, 99–101
hip flexion manual muscle test,
  145–146
hip flexion to 60 degrees, 52–53
hip flexor isometric, 155–156
hip flexors, 129–130
hip hinge, 77–80
hip impingement (FAI), 44, 130
hip injuries
  greater trochanter bursitis/
    glute medius strain,
    132–135
  groin strain, 128–129
  hamstring strain, 138–139
  hamstring tendinopathy,
    136–137
  hip flexor strain/tendinopathy,
    129–130
  hip impingement (FAI), 130
  piriformis syndrome, 135–136
  sports hernia, 131
hip mobility assessment, for
  back pain, 52–54
hip pain
  about, 120–121
  anatomy of hips, 121–127
  hip injuries, 128–139
  mobility assessment for,
    141–143
  rebuilding process for,
    148–165
  relationship with back pain,
    147

screening, 139–148
  stretching and, 152–154
hip socket (acetabulum), 43, 121,
  123–124, 130
hip thrust, for rebuilding strength
  after hip pain, 157
hips
  assessing mobility of,
    190–191
  barbell clean with twisted, 32
  external rotation, 53
  internal rotation, 53, 143,
    190–191
  screening for problems with
    rotation of, 52–53
Horschig, Aaron, personal story
  of, 10
HSR training. See heavy slow
  resistance (HSR) training
humeral retroversion, 282
humerus, 235, 236, 237, 238, 241,
  243, 247, 313, 316
hypermobility, 245

I

IASTM (instrument-assisted
  soft tissue mobilization), 225,
  359–360
ice
  about, 386–387
  after workouts, 384–386
  inflammation and, 377–378
  scientific research on use of,
    380–382
  swelling and, 378–380
  use of, 374–376
Iced! The Illusionary Treatment
  Option (Reinl), 376
IGF–1 (insulin–like growth factor
  1), 377–378
iliac crest, 121, 243
iliacus, 128–129
iliocostalis, 64, 66
iliopsoas, 129
iliopsoas bursa, 129
iliotibial (IT) band, 132, 134, 174,
  176, 177
iliotibial band syndrome (ITBS),
  174–176
ilium, 121
imaging, abnormalities and back
  pain, 16–18
imbalances, shoulder, 241–247

impingement, 241–243
increased sarcomeres in series,
  107
inferior coracoid bursa, 236
inferior pole of the patella, 182
inferior vena cava, 379
inflammation, 34, 377–378
infrapatellar fat pad, 176
infraspinatus, 260, 318
infraspinatus fascia, 260
injuries
  Achilles tendon, 343–349
  back, 19–35
  disc bulges, 22–28
  elbow, 313–319
  facet, 31–32
  greater trochanter bursitis/
    glute medius strain,
    132–135
  groin strain, 128–129
  hamstring strain, 138–139
  hamstring tendinopathy,
    136–137
  herniation, 22–28
  hip flexor strain/tendinopathy,
    129–130
  hip impingement (FAI), 130
  imbalances and instability,
    241–247
  knee, 172–184
  mechanism of, 34–35
  muscle pain, 34
  nerve, 319
  nerve pain, 34
  patellar/quad tendinopathy,
    177–183
  patellofemoral pain syndrome
    (PFPS), 172–174
  piriformis syndrome, 135–136
  shoulder, 241–250
  spondylolysis, 32–33
  sports hernia, 131
  vertebral end–plate fracture,
    28–30
insertional injury, for Achilles
  tendon, 348
instability, shoulder, 241–247, 259
instrument-assisted soft tissue
  mobilization (IASTM), 225,
  359–360
insulin–like growth factor 1
  (IGF–1), 377–378
internal impingement, 241–242
internal oblique, 65, 66

internal rotation
    about, 286
    of hips, 125–127, 143
    improving, 280–283
intervertebral disc, 23
intra-abdominal pressure (IAP),
    95–96
inverted row, for core stability,
    85–86
ischial tuberosity, 136
ischium, 121
isolated strengthening, 332–335
isometric squat hold, for back
    pain, 76
isometrics
    about, 64
    decreasing ankle pain with,
        361–363
    early strengthening with,
        154–156
    for knee pain rehab, 212–213
    muscle contraction and,
        382–383
isotonic movement, 215
isotonics
    for ankle pain rehab, 363–366
    for knee pain rehab, 214–215
ITBS (iliotibial band syndrome),
    174–176

J

Janda, Vladimir, 50
joint mobility, hip pain and,
    149–151

K

kettlebells
    Bulgarian split squat with, 219
    kettlebell swing, 101
    kettlebell Turkish get-up,
        296–298
    suitcase carry with, 334
    weight shift of, for hip pain,
        153–154
kinesiopathologic model (KPM),
    36, 140
kinetic chain screening,
    324–329
knee cave squat, 173
knee injuries
    about, 172
    mechanisms of, 183–184

patellar/quad tendinopathy,
    177–183
patellofemoral pain syndrome
    (PFPS), 172–174
knee pain
    about, 170–171
    box squat, 216–218
    Bulgarian split squat,
        218–228
    knee injury anatomy, 171–184
    mobility assessment for,
        190–192
    rebuilding process for,
        195–215
    screening, 184–194
knee sleeves/wraps, 226–228
knees to chest stretch, 73
Konstantinov, Konstantin, 27
KPM (kinesiopathologic model),
    36, 140

L

"L" screen, 254
labrum, 130, 247
lacrosse ball posterior shoulder,
    285
lacrosse ball soft tissue
    mobilization on wrist flexors,
    336
lacrosse ball to lats standing
    against wall, 273
lat flexibility, 243, 272
lat stretch, 274
lateral band joint mobilization,
    335–336
lateral band walk, 204
lateral banded joint
    mobilizations, 150
lateral cord, 319
lateral elbow, 314–316
lateral patellar ligament, 182
lateral patellar retinacular fibers,
    174
lateral wall sit, as glute medius
    isometric, 156
latissimus dorsi, 66, 237, 243, 260
lat/teres major flexibility
    screening, 256
levator scapulae, 260
ligaments, shoulder joint, 236
load, posture (aka "position")
    assessment with added,
    40–43

load intolerance, 49, 60
load testing
    for Achilles tendon injury,
        350–352
    for back pain, 49–50
    for hip pain, 145–147, 164
    for knee pain, 192–194
load tolerance testing, 193–194,
    211–215
"local" approach, 332
long piriformis syndrome, 136,
    143
long plantar ligament, 343
long thoracic, 319
longissimus thoracis, 64, 66
lower body, enhancing control
    of, 209–210
lumbar lordosis, 33
lumbar vertebrae, 121
lymph nodes, 379
lymphatic system, 379

M

macrophages, 380
malleolar surface of talus, 357
marching resisted bridge, for hip
    pain rehab, 158
material banded joint
    mobilization, 54
McGill, Stuart, 27–28, 36, 40,
    51, 58, 62, 159, 160. See also
    Big Three exercises, for core
    stability
    Back Mechanic, 20
    Gift of Injury, 29
    Ultimate Back Fitness and
        Performance, 20
McGill curl-up, 69
mechanical model, 106–107
medial cord, 319
medial elbow, 316–317
medial epicondyle, 316, 321
medial patellar ligament, 182
medial patellar retinacular fibers,
    174
median nerve, 319
mediastinal lymph nodes, 379
metatarsal, 343
microfibril, 349
mid-back, 240, 266
mid-tendon injury, for Achilles
    tendon, 347–348
Milo of Croton, 8–12

Mirkin, Gabe, 376
mobility
    core stability work and
        restrictions with, 67–68
    kinetic chain screening and,
        325–327
    of thoracic spine, 265
mobility assessment
    for hip pain, 141–143
    for knee pain, 190–192
    for shoulder pain, 253–259
mobility exercises, for ankle
    pain, 357–358
mobilization with movement
    (MWM), 335
modified Thomas test, 144
movement
    about, 139–140
    assessing for back pain,
        43–48
    assessment for shoulders,
        251–252
    retraining, 159–164
    screening for hip pain,
        140–141
    screening for knee pain,
        184–189
    shoulder, 247–250
multifidus, 64, 66
muscle pain, 34
muscles
    adductor, 128–129
    back, 260
    chest, 260
    piriformis, 135
    reducing swelling with
        contraction of, 382–383
muscular imbalances, 286
musculocutaneous nerve, 319
MWM (mobilization with
    movement), 335

N

National Athletic Trainers'
    Association (NATA), 386–387
nerve gliding, 337–338
nerve injuries, 319
nerve pain, 34
nerve tensioning, 337–338
neural drive, 65
neuromuscular electrical
    stimulation (NMES) unit, 13,
    383–384

neutral spine
    bodyweight squat with, 26
    deadlift with, 25
    side view, 23
newton (N), 214
NMES (neuromuscular electrical
    stimulation) unit, 13, 383–384
nucleus pulposus, 22

O

oblique, 65, 66
O'Brien, Josiah, 9–10
olecranon, 318
Olympic lifts
    after knee rehab, 224–225
    as exercise modification after
        back pain, 90–91
Olympic snatch, 86
omohyoid muscle, 260
one-armed row, for core
    stability, 89–90
"open chain" exercises, 197
optimal motor recruitment
    pattern, 51
osteogenesis, 29
overextended spine, in posture
    (aka "position") assessment,
    39
overhand grip pack hold,
    334–335
overhead coordination,
    improving, 301–302
overhead squat, 248, 249, 327
overhead walking lunge, 249

P

Pallof press
    for core stability, 88–89
    in deep squat, 89
    split stance, 89
palmaris longus, 314
paratenon, 349
pars interarticularis, 32–33
partner pec flexibility test, 257
passive straight-leg raise (SLR)
    test, 104–105
passive treatments
    after ankle rehab, 359–360
    after knee rehab, 225–228
patella, 172, 174, 176, 177, 182
patellar straps, 226
patellar tendon, 176, 177, 182, 197

patellar/quad tendinopathy,
    177–183
patellofemoral groove, 172
patellofemoral joint, 172
patellofemoral pain syndrome
    (PFPS), 172–174
pathomechanics, 242
paused deadlifts, as exercise
    modification after back pain,
    91–92
paused scap pull-up, 330–331
"peanut," 265–266
pec flexibility
    improving, 272, 276–277
    testing while supine, 258
pectineus, 128–129, 197
pectoralis major, 66, 237,
    256–258, 260
pectoralis minor, 66, 256–258
pelvis, 243
peritendon, 349
peritendon injury, for Achilles
    tendon, 349
Peyer's patch, 379
PFPS (patellofemoral pain
    syndrome), 172–174
phalanges of the foot, 343
pigeon stretch, for hip pain, 153
pincer impingement, 44
piriformis, 133
piriformis muscle, 135
piriformis stretch, for hip pain,
    152
piriformis syndrome, 135–136
plastic deformation, 107
plyometrics
    after ankle rehab, 366–370
    after knee rehab, 219–220
pogo hops, 222
popliteal lymph nodes, 379
position, kinetic chain screening
    and, 328–329
posterior cord, 319
posterior elbow, 317–318
posterior humeral circumflex
    artery, 319
posterior talofibular ligament,
    348
posture (aka "position")
    assessment, for back pain,
    38–43
prayer stretch, 267
prayer test, 326
primary bundle, 349

primary stabilizers, 236
pronator quadratus, 314
pronator teres, 314
prone floor angel, 291
prone hip extension with pillow
    under stomach, 42
prone lateral raise, 290
prone lie, 41
psoas major, 128–129
pubic arch, 121
pubic symphysis, 121
push-up plus, 302
PVC pipe wall test, 56–57

Q

quadratus femoris, 133
quadratus lumborum (QL),
    64–65, 66
quadruped downward rotation
    stretch, 268–269
quadruped joint mobilization,
    150
quadruped upward rotation,
    271–272
quads, 197

R

radial collateral artery, 319
radial collateral ligament, 313
radial nerve, 319, 322–323
radial nerve slider, 338
radial nerve test, 323
radial tunnel, 322
radial tunnel syndrome, 322
radius, 313
reactive neuromuscular training
    (RNT)
    about, 162
    for enhancing lower body
        control, 209
    RNT banded squat, 209–210
    RNT split squat, 163, 210
    RNT squat, 162–163
    touchdown, 164
reactive tendinopathy, 137,
    178–182, 346–347
rebuilding process
    for ankle pain, 354–371
    for back pain, 61–90
    for elbow pain, 330–339
    for knee pain, 195–215
    for shoulder pain, 265–308

rectus abdominis, 66
rectus femoris, 177, 182
Reinl, Gary, 381
    *Iced! The Illusionary
        Treatment Option,* 376
Reinold, Mike, 284
repeated bout effect, 385
resisted wrist flexion, 317
rest, ice, compression, elevation
    (RICE) protocol, 376, 380,
    386–387
retroverted hip, 124–125, 127
"reverse tailor" position, 125
rhomboideus major, 260
rhomboideus minor, 260
rhythmic stabilizations, 293–294
RNT. *See* reactive
    neuromuscular training (RNT)
Roman chair, 102–103
Romanian deadlift (RDL)
    about, 46–47
    with barbell, 103
rotation
    with extension intolerance,
        60
    of hips, 53, 125–127, 143,
        190–191
rotator cuff, 236, 237, 239, 301
rounded spine
    deadlift with, 25
    in posture (aka "position")
        assessment, 39
row, 85
row with feet elevated, 86
Russian twist with ball, for core
    stability, 63

S

sacrotiberous ligament, 133
sacrum, 121
sagittal plane, 188
Sahrmann, Shirley, 36
sartorius, 128–129, 177, 182
satellite cells, 382
scapula, 235, 236, 240, 247
scapular raise, 303–304
screening
    ankle pain, 349–353
    back pain, 36–57
    elbow pain, 320–329
    hip pain, 139–148
    for hypermobility, 245
    knee pain, 184–194

movement for hip pain,
    140–141
    shoulder pain, 250–265
seated angel sequence, 305
seated heel raise with weight
    directly over shin, 364
seated knee extension, 198
seated mobility assessments,
    253–254
seated piriformis stretch, for hip
    pain, 152
seated pull test, 40
seated rotation and side bend
    stretch, 270
second degree, for hamstring
    strain, 138
secondary impingement,
    242–243
self-mobilization, 265–266
semimembranosus, 137
semispinalis capitis, 260
semitendinosus, 137
serratus anterior muscle, 244,
    260
serratus posterior inferior, 66
serratus strength test, 264
short piriformis syndrome, 136
shoulder blade movement
    (abduction, pull-up, press), 252
shoulder injuries, 241–247
shoulder internal rotation, 255
shoulder pain
    about, 234–235
    anatomy, 235–240
    injury anatomy, 241–250
    rebuilding process for,
        265–308
    screening, 250–265
side plank
    for core stability, 70–71
    quadratus lumborum (QL) in,
        65
side plank clamshell, for
    rebuilding strength after hip
    pain, 158–159
side-lying clamshell, 200
side-lying external rotation, 287
side-lying leg lift side plank, 71
side-lying straight-leg raise,
    200
single-leg bridge, for
    reawakening glutes, 203
single-leg bridge screen, for
    knee pain, 194

single-leg bridge test, 51, 74, 147
single-leg heel raise
    about, 351
    with toes on plate, 351
    with weight, 365
single-leg hop, 224, 368
single-leg RDL, 161–162
single-leg squat
    about, 47–48
    with forward knee travel, 188
    with good hinge, 189
    learning to, 206–207
    for screening hip pain, 141
    for screening knee pain,
        187–189
single-leg stance
    about, 176
    with knee cave, 176
slant board stretch, 355–356
sled push, for core stability, 82
sleeper stretch, 284–285
snatch from blocks, 91
snatch lift, 283
    soft tissue mobilization
    for elbow pain, 336–337
    for hip pain, 148–149
    for improving lat and teres
        major flexibility, 272–273
    for improving pec flexibility,
        276
soleus, 347
Spanish squat, for knee pain
    rehab, 213
speed, for box squat, 217–218
spinalis thoracis, 64
spine
    about, 19–20
    barbell push press with
        extended, 33
    flexed lumbar spine, 24
    neutral spine side view, 23
    overextended, 39
    rounded, 39
spine of scapula, 260
spleen, 379
splenius capitis, 260
split jerk, 246
split squat, RNT, 163
spondylolisthesis, 33
spondylolysis, 32–33, 36–37
sports hernia, 131
sprinting, as a risk factor of
    hamstring strains, 139
squat hips down side plank, 70

squat hips up side plank, 70
squats
    bodyweight squat technique
        considerations based on
        anatomy, 164–165
    bodyweight squat with butt
        wink, 26
    bodyweight squat with
        neutral spine, 26
    box squat, 216–218
    for core stability, 81–82
    decline board squat, for knee
        pain rehab, 215
    deep squat with isometric
        hold, for back pain, 75–76
    deep squat with plate stretch,
        for back pain, 76
    deep squat with rotation, 271
    overhead squat, 248, 249, 327
    progression of, 199
    RNT, 162–163
    RNT banded, 209–210
    RNT split, 163, 210
    screening for hip pain with,
        141
    single-leg squat, 47–48, 141,
        187–189
    single-leg squat with forward
        knee travel, 188
    single-leg squat with good
        hinge, 189
    Spanish squat, 213
    split squat, RNT, 163
    squat hips down side plank,
        70
    squat hips up side plank, 70
    squatting with chains, 93–94
    touchdown squat, 206–207
    zombie front squat, 92–93
SSC (stretch-shortening cycle),
    220, 366
stability
    improving for knees, 197–210,
        201
    kinetic chain screening and,
        325–327
stage of injury, determining for
    Achilles tendon, 345–347
standing, posture (aka "position")
    assessment while, 39
standing hinge start, 78
standing mobility assessment,
    255
Starrett, Kelly, 11, 36, 38, 337

static forces, 238
static hold, "full can" with, 300
sternocleidomastoid, 260
sternum, 260
stiffness, as a measure of
    elasticity, 106
straps, 226
strength
    assessing for hip pain,
        145–147
    of hamstrings, 139
    imbalance testing, 260–264
    improving after hip rehab,
        154–159
    improving ankle pain with
        isotonics, 363–366
stretching
    for ankle pain, 355–356
    for back pain, 73–74
    box lat stretch, 274
    box stretch, 356
    box T-spine stretch, 268
    cross-body stretch, 285
    deep goblet squat stretch,
        356
    effects of long-term, 107–108
    finding the right stretch,
        284–285
    hip pain and, 152–154
    lat stretch, 274
    pigeon stretch, 153
    piriformis stretch, 152
    prayer stretch, 267
    reasons for, 105–107
    seated piriformis stretch, 152
    supine piriformis stretch, 152
stretch-shortening cycle (SSC),
    220, 366
subacromial bursa, 236, 241
subacromial impingement,
    241–242
subclavian artery, 319
subclavian lymph nodes, 379
subclavian vein, 319
subdeltoid bursa, 236
subfibril, 349
submandibular lymph nodes,
    379
submental lymph nodes, 379
subscapularis, 235, 318
suitcase carry
    for core stability, 86–88
    with kettlebell, 334
sulcus test, 259

sumo deadlift, 84
sumo stance deadlift, 124
superficial inguinal lymph nodes, 379
superficial trochanteric bursa, 132
superior pole of the patella, 182
superior ramus of pubis, 121
superior transverse ligament, 236
superior ulnar collateral artery, 319
superior vena cava, 379
Superman, 159–160
supinator, 322
supine floor angel, 304–305
supine knee to chest, 123
supine piriformis stretch, for hip pain, 152
supine serratus punch, 302
suprascapular nerve, 319
supraspinatus, 260, 318
supraspinatus tendon, 241
suspension trainer row, 292–293
sweep under & touch bird dog, 73
swelling
    ice and, 378–380
    reducing with muscle contraction, 382–383
Swiss ball, rhythmic stabilizations with, 294

T

"T" test, 261–262
talus, 343, 357
technique
    assessment for shoulders, 251–252
    based on anatomy, 164–165
    kinetic chain screening and, 328–329
    shoulder, 247–250
tendinitis, 178, 344
tendinopathy, 178
tendinosis, 178
tendon, 349
tendon disrepair, as a knee injury stage, 178–182
tendon of biceps brachii, 313, 316
tendon of triceps brachii, 313, 316

tennis elbow, 314–315
tensile load, 134
tensor fasciae latae (TFL), 133, 197
teres major, 235, 237, 260, 272–275, 318
teres minor, 237, 260, 318
test-retest method, 142
third degree, for hamstring strain, 138
thixotropy, 110
Thomas test, 144
thoracic spine, 240, 265
thoracic spine mobility assessment, 55–57, 258–259
thoracoacromial artery, 319
thoracodorsal nerve, 319
thymus, 379
tibia, 172, 176, 177, 182, 343
tibial tuberosity, 177, 182
tonsil, 379
touchdown squat, 206–207
touchdown, 164
trabecular bone, 28–30
training program considerations, 280
transverse abdominals (TA), 66
transverse load, 134
trapezius, 260
traversus abdominus, 64
triceps, 318
triceps brachii, 260, 318, 321
triceps lateral head, 237
triceps long head, 237
triceps medial head, 237
triceps surae, 343
triceps tendon, 318
triggers, for back pain, 37–38
tripod, 201
tropocollagen, 349
Tsatsouline, Pavel, 101
T-spine rotation, 258–259

U

ulna, 313, 316
ulnar collateral ligament, 316
ulnar nerve, 319, 321–322
ulnar nerve slider, 338
ulnar nerve test (biceps curl with over-pressure), 322
Ultimate Back Fitness and Performance (McGill), 20
ultrasound imaging, 178, 359

unilateral abduction, 205
upside-down kettlebell carry, 87–88

V

vastus intermedius, 177, 197
vastus lateralis, 182, 197
vastus medialis, 177, 182
vastus medialis oblique (VMO), 174, 197
Vaughn, Chad, 248
veins, 379
velocity, 21
vertebral end-plate fracture, 28–30
viscoelastic deformation, 106
Viscott, David, 11
Voight, Michael, 162, 209

W

wall handstand, 279
wall screen, 253–254
wall sit, for knee pain rehab, 213
wall slide, 305–307
warm-up, 110–111
weight, for box squat, 217
weightlifting belts, 95–98
Wilson, E. O., 6–7
Woods, Tiger, 21
workouts, icing after, 384–386
wrist extension isometric, 332–333
wrist extension stretch, 317
wrist extension with movement, 333–334

Y–Z

"Y" test, 261–262
zombie front squat, as exercise modification after back pain, 92–93